Frontiers in Cardiovascular Drug Discovery

(*Volume 5*)

Edited by

Atta-ur-Rahman, *FRS*

Kings College,
University of Cambridge,
Cambridge,
UK

&

M. Iqbal Choudhary

H.E.J. Research Institute of Chemistry,
International Center for Chemical and Biological Sciences,
University of Karachi, Karachi,
Pakistan

Frontiers in Cardiovascular Drug Discovery

Volume # 5

Editor: Atta-ur-Rahman, *FRS* & Muhammad Iqbal Choudhary

ISSN (Online): 1879-6648

ISSN (Print): 2452-3267

ISBN (Online): 978-981-14-1324-7

ISBN (Print): 978-981-14-1323-0

need for a court order if at any point you breach any terms of this License Agreement. In no event will any delay or failure by Bentham Science Publishers in enforcing your compliance with this License Agreement constitute a waiver of any of its rights.

3. You acknowledge that you have read this License Agreement, and agree to be bound by its terms and conditions. To the extent that any other terms and conditions presented on any website of Bentham Science Publishers conflict with, or are inconsistent with, the terms and conditions set out in this License Agreement, you acknowledge that the terms and conditions set out in this License Agreement shall prevail.

Bentham Science Publishers Pte. Ltd.
80 Robinson Road #02-00
Singapore 068898
Singapore
Email: subscriptions@benthamscience.net

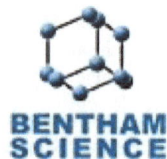

**BENTHAM
SCIENCE**

CONTENTS

PREFACE i

LIST OF CONTRIBUTORS iii

CHAPTER 1 THE LIPID HYPOTHESIS: FROM RESINS TO PROPROTEIN CONVERTASE SUBTILISIN/KEXIN TYPE-9 INHIBITORS 1
Sudarshan Ramachandran, Mithun Bhartia and *Carola S. König*
   INTRODUCTION 2
   CHOLESTEROL 3
      Early Evolution of the Relationship between Cholesterol and Atherogenesis 3
   LONGITUDINAL PROSPECTIVE OBSERVATIONAL STUDIES AND CVD RISK ALGORITHMS 5
   INTERVENTIONAL STUDIES WITH CLINICAL EVENTS AS OUTCOMES 10
      Randomised Controlled Bile Sequestrants Trials 12
      Randomised Controlled Statin Trials 13
      Randomised Controlled Ezetimibe Trials 19
      Randomised Controlled PCSK9 Inhibitor Trials 20
   THE RECENT CASE AGAINST THE LIPID HYPOTHESIS 21
   ROLE OF OTHER LIPID LOWERING AGENTS 21
   ROLE OF ANTI-INFLAMMATORY THERAPY 22
   REFINING THE LIPID HYPOTHESIS: IDENTIFICATION OF SUBGROUPS DEMONSTRATING EVEN GREATER BENEFIT 23
   CONCLUSION 24
   DISCLOSURE STATEMENT 24
   CONSENT FOR PUBLICATION 24
   CONFLICT OF INTEREST 24
   ACKNOWLEDGEMENTS 25
   REFERENCES 25

CHAPTER 2 THE ROLE OF SGLT2I IN THE PREVENTION AND TREATMENT OF HEART FAILURE 36
Hasan AlTurki, Ahmed AlTurki, Mark Sherman, Abhinav Sharma and *Thao Huynh*
   INTRODUCTION 36
   HEART FAILURE 37
   MECHANISMS OF ACTION OF SGLT2 AND SGTL2I 38
      Glucose Homeostasis 39
      Cardiovascular Effects of SGLT2i 40
      Nephroprotective Effects of SGLT2I 41
   CV OUTCOMES IN PATIENTS WITH T2DM 41
   RENAL OUTCOMES IN PATIENTS WITH T2DM AND CHRONIC KIDNEY DISEASE (CKD) 45
   HEART FAILURE 46
   PERIPHERAL ARTERIAL DISEASE 47
   ACUTE HEART FAILURE 48
   REAL-WORLD DATA 49
   CURRENT SGLT2I USES 49
   CURRENT USE OF SGLT2 INHIBITORS IN CLINICAL PRACTICE 52
   PRACTICAL CONSIDERATIONS WITH SGLT2I PRESCRIPTION 52
   FUTURE DIRECTIONS AND ONGOING TRIALS 54
   CONCLUSIONS 55

CONSENT FOR PUBLICATION 55
CONFLICTS OF INTEREST 56
ACKNOWLEDEGEMENTS 56
REFERENCES 56

CHAPTER 3 NATURAL PRODUCTS AND SEMI-SYNTHETIC COMPOUNDS AS ANTITHROMBOTICS: A REVIEW OF THE LAST TEN YEARS (2009-2019) 65
Angelo Piato and *Cedric Stephan Graebin*
INTRODUCTION 65
NATURAL PRODUCTS WITH ANTITHROMBOTIC ACTIVITY 68
    Antithrombotic Molecules Obtained from Marine-based Sources 68
        Antithrombotics from microorganisms 73
    Antithrombotics from Plant-based Sources 77
    Semi-synthetic compounds with antithrombotic activity 92
CONCLUSION 97
ABBREVIATIONS 99
CONSENT FOR PUBLICATION 100
CONFLICT OF INTEREST 100
ACKNOWLEDGEMENT 100
REFERENCES 100

CHAPTER 4 TRANSIENT RECEPTOR POTENTIAL CHANNELS: THERAPEUTIC TARGETS FOR CARDIOMETABOLIC DISEASES? 108
Leidyanne Ferreira Gonçalves, Thereza Cristina Lonzetti Bargut and *Caroline Fernandes-Santos*
INTRODUCTION 108
TRP CHANNELS 109
    TRPA (ankyrin) Family 110
    TRPC (canonical) Family 111
    TRPM (melastatin) Family 112
    TRPML (mucolipin) Family 113
    TRPP (polycystin) Family 114
    TRPV (vanilloid) Family 114
TRP CHANNELS AND CARDIOVASCULAR DISEASES 116
    TRP Expression 117
        TRPA1 117
        TRPC 117
        TRPM 120
        TRPV 122
    Evidence of TRP Modulation in the Cardiovascular System 129
        TRPC 129
        TRPV 130
        Doxorubicin-induced Cardiotoxicity 131
OBESITY AND DIABETES 132
    TRP Expression 133
        TRPA1 133
        TRPC 134
        TRPM 134
        TRPML and TRPP 136
        TRPV 136
    Modulation of TRP Expression in the Adipose Tissue and Endocrine Pancreas 143
        TRPA1 143

TRPC		144
TRPM		144
TRPV		145
FUTURE PERSPECTIVES		146
CONCLUSION		147
CONSENT FOR PUBLICATION		148
CONFLICT OF INTEREST		148
ACKNOWLEDGEMENTS		148
REFERENCES		148
CHAPTER 5 **TREATMENT OF RAYNAUD'S PHENOMENON**		164
Sevdalina Nikolova Lambova		
PRIMARY RAYNAUD'S PHENOMENON		166
Ginkgo Biloba		167
Pharmacology		167
Clinical Trials		167
SECONDARY RAYNAUD'S PHENOMENON IN SYSTEMIC SCLEROSIS		167
Calcium Channel Blockers		169
Pharmacology		169
Clinical Data		170
Safety Profile		171
Pentoxifyllin		171
Pharmacology		171
Clinical Data		172
Safety Profile		173
Nitric Oxide Pathway		173
Phosphodiesterase-5 Enzyme Inhibitors		173
Topical Glyceryl Trinitrate		175
Prostacyclin Pathway		176
Iloprost		177
Epoprostenol		179
Prostaglandin E1 (Alprostadil)		180
Treprostinil		180
Oral Prostanoids		181
Serotonin Inhibition – Fluoxetine		183
Pharmacology		183
Clinical Data and Safety Profile		184
Endothelin Pathway and Endothelin-Receptor Antagonists		184
Endothelin Pathway		184
Clinical Data		186
Safety Profile		187
Renin-Angiotensin System		188
Angiotensin II Receptor Blocker – Losartan		188
Angiotensin-Converting enzyme Inhibitors		189
Alpha-Adrenergic Blockers		190
Prazosin		190
Alpha-2c Adrenergic Receptor Antagonists		191
Statins		191
Pharmacology		191
Clinical Data		193
Safety Profile		193

Antiplatelet Therapy and Anticoagulants 193
Treatment of Digital Ulcers in Severe RP in SSc 195
Combination Therapy in Severe Peripheral Vascular Syndrome with Digital Ulcers in SSc   196
Other Treatments 197
    Botulinum Toxin 197
    Rho-Kinase Inhibitors 198
CONCLUSION 199
CONFLICT OF INTEREST 199
ACKNOWLEDGEMENTS 199
REFERENCES 199

CHAPTER 6 TRADITIONAL MEDICINE BASED CARDIOVASCULAR THERAPEUTICS   211

Sriram Kumar, Rekha Ravindran, Sakthi Abbirami Gowthaman, Sujata Roy and *Johanna Rajkumar*

INTRODUCTION 212
  Cardiovascular Diseases 212
  Pathophysiology of CVD 212
  Different Types of CVD 213
INDIAN CARDIOVASCULAR THERAPEUTICS 213
  Ambrex 213
  Abana 214
  Arjunarishta 214
  Arogh 215
  BHUx 215
  Lipistat 216
  Liposem 216
  Marutham 216
  Triglize 217
TRADITIONAL CHINESE MEDICINE 217
  Bushen Kangle 217
  Dang Gui Long Hui Wan 217
  Er Chen Wan 218
  Fu Fang Dan Shen 218
  Fu Fang Ge Qing 218
  Jiang Zhi Ling 218
  Jin Kui Shen Qi Wan 219
  Ke Chuan 219
  Qing Nao Jiang Ya 219
  Sheng Mai Yin 219
  Su He Xiang Wan 220
  Tian Wang Bu Xin Dan 220
  Tong Xin Luo 221
  Xie Qing Wan 221
  Xin Bao Wan 221
  Yang Xin Yin 221
INFORMATICS IN CVDD 222
  Herboinformatics in CVDD 222
  Pharmacoinformatics in CVDD 222
  Toxicoinformatics in CVDD 223
CELLULAR MODELS FOR IN-VITRO RESEARCH 225
  Human Cardiac Myocytes 225

Human Aortic Endothelial Cells 225
Human Coronary Artery Endothelial Cells 226
Human Pulmonary Artery Endothelial Cells 226
Human Cardiac Microvascular Endothelial Cells 227
Human Pulmonary Microvascular Endothelial Cells 227
Human Dermal Microvascular Endothelial Cells 228
CONCLUSION 228
CONFLICT OF INTEREST 228
ACKNOWLEDGEMENT 228
REFERENCES 228

CHAPTER 7 CARDIOVASCULAR DISEASE: A SYSTEMS BIOLOGY APPROACH 234
Sujata Roy and *Ashasmita S Mishra*
INTRODUCTION 235
Cell-based Cardiac Disease Models and Animal Models 235
Post-genomic Era and Systems Biology Concept 236
SYSTEMS BIOLOGY 239
What is a Network and How to Construct? 239
From Network to Modules and Models 239
SYSTEMS GENETICS 241
Genomic Study and Genome-wide Association in Cardiovascular Traits 241
SYSTEMS MEDICINE 242
Integrative Biology 242
DISEASE COMORBITIES AND NETWORK BIOLOGY 243
TOOLS AND DATABASES 245
Public Data Sources, Prior Knowledge, and Data Integration 245
CONCLUSION 248
CONSENT FOR PUBLICATION 249
CONFLICT OF INTEREST 249
ACKNOWLEDGEMENTS 249
REFERENCES 249

SUBJECT INDEX 251

PREFACE

According to the World Health Organization, cardiovascular diseases (CVDs) are globally the number one cause of death. Over 18 million lives are lost globally due to heart attack alone. CVDs range from benign arrhythmias to massive heart failures and from chronic hypertension to ischemic strokes. They occupy a central place in non-communicable diseases, and they are often the result of complex chronic metabolic disorders. Extensive researches are been conducted on the causes and treatments of CVDs. Changing lifestyle with high calories diets, sedentary life style, and smoking are among the key causes. Volume 5 of the book series *"Frontiers in Cardiovascular Drug Discovery"* covers 7 comprehensive reviews contributed by leading researchers. These reviews broadly cover various drug targets and new classes of therapies for the prevention or treatment of cardiovascular diseases.

The review by Ramachandran *et al* focusses on a fiercely debated topic in CVD, *i.e.* lipid hypothesis. Cholesterol and LDLs have since long been considered as risk factors of cardiovascular diseases. However, there is mounting evidence that challenge this dogma. The authors have carefully reviewed the scientific literature and conclude that the theory stands valid. Huynh *et al* present exciting new advancements of SGLT2i (Sodium-glucose cotransporters 2) inhibitors as an important new class of drugs. These inhibitors increase renal glucose excretion, and lead to natriuresis and glycosuria with subsequent reduction in blood glucose and associated CVDs in diabetic patients Platelet aggregation and thrombosis are the major causes of morbidity and mortality worldwide. Piato and Graebin have the reviewed recent literature on the development of antithrombotic agents of natural and semi-synthetic origins, with a higher level of safety. Santos *et al* have contributed a chapter on the significance of transient receptor potential (TRP) channels as potential drug targets against cardiometabolic diseases. Mutations in some of the TRP channels are implicated in various metabolic and cardiovascular disorders, and thus activations of TRP channels through natural products may lead to the development of a new class of drugs.

Raynaud's phenomenon (RP), vasospasm due to cold exposure and emotional stress, is a common disorder. Lambova discuss various molecular approaches towards the treatment of RP. Traditional medicines have played an important role in the treatment of human diseases, including cardiovascular disorders. Ravindran *et al* have reviewed pharmacological, toxicological, and informatics studies, carried on various polyherbal formulations, in order to scientifically validate their efficacy against CVDs. The chapter by Roy and Mishra is focused on the applications of system biology approach in developing a better understanding of the molecular basis of the CVDs and its comorbidities. Special emphasis is paid to the identification of biomarkers for early diagnosis of CVD for a better management of the disease states.

We would like to express our gratitude to all the authors of above cited review articles for their excellent contributions in this dynamic and exciting field of biomedical and pharmaceutical research. The efforts of the team of Bentham Science Publishers, particularly Ms. Mariam Mehdi (Assistant Manager Publications), and Mr. Mahmood Alam (Director Publications) are deeply appreciated.

Atta-ur-Rahman *FRS*
Kings College, University of Cambridge
Cambridge
UK

&

M. Iqbal Choudhary
H.E.J. Research Institute of Chemistry
International Center for Chemical and Biological Sciences
University of Karachi
Karachi
Pakistan

List of Contributors

Ahmed AlTurki Division of Cardiology, McGill University Health Center, Montreal, Canada

Abhinav Sharma Division of Cardiology, McGill University Health Center, Montreal, Canada

Angelo Piato Departamento de Farmacologia, Instituto de Ciências Básicas da Saúde, Universidade Federal do Rio Grande do Su, Porto Alegre, Brasil

Ashasmita S. Mishra Department of Biotechnology, Rajalakshmi Engineering College, Rajalakshmi Nagar, Thandalam, Chennai-602105, Tamil Nadu, India

Cedric Stephan Graebin Departamento de Química Orgânica, Instituto de Química, Universidade Federal Rural do Rio de Janeiro, Seropédica, Brasil

Carola S. König College of Engineering, Design & Physical Sciences, Brunel University London, London, United Kingdom

Caroline Fernandes-Santos Instituto de Saude de Nova Friburgo, Universidade Federal Fluminense, Nova Friburgo, Rio de Janeiro, Brazil

Hasan AlTurki Department of Medicine, University of British Columbia,, Vancouver, Canada

Johanna Rajkumar Department of Biotechnology, Rajalakshmi Engineering College, Rajalakshmi Nagar, Thandalam, Chennai-602105, Tamil Nadu, India

Leidyanne Ferreira Gonçalves Instituto de Saude de Nova Friburgo, Universidade Federal Fluminense, Nova Friburgo, Rio de Janeiro, Brazil

Mark Sherman Division of Endocrinology, McGill University Health Center, Montreal, Canada

Mithun Bhartia Apollo Hospitals, International Hospitals, Guwahati, Assam, India
Dr Bhartia's Diabetes and Thyroid Clinic, Guwahati, Assam, India

Rekha Ravindran Department of Biotechnology, Rajalakshmi Engineering College, Rajalakshmi Nagar, Thandalam, Chennai-602105, Tamil Nadu, India

Sudarshan Ramachandran Department of Clinical Biochemistry, University Hospitals Birmingham NHS Foundation Trust, West Midlands, United Kingdom
Department of Clinical Biochemistry, University Hospitals of North Midlands/Faculty of Health Sciences, Staffordshire University/Institute of Science and Technology, Keele University/Staffordshire, United Kingdom
College of Engineering, Design & Physical Sciences, Brunel University London, London, United Kingdom

Sevdalina Nikolova Lambova Medical University - Plovdiv, Faculty of Medicine, Department of Propaedeutics of Internal Disease, Bulgaria

Sriram Kumar Department of Biotechnology, Rajalakshmi Engineering College, Rajalakshmi Nagar, Thandalam, Chennai-602105, Tamil Nadu, India

Sakthi Abbirami Gowthaman Department of Biotechnology, Rajalakshmi Engineering College, Rajalakshmi Nagar, Thandalam, Chennai-602105, Tamil Nadu, India

Sujata Roy	Department of Biotechnology, Rajalakshmi Engineering College, Rajalakshmi Nagar, Thandalam, Chennai-602105, Tamil Nadu, India
Thereza Cristina Lonzetti Bargut	Instituto de Saude de Nova Friburgo, Universidade Federal Fluminense, Nova Friburgo, Rio de Janeiro, Brazil
Thao Huynh	Division of Cardiology, McGill University Health Center, Montreal, Canada
Thereza Cristina Lonzetti Bargut	Instituto de Saude de Nova Friburgo, Universidade Federal Fluminense, Nova Friburgo, Rio de Janeiro, Brazil
Thao Huynh	Division of Cardiology, McGill University Health Center, Montreal, Canada

The Lipid Hypothesis: From Resins to Proprotein Convertase Subtilisin/Kexin Type-9 Inhibitors

Sudarshan Ramachandran[1,2,3], **Mithun Bhartia**[4,5] and **Carola S. König**[3]

[1] Department of Clinical Biochemistry, University Hospitals Birmingham NHS Foundation Trust, West Midlands, United Kingdom

[2] Department of Clinical Biochemistry, University Hospitals of North Midlands / Faculty of Health Sciences, Staffordshire University / Institute of Science and Technology, Keele University / Staffordshire, United Kingdom

[3] College of Engineering, Design & Physical Sciences, Brunel University London, United Kingdom

[4] Apollo Hospitals, International Hospitals, Guwahati, Assam, India

[5] Dr Bhartia's Diabetes and Thyroid clinic, Guwahati, Assam, India

Abstract: The validity of the lipid hypothesis has been debated recently in both, the media and the medical press. In this chapter we review the relevant evidence to evaluate whether it is still applicable in cardiovascular prevention. After a brief description of developments leading to the lipid hypothesis we consider prospective epidemiological studies, paying particular attention to the Framingham Heart Study as it was conceived at a time when lipid lowering therapy was unavailable. We also present the predictive factors of the other commonly used cardiovascular risk scoring models. All the algorithms show cholesterol (total or low density lipoprotein – cholesterol) and high density lipoproteins to predict cardiovascular disease. Our own data from the Whickham Study where subjects were recruited in the pre-statin era also show total cholesterol to be significantly associated with coronary heart disease. We then discuss intervention randomised controlled studies using agents that lower low density lipoprotein – cholesterol (resins, statins, ezetimibe and Proprotein convertase subtilisin/kexin type 9 inhibitors) paying particular attention to studies not demonstrating reduction in cardiovascular outcomes. Apart from patients with heart failure and possibly on dialysis the lipid hypothesis appears to be true. This is reinforced by a meta-analysis carried out by the Cholesterol Treatment Trialists' Collaboration. We do not feel that outcomes from cohort studies consisting of patients subject to multiple guideline driven treatments can be used as good quality evidence against the lipid hypothesis. We do acknowledge that more research is required rega-

---

* **Corresponding author Dr. S. Ramachandran:** Department of Clinical Biochemistry, University Hospitals Birmingham NHS Foundation Trust, Good Hope Hospital, Rectory Road, Sutton Coldfield, West Midlands B75 7RR, United Kingdom; Tel: +44-121-424 7246; Fax: +44-121-311 1800; E-mail: sud.ramachandran@heartofengland.nhs.uk

Atta-ur-Rahman & M. Iqbal Choudhary (Eds.)

rding heterogeneity and describe a non-invasive way in which atherogenesis of the individual may be measured. We would like future randomised controlled trials to incorporate study of disease mechanism(s) within the study design.

Keywords: Cardiovascular disease, Cardiovascular disease prediction, Coronary heart disease, Ezetimibe, Framingham Heart Study, Lipid hypothesis, LDL-cholesterol, Peak systolic velocity, Proprotein convertase subtilisin/kexin type 9 inhibitors, Randomised Controlled Trials, Statins, Total cholesterol, Whickham study.

INTRODUCTION

Atherosclerotic obstruction of arteries by plaque formation leading to cardiovascular disease (CVD) is one of the most common causes of mortality globally. Although the incidence has been decreasing [1], CVD still remains a leading cause of death in the United Kingdom [2]. Interestingly the prevalence of CVD has remained constant at about 3% [3] even though incidence has decreased, perhaps due to a fall in mortality. Thus, incidence and mortality rates and not prevalence may be the best indicators to evaluate CVD prevention measures. The Cholesterol Treatment Trialists' (CTT) Collaboration carried out meta-analyses of randomised controlled trials (RCTs) with a minimum of 1000 participants and concluded that a 1 mmol/l reduction in low density lipoprotein (LDL) - cholesterol was associated with a reduction in myocardial infarction, revascular-isation and ischaemic stroke by just over 20% [4]. The lipid hypothesis describes this widely observed association between CVD risk and raised serum total cholesterol and LDL- cholesterol. Thus, a recent editorial in the New England Journal of Medicine describing the results of the IMPROVE-IT study, convincingly supported the hypothesis on the basis of prospective longitudinal studies showing significant decreases in CVD following use of LDL-cholesterol reducing agents, such as statins and ezetimibe [5].

However, there are publications arguing against the causative effect of cholesterol and LDL-cholesterol in the pathogenesis of atheroma and these have raised doubts regarding the benefit of lipid lowering therapy and indeed, the validity of the lipid hypothesis [6, 7]. This view contrasts with data showing statistically significant reductions in CVD using drugs that reduce LDL-cholesterol by different mechanisms. We speculate that the prevalent guideline culture in clinical medicine requires complex diseases to be simplified to aid the use of treatment pathways. Heterogeneity of populations, based on the degree of risk and mechanisms leading to risk, is often not considered [8]. After describing the history of the development of the lipid hypothesis we will consider epidemiology and interventional trials and how they fit in with the lipid hypothesis. In this chapter it is not our intention to list details of the various trials, but to discuss and place the lipid hypothesis in the context of CVD prevention.

CHOLESTEROL

Cholesterol is found in body tissues and plasma of animals and is a ubiquitous constituent of cell membranes. It is a precursor of bile acids, vitamin D and steroid hormones such as cortisol, aldosterone, testosterone, oestrogens and progesterone. Further, it is important in the development / functioning of the nervous system, and is involved in signal transduction and sperm development. The structure of cholesterol is shown in Fig. (**1**) and the molecule can exist in either free or esterified (a fatty acid covalently attached to the hydroxyl group at position 3 of the ring) forms.

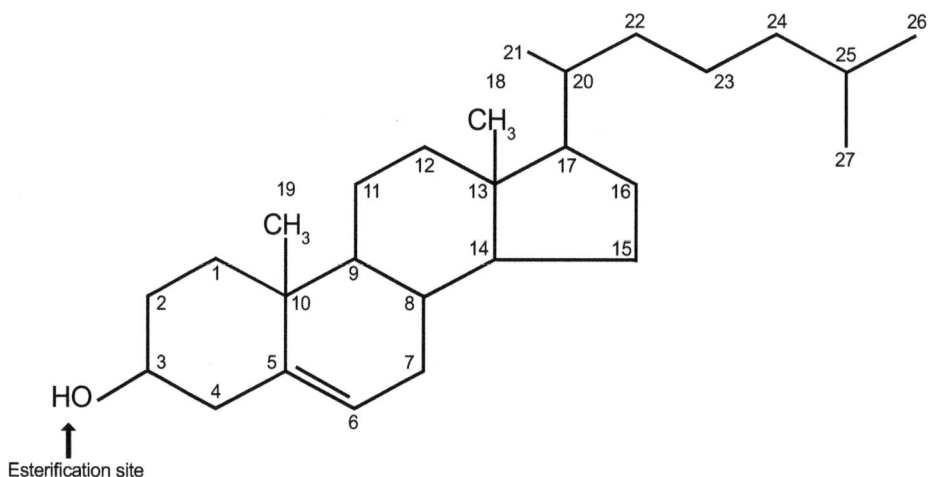

Fig. (1). Structure of cholesterol with the point of esterification highlighted.

Early Evolution of the Relationship between Cholesterol and Atherogenesis

We now consider major historical landmarks in the evolution of the lipid hypothesis, including the advent of evidence-based medicine *via* clinical trials. Controversy regarding the lipid hypothesis has ranged ever since Nikolai Anitschkow in 1913 demonstrated that rabbits when fed with purified cholesterol dissolved in sunflower oil developed vascular lesions similar to atheroma, this not being the case when the animals were fed just sunflower oil [9]. Anitschkow's findings were not confirmed in rats or dogs, hence the observation was considered to be specific to the rabbit model and cast aside. The fact that dietary cholesterol in rats and dogs did not translate into elevated serum cholesterol, perhaps due to high conversion of cholesterol to bile acids as suggested by Anitschkow, was not considered. That atherogenesis in the rabbit model was a two-step process (ongoing feeding of cholesterol followed by elevation of blood cholesterol levels in lipoproteins) and was not recognised at the time [9]. Further, the serum cholesterol level in the rabbit was significantly higher than in humans cast doubts on the clinical relevance of Anitschkow's work. However, continuing research confirmed the association between CVD and lipids and provided an understanding of the metabolism and transport of lipids.

The relationships between xanthomatosis, hypercholesterolemia (familial hypercholestrolaemia) and CVD were described between 1925-1938 by Francis Harbitz and Carl Müller [10]. Interestingly Müller suggested that reducing cholesterol levels may improve the prognosis [10]. John Oncley, used Cohn fractionation and electrophoresis to identify and separate the lipoproteins; their classification was based on their migration with the globulins, hence the nomenclature of alpha, prebeta and beta lipoproteins [11]. Gofman, an American scientist was convinced of the validity of Anitschkow's experimental observations and focused on the key issue of cholesterol transport in the blood [12, 13]. This led to him to use ultracentrifugation to identify and quantify lipoproteins, the particles transporting lipids in blood and then to associate them with atherosclerosis. Further work by Fredrickson and Gordon (1958) [14] and Olson and Vester (1960) [15] resulted in some clarity of lipid transport pathways. Integrating physiology of organs such as gut, liver and adipose tissue with isotopic studies of lipoprotein metabolism led them to conclude that triglycerides were transported by chylomicrons from the gut to adipose tissue, and by very low density lipoprotein (VLDL) from the liver to adipose tissue; both processes requiring lipoprotein lipase and local uptake of free fatty acids by fat cells. Apoproteins (Apo), the protein components of lipoproteins following delipidation and fractionation of lipoproteins, was characterised by Fredrickson *et al.,* (1967) based on size shape and amino acid composition [16]. Four families of Apo, each containing isoforms and determining metabolism of lipoproteins were identified by Jackson *et al.,* in 1976; Apo A primarily associated with the α-lipoproteins (HDL), Apo B and Apo E with β-lipoproteins (VLDL, Intermediate Density Lipoproteins (IDL) and LDL) and chylomicrons, and Apo C with all lipoproteins other than LDL [17]. Apo B has 2 forms; Apo B 100 found in VLDL, IDL and LDL and the truncated Apo B 48 form, synthesised in the intestine following editing of mRNA, in chylomicrons [17]. Apo E has 3 isoforms (E2, E3 and E4) with E2 and E4 resulting from mutations of the E3 isoform. Both, Apo B100 (Apo B 48 is devoid of the LDL-receptor (LDLR) binding site) and Apo E are integral to lipoprotein clearance with mutations of apoproteins or receptors affecting clearance and hence, accumulation of lipoproteins. Goldstein and Brown are credited with identifying the LDLR found in coated pits of most cells, which includes a ligand binding domain for Apo B 100 and Apo E, and characterising its functional role of endocytosis of the LDL particle [18, 19]. The LDL-LDLR complex is internalised and fused with a lysosome leading to degradation of apoproteins and lipids and disorder in this process was associated with familial hypercholesterolaemia and CVD. Over a period of nearly 70 years we moved from Anitschkov's observation to an understanding of LDL / LDLR and CVD based on a mechanistic framework devised by Goldstein and Brown. Current research is largely based on three approaches; 1. Basic science increasing our understanding of the mechanisms (*e.g.* lipoproteins, apoproteins and lipids) that leads to CVD, thus furthering drug development, 2. Large population based prospective studies establishing risk factors and at-risk populations, and 3. Intervention trials using therapeutic agents acting *via* different mechanisms resulting in the development of management guidelines. In this chapter we will mainly focus on the Framingham Heart Study and unpublished data from the Whickham study, both prospective studies, and interventional trials with LDL-cholesterol lowering agents that have led to the lipid hypothesis.

LONGITUDINAL PROSPECTIVE OBSERVATIONAL STUDIES AND CVD RISK ALGORITHMS

Current longitudinal studies studying complex pathologies with numerous risk factors have inherent problems due to the holistic management approach adopted. Since Scandinavian Simvastatin Survival Study (4S) [20] and West of Scotland Coronary Prevention Study (WOSCOPS) [21], statin treatment has been built into cardiovascular prevention guidelines. Thus, high risk populations would likely be on statins whose LDL-cholesterol efficacy would vary depending on the individual drug and dose. The pharmacokinetic and pharmacodynamic properties of the available statins vary. Similarly, other CVD risk factors would be treated according to national and professional organisation guidelines. This would, in our view make it very difficult to estimate the impact of individual risk factors over a long period. Thus, in this section we will primarily examine the Framingham Heart Study in depth, selected in view of it being initiated when lipid lowering therapy was not available, its length of follow-up, subsequent inclusion of children and grandchildren of the original cohort and study extension to widen the ethnicity of the original study population (https://www.nih.gov/sites/default/files/about-nih/impact/framingham-heart-study.pdf).

The initial objectives of the study when launched in 1948 were to identify factors associated with CVD with 5,209 men and women recruited between the ages of 30 and 62 with no evidence of CVD residing in the town of Framingham in Massachusetts, USA with lifestyle details noted and physical examinations carried out (https://crimsonpublishers.com/iod/pdf/IOD.000505.pdf). Following recruit-ment, a cardiovascular focused physical examination was carried out together with updates on medical history, blood test results at 2 – 4 year intervals [22]. Importantly recruitment of children and their spouses (Offspring-Spouse Cohort) and grandchildren (Third Generation Cohort) of the original cohort was initiated in 1971 and 2002, respectively. Heterogeneity was recognised with the Framingham OMNI 1 and OMNI 2 cohorts comprising ethnic minority residents in Framingham were included in 1994 and 2003, respectively, to reflect the changing diversity [22]. In order to identify genotypes related to CVD the Framingham investigators collaborated with the Jackson Heart Study and the American Heart Association and whole genome sequencing was carried out in 4200 of the subjects [22]. The outcomes from the Framingham Heart Study also gradually evolved; the original aim was to identify factors that were associated with CVD in the study population. With the original cohort aging, outcomes expanded to include osteoporosis, cognitive decline, dementia, Alzheimer's disease, Parkinson's disease and atrial fibrillation [22].

Identification of factors associated with CVD was gradual. Dawber *et al.,* in 1957 identified that the incidence of coronary heart disease (CHD) was nearly double in men compared to women [23]. Further, increased cholesterol, body weight and blood pressure were independently associated with the development of CHD in men between 45 and 62 years of age over a 4 year follow-up period [23]. Subsequently in 1961 Kannel *et al.,* showed CHD to be related to male gender, diabetes, left ventricular hypertrophy and increased age, cholesterol and blood pressure [24]. A year later cigarette smoking was shown to be related to CHD (the analysis was carried out on combined data from the Framingham Heart Study and the Albany Cardiovascular Health Study (http://www.epi.umn.edu/cvdepi/ study-synopsis/albany-cardiovascular-health-center-study/) [25]. Following measure-ment of lipoprotein fractions by ultracentrifugation, it became apparent that CHD was associated with increased LDL-cholesterol and decreased HDL-cholesterol levels, and this led to a ratio of total cholesterol to HDL-cholesterol being incorporated subsequently in the Framingham Risk Score [26]. Subsequently serum total cholesterol was also found to be a predictor of all-cause mortality [27]. Diabetes was in 1979 established to increase risk of CHD, cerebrovascular disease, peripheral vascular disease and heart failure [28]. Interestingly in 1996 lipoprotein (a) was identified to be an independent risk factor of CVD [29].

In addition to smoking other lifestyle factors were also recognised as risk factors. Physical inactivity was inversely and independently associated with mortality due to CVD in men, but not women [30]. When investigating the effects of nutrition the Framingham investigators compared CVD risk in the Framingham Offspring Spouse cohort with that of the second National Health and Nutrition Examination Survey (NHANES 2) and recommended that national nutrition strategies should target weight reduction with recommendations including reducing of foods rich in animal and plant fats and salt together with increases in complex carbohydrates and fibre [31].

The initial hypothesis of the Framingham Heart Study was that CVD was multifactorial and the findings described above have shown this to be correct. CHD and CVD risk function scores have also evolved since the 1960's [32 - 40]. Currently separate risk models have been derived for CVD (10 and 30 year risk), CHD, congestive heart failure, stroke and intermittent claudication in individuals without prior disease (https://www.framinghamheartstudy.org/fhs-risk-functions/cardiovascular-disease-10-year-risk/). The factors associated with these conditions in are presented in Table **1**. Interestingly, total cholesterol and HDL-cholesterol are risk factors predicting CVD (10 and 30 year models) and CHD, but not stroke, intermittent claudication and congestive heart failure (Table **1**). It is worth speculating that this may be due to stroke, intermittent claudication and congestive heart failure being associated with previous CVD / CHD as both these conditions are predicted by total cholesterol and HDL-cholesterol (hence, total cholesterol and HDL-cholesterol may have lost significance when statistical models included previous CVD / CHD). It is very evident from the hazard ratios in each of the models (https://www.framing hamheartstudy.org/fhs-ris--functions/cardiovascular-disease-10-year-risk/) that all these outcomes are multifactorial with each factor being weighted differently. Heterogeneity is also hinted at as separate algorithms were derived for men and women when CVD (10 year risk), CHD and stroke were outcomes. The omission of triglycerides as a risk factor is interesting. Triglyceride levels (above 150mg/dl) along with age, gender, fasting glucose levels, HDL-cholesterol, hypertension and parental history of diabetes, predict the development of diabetes (not shown in Table **1**). It could be that triglycerides levels by predicting diabetes are included in the outcomes predicted by diabetes (CVD, stroke and intermittent claudication). Receiver operated characteristic curves plotting true positive (sensitivity) against false positive rates (1- specificity) for CHD shows area under the curve of 0.79 for men and 0.83 for women [41]. The area under the receiver operated characteristic curves indicates the discriminatory ability of the models. We would consider area under the curve values of 0.9 -1.0, 0.8 - 0.9, 0.7 - 0.8 and 0.6 - 0.7 to be excellent, good, fair and poor, respectively (http://gim.unmc.edu/dxtests/roc3.htm). The values seen with the CHD predictive models also suggest that further study is required to identify new risk factors and / or to repeat the analysis for subgroups where these factors may be more strongly associated with the outcome in view of probable heterogeneity. Integrating genetic and epigenetic factors into the prediction model could potentially improve the discriminatory ability [42].

In addition to the Framingham Heart Study risk score there are numerous CVD / CHD risk calculators that are in clinical use (Table **2**) [43 - 46]. Details of the studies which gave rise to the risk algorithms are provided in Tables **1** (Framingham Heart Study) and Table **2**. Significantly all the risk algorithms presented based on observational studies include Total or LDL-cholesterol and HDL-cholesterol values. The Framingham Heart Study has many strengths including prospective recruitment at a single centre at a time when most patients were not on lipid lowering and antihypertensive treatment [47]. As all risk scores are strictly speaking only applicable to the study cohort, validation in other populations is essential. The Framingham risk algorithm has been validated in different countries with varying results. Interestingly, the scores derived appear to depend on the underlying CHD risk of the population. Whilst reasonable in non-American populations with similar CHD rates [48, 49] it appears to overestimate risk in European and Chinese populations at lower risk levels [50 - 54]. This was the pattern that we observed when comparing predicted and actual CHD rates in 2471 individuals during a 20 year follow-up in the Whickham Study [55] in Northeast England which has been cited in the latest NICE guidelines; CG 181 (Fig. **7** of this document) (https://www.ncbi.nlm.nih.gov/ books/ NBK248067/ pdf/ Bookshelf_NBK248067.pdf). Our results confirm that the Framingham model predicted the absolute risk of heart disease in 1700 men and women (where the Framingham risk score could be obtained) aged between 35 – 70 years without prior CVD in the United Kingdom when the annual CHD risk was above 1.5% (the observed risk falling within the 95% confidence intervals of the calculated risk using the Framingham algorithm), but underestimated the risk when the absolute risk was lower [55]. Of the 1700 participants, 529 (31.1%) developed heart disease during the 20 year follow-up. Logistic regression of the subgroup showed that CHD was significantly associated with age, male gender, smoking, diabetes, total cholesterol (also total cholesterol: HDL-cholesterol ratio using mean HDL-cholesterol values of 1.15 mmol/l and 1.4 mmol/l in men and women, respectively [56]) and systolic blood pressure, these results similar to the Framingham model (Table **3**); unpublished data from [55]. Unlike in the Framingham model (Table **1**) left ventricular hypertrophy was associated with CHD. Significantly, whilst triglycerides levels and diastolic blood pressure were not significantly associated with CHD, baseline HDL-cholesterol could not be considered as it was not routinely measured during the period of recruitment. The association between baseline cholesterol levels (stratified) and CHD in the total cohort is shown in Fig. (**2**); unpublished data from [55]. It is clear that a strong near linear association exists with no hint of CHD rates rising at the lower end or falling at the upper end of the cholesterol range. Importantly, the mean age of the stratified baseline cholesterol categories varied, cholesterol level was associated with age (linear regression analysis: c: 0.02, 95% CI: 0.02 – 0.03, p<0.001), hence it is important to be cautious with a univariate analysis. We include this figure only to demonstrate no evidence of a J or U shaped association between cholesterol and CHD, this data possibly important in the current cholesterol debate. Logistic regression analysis with age (OR: 1.04, 95% CI: 1.03 – 1.05, p<0.001) and baseline cholesterol (OR: 1.11, 95% CI: 1.02 – 1.21, p=0.015) as continuous variables included as independent variables in a single model showed both factors were independently associated with CHD. The strength of our validation was that baseline measurements were gathered between 1972 - 4 and therapeutic intervention would have been minimal with statins being unavailable for most of the follow-up period, similar to that in the Framingham Heart Study.

Table 1. Risk factors associated with the various cardiovascular outcomes obtained from the Framingham Heart Study.

	CVD		CHD	Stroke	Intermittent Claudication	Congestive Heart Failure
	10 year risk	30 year risk	10 year risk	10 year risk	4 year risk	4 year risk
Age	Yes	Yes	Yes	Yes	Yes	Yes
Male gender	Yes (separate model)	Yes	Yes (separate model)	Yes (separate model)	Yes	NA
Diabetes	Yes	Yes	No	Yes	Yes	Yes
Smoking	Yes	Yes	Yes	Yes	Yes	No
Hypertension	NA	NA	NA	NA	Yes	Yes
Systolic BP - untreated	Yes	Yes	Yes	Yes	NA	NA
Systolic BP - treated	Yes	Yes	Yes	Yes	NA	NA
Total cholesterol	Yes	Yes	Yes	No	Yes	No
HDL-cholesterol	Yes	Yes	Yes	No	No	No
Atrial Fibrillation	No	No	No	Yes	No	No
Left venriculat hypertrophy	No	No	No	Yes	No	Yes
Prior CHD / CVD	NA	NA	NA	Yes	Yes	Yes
Heart rate	NA	NA	NA	NA	NA	Yes
Body mass index	NA	NA	NA	NA	NA	Yes
Coronary valve disease	NA	NA	NA	NA	NA	Yes

It is not within the scope of this chapter to analyse the use of CHD and CVD risk algorithms. As previously stated lipid levels have been significantly associated with CHD and CVD in all the major risk predictive models [38, 39, 43 - 46]. We have described the Framingham Heart Study in some depth as it commenced in the pre lipid lowering era and will continue to remain relevant as it is evolving with the addition of genetic data *etc*. We have also shown that total cholesterol levels were independently associated with CHD in a United Kingdom population also in the pre-intervention era. In our view it is very difficult to establish the role of lipids in the aetiology of CVD in the current climate. Non-lipid lowering strategies have also demonstrated significant CHD and CVD reduction. The Heart Outcomes Prevention Evaluation (HOPE) [57, 58], Captopril Prevention Project (CAPP) [59] and Appropriate Blood Pressure Control in Diabetes (ABCD) [60] trials showed antihypertensives resulting in cardiovascular benefits, often far greater than that could be expected from their effect on blood pressure in different cohorts. More recently the sodium glucose cotransporter 2 inhibitor empagliflozin reduced CVD and CVD associated mortality in patients with type 2 diabetes [61]. Observational studies have shown Phosphodiesterase type 5-inhibitors to reduce myocardial infarction [62] and all-cause mortality [63]. The above examples demonstrate the difficulty of studying in isolation, the impact of lipids and lipid lowering therapy on CVD, in view of its multifactorial aetiology. Heterogeneity of aetiology is also problematic as study results may only be applicable to the characteristics of the cohort studied [8].

Table 2. CVD and CHD risk scores in general use with study details.

	PROCAM	WHO / ISH	SCORE	QRISK
Publication year [ref]	2002 [41]	2003 [42]	2003 [43]	2008 [44]
Study characteristics				
Outcomes	CHD	CHD and stroke	Fatal CVD	CVD
Recruitment	1985	NA	1972 - 1991	1995 - 2007
Follow-up (years)	10	NA (incidence rate of outcome)	Variable	variable
Number of individuals	5389	NA	205,178	1,200,000
Age range	40 - 65	40 - 70	45 - 64	35 - 74
Gender	Males	Males / Females	Males / Females	Males / Females
Identified Risk Factors				
Age	Yes	Yes	Yes	Yes
Gender	NA	No	Yes	Yes
Smoking status	Yes	Yes	Yes	Yes
systolic blood pressure	Yes	Yes	Yes	Yes
Total / LDL - cholesterol	Yes	Yes	Yes	Yes
HDL-cholesterol	Yes	Yes	Yes	Yes
Triglycerides	Yes	No	No	Yes
Diabetes	Yes	Yes	No	No
Familiy History of CVD / CHD	Yes	No	No	Yes
Left ventricular hypertrophy	No	No	No	Yes
Body mass index	No	No	No	Yes
Anto hypertensive therapy	No	No	No	Yes

INTERVENTIONAL STUDIES WITH CLINICAL EVENTS AS OUTCOMES

The above observational studies have clearly shown an association between lipids and CVD. In 1965, Sir Austin Bradford Hill gave the first President's Address to the newly formed Section on Occupational Medicine discussing criteria whereby an observed association could be stated as causative [64]. The criteria consisted of strength of association, consistency, specificity, temporality, biological gradient, plausibility, coherence, experiment, and analogy. Schade *et al.,* in 2017, after examining the association between LDL-cholesterol and CVD, concluded that LDL is the primary cause of atherosclerotic CVD [65]. This review concluded that the data studied complemented the results of RCTs in humans demonstrating that the reduction of LDL-cholesterol resulted in not only a reduction but a reversal of atherosclerosis. They rightfully acknowledged that LDL-cholesterol was not the sole factor. The progression of atherosclerosis may be accelerated by hypertension, smoking, diabetes, and obesity. They also controversially stated that without the contribution of LDL-cholesterol, clinically significant plaques would not be formed [65]. It is acknowledged that RCTs have inherent limitations and it can be often difficult to gain an understanding of a treatment in an individual patient as opposed to the study population [66]. Reporting has improved with standardisation protocols such as CONsolidated Standards Of Reporting Trials (CONSORT) [67 - 70]. Further, strategies have been devised for integrating the results *via* guidelines into clinical practice [71].

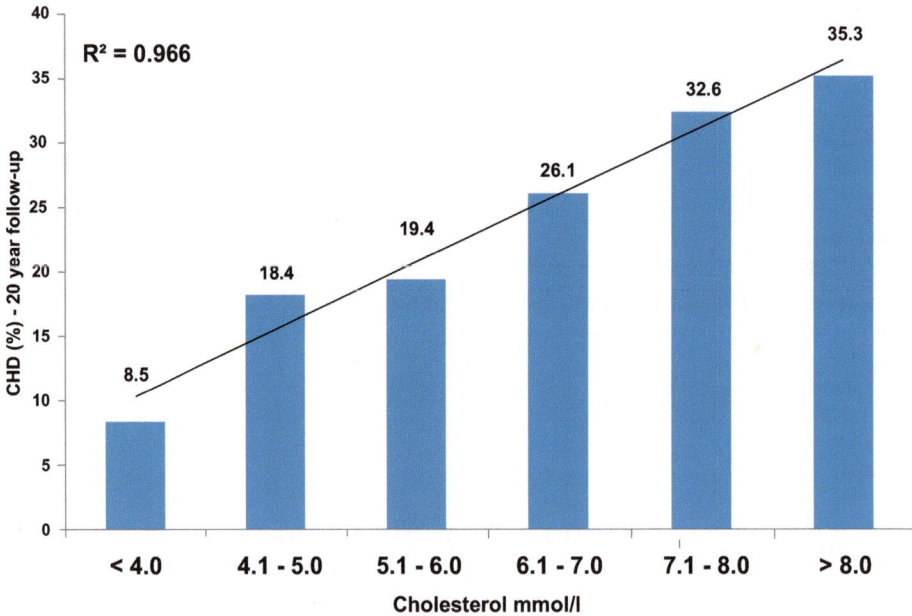

Baseline Cholesterol (mmol/l)	Individuals screened	Mean age ± SD (years)	% CHD (20 years follow-up)
< 4.0	47	36.0 ± 18.5	8.5
4.1 - 5.0	456	38.7 ±15.9	18.4
5.1 - 6.0	871	43.8 ± 15.3	19.4
6.1 - 7.0	690	48.7 ± 15.0	26.1
7.1 - 8.0	285	53.0 ±14.1	32.6
>8.0	122	54.5 ± 14.2	35.3

Fig. (2). Association between CHD during 20 years of follow-up and baseline cholesterol stratified in the total Whickham cohort. Mean age is provided in the attached table to demonstrate the importance of adjusting any analysis for age in view of its association with cholesterol concentrations (linear regression analysis: c: 0.02, 95% CI: 0.02 – 0.03, p<0.001). (Unpublished data from Ramachandran S, French JM, Vanderpump

MP, Croft P, Neary RH. Using the Framingham model to predict heart disease in the United Kingdom: retrospective study. BMJ 2000; 320: 676 – 677).

We will now move onto RCTs evaluating the effects of various cholesterol (and LDL-cholesterol) lowering drugs have on clinical endpoints. Resins, statins and ezetimibe lower cholesterol and LDL-cholesterol *via* varied mechanisms.

Table 3. Association between CHD during 20 years of follow-up and baseline factors measured in the Whickham Study cohort in a single logistic regression model. All factors were significant in separate regression models and remained significant when included in a single regression model. HDL-cholesterol concentrations were not measured at baseline, hence values of 1.15 mmol/l were used for men and 1.4 mmol/l for women were used in calculating the cholesterol / HDL-cholesterol ratio. (unpublished data from Ramachandran S, French JM, Vanderpump MP, Croft P, Neary RH. Using the Framingham model to predict heart disease in the United Kingdom: retrospective study. BMJ 2000; 320: 676 – 677). The corresponding author (Dr R H Neary) provided consent to use this previously unpublished data.

Risk Factor	Odds Ratio	95% CI	p
Age (years)	1.02	1.01 - 1.04	<0.001
Male Gender	1.42	1.08 - 1.85	0.011
Smoking	1.47	1.18 - 1.83	0.001
Systolic blood pressure (mm Hg)	1.01	1.01 - 1.02	<0.001
Diabetes	3.11	1.04 - 9.27	0.042
Cholesterol:HDL cholesterol	1.16	1.03 - 1.30	0.015
Left ventricular hypertrophy	4.76	1.20 - 18.82	0.026

Randomised Controlled Bile Sequestrants Trials

Bile acid sequestrants (anion exchange resins) were developed in the 1970s and by binding gut bile acids, reduced the entero-hepatic recirculation of bile acids and decreased LDL- cholesterol by 10 - 15% [72]. Most data are derived from use of cholestyramine and colestipol, but the more recently introduced colesevelam, possibly has fewer side effects [73]. The Lipid Research Clinics Coronary Primary Prevention Trial (LRC-CPPT) a double-blinded RCT studied the association between cholestyramine treatment and CHD (primary end point: composite of death due to CHD and myocardial infarction) in 3,806 asymptomatic middle-aged men with hypercholesterolemia over a mean follow-up of 7.4 years [74]. All patients followed a moderate cholesterol lowering diet. A significant reduction in the primary outcome was observed in form of a 19% relative risk reduction with cholestyramine treatment (events: 7.0%) compared to placebo (events: 8.6%). Further, the cholestyramine treatment was associated with 25%, 20%, and 21% lower rates for positive exercise stress tests, angina, and coronary bypass surgery, respectively. All-cause mortality was not significantly different in the two study arms. The LRC-CPPT showed that reducing total cholesterol and LDL-cholesterol levels significantly decreased CHD morbidity and mortality in men with elevated LDL-cholesterol levels [74]. Despite the above outcome this therapy is a minor player in lipid lowering because of low tolerability with gastrointestinal side effects and high price in the case of the better tolerated colesevalem (£0.97 - £2.91 per day: https://www.nice.org.uk/ advice/ suom22/ chapter/ evidencereview-economic-issues#cost). Further, more evidence from RCTs is required to establish benefits when bile acid sequestrants are added to statins as most statin treated patients would be expected to have lower lipid levels.

Randomised Controlled Statin Trials

Cholesterol is synthesised *via* a multistep pathway from acetyl-CoA taking place in the cytosol and endoplasmic reticulum [75]. From the endoplasmic reticulum it is transported to the plasma membrane and other organelles such as mitochondria, and lipid droplets. Fig. (**3**) shows many of the enzymes involved in the synthetic pathway with HMG-CoA reductase (targeted by statins) catalysing the rate-limiting step converting HMG-CoA to mavelonic acid [76]. This was demonstrated by the Japanese biochemist Akira Endo in the 1970s using citrinin produced by the fungus Pythium ultimum to inhibit cholesterol synthesis in rats [77]. Since then we have had lovastatin (1987), simvastatin, a semi synthetic derivative of lovastatin (1987), pravastatin (1991), fluvastatin (1994), atorvastatin (1997), cerivastatin (1998: withdrawn in 2001), rosuvastatin (2003) and pitavastatin (2003) [78].

The expression of genes encoding HMG-CoA reductase is regulated by the sterol response element binding protein (SREBP), a membrane protein residing in the endoplasmic reticulum, binding to upstream sterol response elements sequences and activating transcription. SREBP contains two transmembrane domains and two cytosol facing DNA-binding domains and is held in the endoplasmic reticulum via interactions with other proteins containing a sterol-sensing domain. Binding of this domain and cholesterol determines regulation of HMG-CoA reductase; following association with cholesterol the conformation allows other parts of the protein to interact with SREBP. However, when cholesterol levels decrease, interaction between the sterol-sensing domain and cholesterol is lost leading to a change in the structure resulting in disassociation of the protein from SREBP. Free SREBP is transported to the Golgi where DNA-binding domains are released into the cytosol following the actions of proteases. In the nucleus, the DNA-binding domains bind sterol response elements and activate genes transcription promoting cholesterol synthesis and uptake [74].

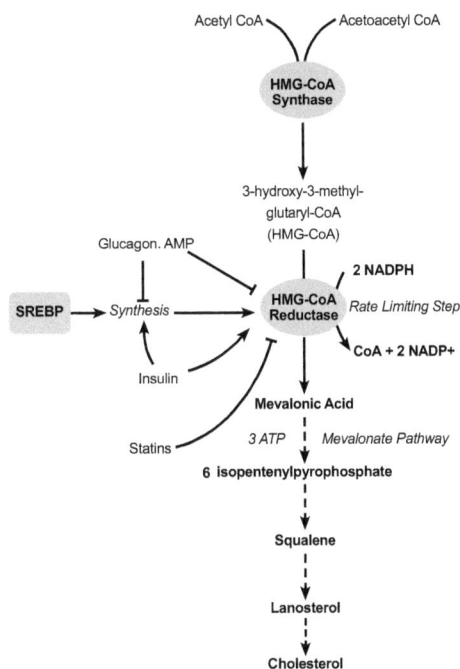

Fig. (3). Pathway leading to cholesterol synthesis.

Since 4S in 1994 there have been numerous RCTs conducted to study the effect of reducing LDL-cholesterol on clinical outcomes. We picked the RCTs including >1000 individuals from Pubmed (Fig. **4**, abbreviations of the trials are provided in the footnote of the figure) to discuss further [5, 20, 21, 78 - 109]. Whilst many of the trial cohorts comprised only individuals with established CVD (secondary prevention) some trials had individuals with no previous CVD (primary prevention). The proportion of individuals without previous CVD includes WOSCOPS: 92% [21], AFCAPS/TEXCAPS: >99% [81], HPS: 15% [85], PROSPER: 56% [88], ALLHAT-LLT: 78% [89], ASCOT-LLT: 86% [90], ALERT: 81% [91], CARDS: 96% [92], 4D: 27% [97], MEGA: 99% [99], JUPITER: 100% [103] and AURORA: 60% [104]. Fig. (**4**) shows the RCTs that did not show benefit regarding the clinical CVD outcomes (trials with red backgrounds). We consider these to see if cohort properties (*e.g.* underlying risk, type of dyslipidaemia *etc*) or scale of LDL-cholesterol reduction could contribute to them not achieving significant CVD reduction. RCTs showing statins reducing CVD outcomes are assumed to adhere to the lipid hypothesis and will not be discussed.

The **post CABG trial** included 1351 individuals who had undergone coronary artery bypass grafting with LDL- cholesterol between 3.4 – 4.5 mmol/l and triglycerides < 3.4 mmol/l randomised to either intensive (to achieve LDL-cholesterol of 1.6 – 2.5 mmol/l) or standard (> 2.5 mmol/l) lipid lowering therapy (lovastatin ± cholestyramine if required) and warfarin or placebo over a mean 4.3 years and an extended follow-up of 3 further years [80]. The progression of atherosclerosis was significantly reduced in the intensive lipid lowering arm. Though the clinical CVD end-points were lower they did not achieve statistical significance in the intensive lipid lowering arm at the end of the follow-up [80]. However, at the end of the extended follow-up both end points were significantly lower in the intensive lipid lowering arm [110]. Thus, though the study did not meet strict statistical criteria, it did suggest lowering LDL-cholesterol was beneficial. Interestingly, warfarin did not demonstrate any benefit.

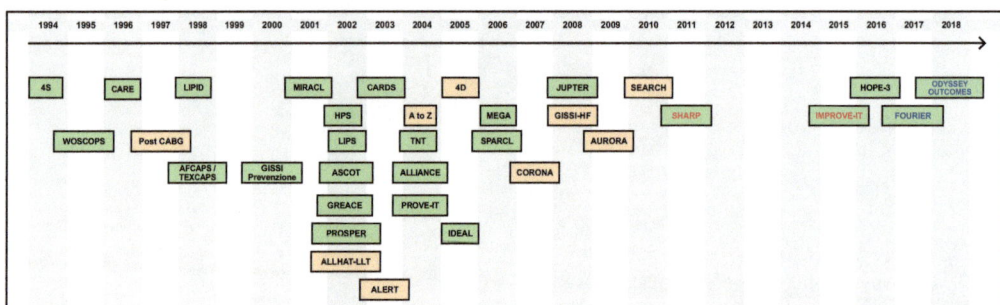

Fig. (4). Time line of RCTs with LDL-cholesterol reducing agents (statins, ezetimibe and PCSK9 inhibitors) and CVD reduction since the 4S in 1994.

The RCTs significantly achieving and not achieving reduction in CVD outcomes are coloured green and red respectively. Statin RCTs are denoted in black print whilst ezetimibe RCTs (SHARP, IMPROVE-IT) are in red and PCSK9 inhibitor RCTs (FOURIER, ODYSSEY OUTCOMES) are in blue print.
4S: Scandinavian Simvastatin Survival Study [18]
4D: Die Deutsche Diabetes Dialyze Studie [95]
A to Z: Aggrastat-to-Zocor Trial [93]
AFCAPS/TEXCAPS: Air Force/Texas Coronary Atherosclerosis Prevention Study [79]
ALERT: Assessment of Lescol in Renal Transplantation [89]
ALLHAT-LLT: Antihypertensive and Lipid-Lowering Treatment to Prevent Heart Attack Trial Lipid-Lowering Trial [87]
ALLIANCE: Aggressive Lipid-Lowering Initiation Abates New Cardiac Events [91]
ASCOT: Anglo-Scandinavian Cardiac Outcomes Trial [88]
AURORA: A Study to Evaluate the Use of Rosuvastatin in Subjects on Regular Hemodialysis: An Assessment of Survival and Cardiovascular Events [102]
CARDS: Collaborative Atorvastatin Diabetes Study [90]
CARE: The Cholesterol and Recurrent Events Trial [77]
CORONA: The Controlled Rosuvastatin Multinational Trial in Heart Failure [99]
FOURIER: Further Cardiovascular Outcomes Research with PCSK9 Inhibition in Subjects with Elevated Risk [106]
GISSI HF: The Gruppo Italiano per lo Studio della Sopravvivenza nell'Insufficienza cardiac [100]
GISSI Prevenzione: The Gruppo Italiano per lo Studio della Sopravvivenza nell'Infarto Miocardico [81]
GREACE: The Greek Atorvastatin and Coronary Heart-disease Evaluation Study [85]

HOPE-3: Heart Outcomes Prevention Evaluation – 3 [105]
HPS: Heart Protection Study [83]
IDEAL: Incremental Decrease in End Points Through Aggressive Lipid Lowering study [96]
IMPROVE-IT: Improved Reduction of Outcomes: Vytorin Efficacy International Trial [5]
JUPITER: Justification for the Use of Statins in Prevention: an Intervention Trial Evaluating Rosuvastatin [101]
LIPID: The Long-Term Intervention with Pravastatin in Ischemic Disease [80]
LIPS: The Lescol Intervention Prevention Study [84]
MEGA: Management of Elevated Cholesterol in the Primary Prevention Group of Adult Japanese study [97]
MIRACL: The Myocardial Ischemia Reduction with Aggressive Cholesterol Lowering study [82]
ODYSSEY OUTCOME: A Randomized, Double-Blind, Placebo-Controlled, Parallel-Group Study to Evaluate the Effect of Alirocumab on the Occurrence of Cardiovascular Events in Patients Who Have Recently Experienced an Acute Coronary Syndrome [107]
Post CABG: coronary artery bypass graft [78]
PROSPER: The Prospective Study of Pravastatin in the Elderly at Risk [86]
PROVE IT: The Pravastatin or Atorvastatin Evaluation and Infection Therapy study [92]
SEARCH: Study of the Effectiveness of Additional Reductions in Cholesterol and Homocysteine [103]
SHARP: Study of Heart and Renal Protection [104]
SPARCL: The Stroke Prevention by Aggressive Reduction in Cholesterol Levels study [98]
TNT: Treating to New Targets study [94]
WOSCOPS: The West of Scotland Coronary Prevention Study [19]

The **ALLHAT-LLT** investigated a mixed primary (LDL-cholesterol: 3.1 – 4.9 mmol/l) and secondary prevention (LDL-cholesterol: 2.6 – 3.3 mmol/l) multiethnic (38% black, 23% Hispanic) cohort comprising 10,355 individuals aged >55 years and compared the effects of pravastatin 40mg *vs* usual care (in this group 32% and 29% of individuals with and without CHD were commenced on lipid lowering therapy) over a mean 4.8 years [89]. All-cause mortality was similar in the groups (pravastatin: 14.9%, usual care: 15.3%) and though CHD was lower in the pravastatin subjects (pravastatin: 9.3%, usual care: 10.4%) risk reduction did not achieve significance (RR: 0.91, 95% CI: 0.79 – 1.04, p=0.16). This non-significant outcome may be due to the modest LDL-cholesterol difference (16.7%) between the 2 arms.

The **ALERT trial** compared fluvastatin and placebo treatments in 2102 renal transplant recipients with total cholesterol values between 4.0 – 9.0 mmol/l [91]. Although major adverse cardiac events were lower in the fluvastatin arm compared to the placebo arm statistical significance was not achieved (RR: 0.83, 95% CI: 0.64 – 1.06, p=0.14). However, it is important to note that fewer cardiac deaths and non-fatal myocardial infarctions, a secondary outcome, were seen in the fluvastatin arm (RR: 0.65, 95% CI: 0.48 – 0.88, p=0.005).

The **A to Z trial** compared patients commenced on simvastatin 40mg, increased after 1 month to 80mg arm (LDL-cholesterol after 8 months was 1.63 mmo/l) with those on placebo who were converted after 4 months to simvastatin 20mg (LDL-cholesterol after 8 months was 1.99 mg) in 4497 individuals [95]. The primary outcome was a composite of cardiovascular death, non-fatal myocardial infarction hospitalisation with acute coronary syndrome and stroke over 6 – 24 months and this was not achieved; simvastatin event rate: 14.4%, placebo / simvastatin event rate: 16.7% (HR: 0.89, 95% CI: 0.76 – 1.04, p=0.14). Primary outcome events after the initial 4 months of follow-up, showed a significant reduction in the simvastatin arm (HR: 0.75, 95% CI: 0.60 – 0.95, p=0.02). In our view, this study with a relatively short follow-up and results that do not reach statistical significance does not disprove the lipid theory.

The **SEARCH study** included 12,064 patients aged 18 – 80 years with a history of myocardial infarction were randomised to either simvastatin 20mg or 80mg for a mean follow-up of 6.7 years [105]. The primary endpoint consisted of major vascular events; coronary death, non-fatal myocardial infarction, stroke, or arterial revascularisation. The LDL-cholesterol difference between the groups was a modest 0.35mmol/l. This probably accounted for the primary outcome not being significantly different between the simvastatin 80mg (24.5%) and simvastatin 20mg (25.7%) groups; RR: 0·94, 95% CI: 0·88 – 1·01, p=0·10.

The **4D study** included 1255 subjects with type 2 diabetes receiving haemodialysis randomised to atorvastatin 20mg or placebo [97]. The primary end point was a composite of cardiovascular death, nonfatal myocardial infarction, and stroke. Primary outcome event rate in the total cohort after a median follow-up of 4 years was high at 37% (atorvastatin arm: 37%, placebo arm: 38%, RR: 0.92, 95% CI: 0.77 – 1.10, p=0.37). It is also worth stating that fatal strokes were more common in the atorvastatin arm (4.0%) than the placebo arm (2.0%); RR: 2.03, 95% CI: 1.05 – 3.93, p= 0.04), this result not driven by haemorrhagic stroke as was seen in the SPARCL study [100]. When all cardiac events such as death from CVD, non-fatal myocardial infarction, and interventions were combined (secondary outcome), the atorvastatin arm showed benefit (33%) compared to placebo (39%); HR: 0.82, 95% CI: 0.68 – 0.99, p=0.03. The **AURORA study** included 2776 patients between 50 – 80 years of age receiving haemodialysis randomised to either rosuvastatin 10mg or placebo during a median follow-up of 3.8 years [104]. The primary end point was a composite of death from cardiovascular causes, nonfatal myocardial infarction and nonfatal stroke. No significant difference was observed in the primary end-point with between the rosuvastatin group (9.2 events / 100 patient years) and the placebo group (9.5 events / 100 patient years); HR: 0.96; 95% CI: 0.84 - 1.11; p=0.59. We speculate that the reason for the primary outcome not being reached could be related to cohort characteristics (*e.g.* renal failure, dialysis *etc*). However, this speculation is not supported by the **SHARP study** which included 9270 individuals with renal impairment showing the primary outcome of the first major cardiovascular event was significantly lower in the simvastatin + ezetimibe group (11.3%) compared to the simvastatin + placebo group (13.4%) during a median follow-up of 4.9 years;

RR: 0·83, 95% CI: 0·74–0·94, p=0·0021 [106]. Importantly, 27% of patients in both arms were receiving haemodialysis. Interestingly patients on dialysis were not treated as a subgroup. However, it must be emphasised that the LDL-cholesterol difference between the groups was a result of ezetimibe and not statin therapy.

The **CORONA study** included 5011 patients > 60 years of age with heart failure (New York Heart Association class 2 – 4) who were randomised to receive either rosuvastatin 10mg or placebo over a median follow-up of 32.8 months [101]. The primary outcome was a composite of death from cardiovascular causes, nonfatal myocardial infarction and nonfatal stroke. No significant difference (HR: 0.92, 95% CI: 0.83 – 1.02, p=0.12) in primary outcome was evident between the rosuvastatin (11.4%) and placebo (12.3%) arms. The **GISSI-HF trial** was carried out in 4574 patients > 18 years of age with heart failure (New York Heart Association class 2 – 4) over a median follow-up of 3.9 years [102]. Primary endpoints consisted of time to death, and time to death or admission to hospital for cardiovascular reasons. No benefit was observed with rosuvastatin therapy regarding either end-point. In the rosuvastatin group 29% patients died from any cause and in the placebo group 28% (HR: 1·00, 95% CI: 0·90 – 1·12, p=0·94). The second end-point of death or hospital admission for cardiovascular reasons was seen in 57% and 56% of patients rosuvastatin and placebo, respectively (HR: 1·01, 99% CI: 0·91 – 1·11, p=0·90). The above 2 trials (CORONA and GISSI-HF) raise the question whether rosuvastatin (it is important to further study whether this phenomenon is a class effect or not) treatment is of any benefit in patients with heart failure, although it must be emphasised that in neither study did it result in any harm. Once again we speculate whether lipid lowering therapy is of benefit in patients with heart failure.

Fig. (4) shows most RCTs led to significant reduction in CVD, the primary end point in virtually all the studies. It must be emphasised that none of the RCTs showed statins being associated with any increase in CVD. We have also briefly described the studies where the primary outcome was not met. Perhaps the benefit of lipid lowering therapy in patients with heart failure or haemodialysis needs to be reconsidered, although for the latter group the results of the **SHARP study** are perhaps reassuring [106].

We did not consider the **ASPEN** (Atorvastatin Study for Prevention of coronary heart disease Endpoints in Non-insulin dependent diabetes mellitus) as it was originally designed as a secondary cardiovascular prevention trial in patients with prior myocardial infarction or interventions for CVD [111]. However, in view of changing treatment guidelines for patients with CHD, recruitment was compromised which led to a change in protocol after 2 years leading to inclusion of individuals without CVD. Further, all patients with CVD developed either before or during the trial were commenced on active therapy. In view of this we did not include ASPEN in Fig. (**4**).

The CTT Collaboration carried out a meta-analysis of 26 trials (5 trials (39,612 patients) comparing more *vs* less intensive statin therapy and 21 trials (129,526 patients) comparing statins *vs* placebo) [4]. All trials in this meta-analysis, apart from ASPEN are included in Fig. (**4**). The results suggested a 1mmol/l decrease in LDL-cholesterol was associated with a significant (RR: 0.78, 95% CI: 0.76 – 0.80, p<0.0001) 22% reduction in major vascular events. Even the negative studies described above showed event reduction close to what would be predicted from the CTT collaboration meta-analysis. All-cause mortality was reduced by 10% (RR: 0.90, 95% CI: 0.87 – 0.93, p <0.0001), mainly driven by lower CHD deaths. No significant differences were observed in cancer rates or deaths due to non-vascular causes.

Randomised Controlled Ezetimibe Trials

The source of cholesterol in the intestinal lumen is mainly dietary (300 – 500mg/day) and biliary (800 – 1200mg/day). Absorption (about 50-60% of intestinal content, although saturation of absorption takes place at higher cholesterol content) takes place principally in the duodenum and proximal jejunum, the process facilitated by bile salts [112]. Cholesterol and phytosterols are taken up both from the intestinal lumen of the enterocyte (the uptake of cholesterol being greater than phytosterols) by what appears to be a common unidirectional sterol transporter involving a Neiman–Pick C1 Like 1 (NPC1L1) protein in the jejunal brush border membrane [112, 113]. Reverse transport of the sterols into the intestinal lumen is mediated by the ATP-binding cassette (ABC) hemitransporters (ABCG5 and ABCG8) function. Ezetimibe, or 1-(-
-fluorophenyl)-(3R)-[3-{4-fluorophenyl}-{3S}-hydroxyprophyl-
-(4S)-(4-hydroxyphenyl)-(2-azetidinone), inhibits intestinal cholesterol absorption by selectively blocking the NPC1L1 protein [113].

The large RCTs with clinical outcomes assessing the association between ezetimibe and CVD are included in Fig. (**4**); **SHARP** [106] and **IMPROVE-IT** [5], both trials showing results in accordance with the lipid theory. The results of SHARP have been discussed previously. In IMPROVE-IT, 18,144 patients previously hospitalised with acute coronary syndrome were randomised to either simvastatin 40mg + ezetimibe or simvastatin 40mg + placebo groups and followed up for a median 6 years [5]. The primary end point was a composite of cardiovascular death, nonfatal myocardial infarction, unstable angina requiring rehospitalisation, coronary revascularisation or nonfatal stroke. The primary end point after 7 years in the simvastatin + ezetimibe group was 32.7% compared with 34.7% in the simvastatin + placebo group (HR: 0.94, 95% CI: 0.89 - 0.99, p=0.016).

Randomised Controlled PCSK9 Inhibitor Trials

Proprotein convertase subtilisin/kexin type 9 (PCSK9) inhibitors are monoclonal antibodies that bind and inactivate PCSK9, leading to decreased LDLR degradation thus enhancing LDLR recycling back to the liver surface (up to 150 times) and increasing LDL particle uptake [114]. PCSK9 inhibition was identified as a potential modifier of CVD risk, as loss of function mutations in the PCSK9 gene were associated with low LDL-cholesterol and reduced CVD [115].

CVD reduction with PCSK9 inhibitors was suggested by post-hoc analyses of the **OSLER** [116] and **ODYSSEY LONG TERM** [117], both efficacy trials. Similarly in the **GLAGOV** study comprising 970 patients with angiographic coronary artery disease, evolocumab was associated with reduction in atheroma volume (primary outcome) on angiography, with more individuals on it demonstrating plaque regression (64.3% *vs* 47.3%) and fewer developing major adverse cardiac events (12.2% *vs* 15.3%) compared to controls (secondary outcomes) [118].

The **FOURIER** study was the first PCSK9 clinical inhibitor outcome trial comparing evolocumab against placebo in 27,564 patients with CVD with LDL-cholesterol $\geq$ 1.8mmol/l or non-HDL-cholesterol $\geq$ 2.6mmol/l receiving moderate to high intensity statin therapy over a median follow-up of 2.2 years [108]. A statistically significant reduction (HR: 0.85, 95% CI: 0.79 - 0.92, p<0.001) in a composite major adverse cardiac events end point (primary outcome) of cardiovascular death, myocardial infarction, stroke, hospital admission with unstable angina or coronary revascularisation was observed in the evolocumab (9.8%) compared to placebo group (11.3%). Relative risk reduction in the FOURIER trial was in accordance with benefit seen in statin trials [4] when follow-up was taken into account.

The **ODYSSEY OUTCOMES trial** evaluated over 4 years, the primary outcome a composite of mortality associated with coronary heart disease, non-fatal myocardial infarction, fatal or non-fatal stroke or hospitalisation due to unstable angina (primary outcome) in 18,924 patients following alirocumab (75mg, titrated up to 150mg depending on whether target LDL-cholesterol was achieved) or placebo treatment [109]. Inclusion criteria consisted of age $\geq$ 40 years, occurrence of acute coronary syndrome 1 - 12 months prior to randomisation, being on high intensity statins and elevated lipids (LDL-cholesterol $\geq$ 1.8mmol/l, Non HDL-cholesterol $\geq$ 2.6mmol/l or Apo B $\geq$ 80mg/dl). The LDL-cholesterol reductions seen with alirocumab, compared with placebo, were 62.7%, 61.0% and 54.7% after 4, 12 and 48 months, respectively. Alirocumab (9.5%) was associated with fewer primary outcome events (HR: 0.85, 95% CI: 0.78 – 0.93, p=0.0003) compared to placebo (11.1%). Analysis of specified groups suggested that maximum benefit was in the 5629 individuals with a baseline LDL-cholesterol $\geq$ 2.59mmol/l (HR: 0.76, 95% CI: 0.65 – 0.87, p=0.0003).

THE RECENT CASE AGAINST THE LIPID HYPOTHESIS

Recently, Ravnskov *et al.,* suggested a lack of an association or even an inverse association between LDL-cholesterol and mortality in the elderly [7]. The lipid hypothesis is mainly about lowering CVD and not all cause mortality, however it is reasonable to expect some reduction in mortality in view of CVD being a contributor [2]. The CTT Collaboration carried out a meta-analysis of 26 RCTs with about 170,000 individuals showed that LDL-cholesterol reduction was associated with decreased mortality [4]. Cohort studies, especially since the 4S study in 1994 [21] would be compromised by guideline based statin therapy. Care is needed when considering cohort studies as most RCT's (Fig. **4**) have shown that LDL-cholesterol reduction is associated with decreased CVD and in some cases lower mortality as well. Decrease in CVD has been associated with resins, statins, ezetimibe and PCSK9 inhibitors. That is strong evidence for the lipid hypothesis [119]. It is also important to offer explanations as why RCTs showing benefit may be erroneous [7]. Until such an in-depth analysis takes place we believe the lipid hypothesis is true regarding CVD. Further research is required in patients with chronic renal disease on haemodialysis and heart failure.

ROLE OF OTHER LIPID LOWERING AGENTS

Randomised controlled studies using fibrates have not been consistent [120, 121]. Following significant CVD risk reduction with gemfibrozil treatment in the Helsinki Heart Study [122] and Veterans Affairs High-Density Cholesterol Intervention Trial [123], evidence for the usefulness of fibrate therapy has diminished [121]; the three studies not using gemfibrozil studies (Bezafibrate Infarction Prevention study [124], Fenofibrate Intervention and Event Lowering in Diabetes [125] and Action to Control Cardiovascular Risk in Diabetes – LIPID [126]) failed to achieve their primary outcomes. The question remains whether a sub-group of individuals may benefit from fibrate use as inclusion criteria varied amongst the fibrate trials or whether gemfibrozil was different to fenofibrate and bezafibrate [121].

Bruckert *et al.,* analysed individuals with HDL-cholesterol and triglyceride values closest to those of atherogenic dyslipidaemia (HDL-cholestreol <0.91mmol/L (35mg/dl) and triglycerides > 2.2mmol/l (195mg/dl) in the above trials (11% -

33% of the total cohorts) and showed a significant reduction of 28% in CVD whilst the complementary group demonstrated only a non-significant 6% risk reduction [120]. A meta-analysis of fibrates trials carried out by Jun *et al.,* including 18 RCTs comprising 45,058 individuals and significant decreases were observed in major cardiovascular events [127]. Importantly, sub-group analysis demonstrated a greater effect in trials with higher mean triglyceride levels [127]. As there are limitations in the interpreting subgroup data analyses a RCT designed with narrower inclusion criteria is required for the various fibrates.

Although the Framingham Heart Study as seen previously demonstrated an inverse relationship between HDL-cholesterol and CVD this relationship was not evident in the Dallas Heart Study which showed that cholesterol efflux and not HDL-cholesterol was associated with CVD [128]. Further, RCTs with HDL-cholestreol raising agents such as niacin [129] and torcetrapib, a cholesteryl ester transfer protein inhibitor [130] failed to show CVD benefits. In the ILLUMINATE study, torcetrapib increased HDL-cholesterol by 72.1% but significantly increased CVD and mortality [130]. Anacetrapib, another CETP inhibitor, was associated with a small but significant effect on CVD events, but this could have been due to the lowering of Non-HDL-cholesterol rather than the increasing of HDL-cholesterol [131]. In view of the above varying trial outcomes the latest United Kingdom National Institute for Health and Care Excellence lipid modification guidelines issued in 2014 did not recommend fibrates for primary/secondary prevention, chronic kidney disease, T2DM/ T1DM. Fibrates could be considered in mixed dyslipidaemia / hypertriglyceridaemia, especially in individuals with triglycerides between 4.5 - 9.9mmol/L, as statin trials usually recruited subjects with triglycerides < 4.5 mmol/l [132].

ROLE OF ANTI-INFLAMMATORY THERAPY

It has been shown that markers of inflammation such as high sensitivity C-reactive protein and interleukin-6 have been associated with CVD pathogenesis, this relationship being independent of cholesterol [133, 134]. Statins have been seen to reduce levels of inflammation and interestingly CVD reduction has been related to both lipid lowering and reduction in inflammatory marker levels [135, 136]. The Canakinumab Antiinflammatory Thrombosis Outcome Study (CANTOS) Trial was a double blind RCT investigating the effect of 50mg, 150mg and 300mg of canakinumab (a monoclonal antibody administered 3 monthly reducing inflammation by targeting interleukin1β) on CVD in 10,061 patients who had suffered a previous myocardial infarction together with a high sensitivity C-reactive protein ≥ 2mg/l [137]. The trial was important as canakinumab did not alter lipid levels. Interestingly, 150 mg of canakinumab (*vs* placebo), but not the 50mg or 300mg dose was associated with reduced CVD reaching the prespecified threshold for statistical significance regarding the primary outcome (non-fatal myocardial infarction, non-fatal stroke and cardiovascular death); 50mg (HR: 0.93, 95% CI: 0.80 – 1.07, p=0.30), 150mg (HR: 0.85, 95% CI: 0.74 – 0.98, p=0.021), 300mg (HR: 0.86, 95% CI: 0.75 – 0.99, p=0.031). These results suggest that further research has to be directed at the effects of anti-inflammatory therapy with different levels of baseline inflammation.

REFINING THE LIPID HYPOTHESIS: IDENTIFICATION OF SUBGROUPS DEMONSTRATING EVEN GREATER BENEFIT

It is important that enthusiasts of the lipid hypothesis consider other CVD related risk factors and treatments. As suggested in the previous section patients with the atherogenic lipoprotein phenotype (elevated triglycerides, low HDL-cholesterol), the dyslipidaemia characterising the metabolic syndrome may benefit from fibrate therapy [120, 121]. In our view this benefit is not adequately stated in the current NICE guidelines, perhaps due to the focus being entirely on the lipid hypothesis [132]. It is important to be aware of heterogeneity within every cohort that we have described. As previously suggested this is evident in the subgroup of patients with the atherogenic lipoprotein phenotype who may benefit from fibrates. The same may apply to statins with some subgroups benefiting more than others. Reported benefits are mean values and obviously not all individuals treated will benefit [8]. Thus, it would be useful to identify subgroups, perhaps *via* clinical phenotypes and narrow the inclusion criteria and try and confirm maximal benefit. This approach could be allied with markers indicating CVD benefit that could be assessed during treatment. It has been suggested that evaluating endothelial state, a predictor of atherosclerosis may achieve that aim [138]. It has been seen that endothelial function has been associated with vascular flow characteristics [139]. The pathogenesis of atherosclerosis is associated with both, vessel wall injury and other factors, both, systemic and local. It is suggested that atherosclerosis is related to a decrease in nitric oxide synthase production resulting in altered wall shear stress, vasodilation and cell repair [140, 141]. Conventional atherosclerosis risk factors such as diabetes, dyslipidaemia, smoking and hypertension have been seen to alter endothelial cell function [142]. With this in mind we compared differences in blood flow data and computational flow dynamics (https://www.sciencedirect.com/science/article/pii/S1872931217301795) between 27 individuals with established CHD and 30 individuals without any symptoms suggestive of CHD. Our results suggested that peak systolic velocity may be an area of interest. Even with a small number of subjects a significant difference was observed (patients without CHD, mean (SD): 62.8 (16.1) cm/s, patients with CHD, mean (SD): 53.6 (17.3) cm/s, p=0.042). Many other factors such as wall shear stress were associated with peak systolic velocity and these associations must be studied further. Our study is in agreement with other reports suggesting that peak systolic velocity may be a predictor of CVD [143 - 145].

CONCLUSION

Evidence presented above suggests that the lipid hypothesis is valid in most patients, possible exceptions being those with heart failure or dialysis. All CVD risk scoring models and RCTs using therapeutic agents reducing LDL-cholesterol *via* different mechanisms provide evidence for the validity of the lipid hypothesis. Cohort studies of patients on multiple agents do not have the same authority of the Framingham Heart Study or the numerous interventional RCTs. Thus, we are happy to accept the lipid hypothesis in most cohorts at this point.

The degree of CVD risk reduction is an area that has to be made clear. A lot has been made of relative risk reduction. The meta-analysis by the CTT collaboration suggested a 22% reduction in CVD for 1 mmol/l reduction of LDL-cholesterol [4]. In addition patients should be informed of the absolute risk reduction or its derivative 'numbers needed to treat' to prevent 1 CVD event (100/absolute risk reduction) together with available evidence in a cohort closely matching their presentation phenotype. Lifetime risk reduction is another way of presenting the evidence [146]. In our opinion this takes a long-term view which is important when treating conditions such as CVD. This should form the basis of lipid lowering treatment decisions made jointly by the patient and physician. We have previously studied the effect of statins, testosterone and phosphodiesterase 5-inhibitor therapy on the age related probability of death in men with type 2 diabetes and late onset testosterone deficiency using the Gompertz model [147, 148]. This clearly presents relative risk reduction, absolute risk reduction and lifetime risk reduction with clarity [148]. In our view benefits shown by RCTs would be clearer to patients if they were presented in such a manner.

DISCLOSURE STATEMENT

Professor Sudarshan Ramachandran has received educational grants to attend meetings and honoraria for serving as a speaker for Sanofi, Astra Zeneca and Merck Sharp & Dohme. Dr Mithun Bhartia and Dr Carola S König have no disclosures.

CONSENT FOR PUBLICATION

Not applicable.

CONFLICT OF INTEREST

The authors declare that there is no conflict of interest.

ACKNOWLEDGEMENTS

We would like to thank Professor Richard C. Strange for his valuable comments which added balance to the review.

REFERENCES

[1]   Newton JN, Briggs ADM, Murray CJL, *et al.* Changes in health in England, with analysis by English regions and areas of deprivation, 1990-2013: a systematic analysis for the Global Burden of Disease Study 2013. Lancet 2015; 386(10010): 2257-74.
         [http://dx.doi.org/10.1016/S0140-6736(15)00195-6] [PMID: 26382241]

[2]   Townsend N, Bhatnagar P, Wilkins E, *et al.* Cardiovascular disease statistics 2015. London: British Heart Foundation 2015.

[3]   Bhatnagar P, Wickramasinghe K, Wilkins E, Townsend N. Trends in the epidemiology of cardiovascular disease in the UK. Heart 2016; 102(24): 1945-52.
         [http://dx.doi.org/10.1136/heartjnl-2016-309573] [PMID: 27550425]

[4]   Baigent C, Blackwell L, Emberson J, *et al.* Efficacy and safety of more intensive lowering of LDL cholesterol: a meta-analysis of data from 170,000 participants in 26 randomised trials. Lancet 2010; 376(9753): 1670-81.
         [http://dx.doi.org/10.1016/S0140-6736(10)61350-5] [PMID: 21067804]

[5]   Cannon CP, Blazing MA, Giugliano RP, *et al.* Ezetimibe added to statin therapy after acute coronary syndromes. N Engl J Med 2015; 372(25): 2387-97.
         [http://dx.doi.org/10.1056/NEJMoa1410489] [PMID: 26039521]

[6]   DuBroff R, de Lorgeril M. Cholesterol confusion and statin controversy. World J Cardiol 2015; 7(7): 404-9.
         [http://dx.doi.org/10.4330/wjc.v7.i7.404] [PMID: 26225201]

[7]   Ravnskov U, Diamond DM, Hama R, *et al.* Lack of an association or an inverse association between low-density-lipoprotein cholesterol and mortality in the elderly: a systematic review. BMJ Open 2016; 6(6)e010401
         [http://dx.doi.org/10.1136/bmjopen-2015-010401] [PMID: 27292972]

[8]   Ramachandran S, König CS, Hackett G, *et al.* Managing clinical heterogeneity: An argument for benefit based action limits. J Med Diag Ther 2018; 1034701
         [http://dx.doi.org/10.1115/1.4039561]

[9]   Steinberg D. Thematic review series: the pathogenesis of atherosclerosis. An interpretive history of the cholesterol controversy: part I. J Lipid Res 2004; 45(9): 1583-93.
         [http://dx.doi.org/10.1194/jlr.R400003-JLR200] [PMID: 15102877]

[10]   Ose L. Müller-Harbitz disease--familial hypercholesterolemia. Tidsskr Nor Laegeforen 2002; 122: 924-5.
         [PMID: 12082837]

[11]   Oncley JL, Scatchard G, Brown A. Physical-chemical characteristics of certain of the proteins of normal human plasma. J Phys Colloid Chem 1947; 51(1): 184-98.
         [http://dx.doi.org/10.1021/j150451a014] [PMID: 20286398]

[12]   Gofman JW, Lindgren FT, Elliott H. Ultracentrifugal studies of lipoproteins of human serum. J Biol Chem 1949; 179(2): 973-9.
         [PMID: 18150027]

[13]   Gofman JW, Lindgren F, Elliott H, *et al.* The role of lipids and lipoproteins in atherosclerosis. Science 1950; 111(2877): 166-71.
         [http://dx.doi.org/10.1126/science.111.2877.166] [PMID: 15403115]

[14] Fredrickson DS, Gordon RS Jr. The metabolism of albumin-bound C14-labeled unesterified fatty acids in normal human subjects. J Clin Invest 1958; 37(11): 1504-15.
[http://dx.doi.org/10.1172/JCI103742] [PMID: 13587659]

[15] Olson RE, Vester JW. Nutrition-endocrine interrelationships in the control of fat transport in man. Physiol Rev 1960; 40: 677-733.
[http://dx.doi.org/10.1152/physrev.1960.40.4.677] [PMID: 13730906]

[16] Fredrickson DS, Levy RI, Lees RS. Fat transport in lipoproteins--an integrated approach to mechanisms and disorders. N Engl J Med 1967; 276(1): 34-42.
[http://dx.doi.org/10.1056/NEJM196701052760107] [PMID: 5333081]

[17] Jackson RL, Morrisett JD, Gotto AM Jr. Lipoprotein structure and metabolism. Physiol Rev 1976; 56(2): 259-316.
[http://dx.doi.org/10.1152/physrev.1976.56.2.259] [PMID: 180553]

[18] Goldstein JL, Brown MS. Lipoprotein receptors: Genetic defense against atherosclerosis. Clin Res 1982; 30: 417-26.

[19] Brown MS, Goldstein JL. A receptor-mediated pathway for cholesterol homeostasis. Science 1986; 232(4746): 34-47.
[http://dx.doi.org/10.1126/science.3513311] [PMID: 3513311]

[20] Randomised trial of cholesterol lowering in 4444 patients with coronary heart disease: the Scandinavian Simvastatin Survival Study (4S). Lancet 1994; 344(8934): 1383-9.
[PMID: 7968073]

[21] Shepherd J, Cobbe SM, Ford I, *et al.* Prevention of coronary heart disease with pravastatin in men with hypercholesterolemia. N Engl J Med 1995; 333(20): 1301-7.
[http://dx.doi.org/10.1056/NEJM199511163332001] [PMID: 7566020]

[22] Tsao CW, Ramachandran VS. Cohort Profile: The Framingham Heart Study (FHS): overview of milestones in cardiovascular epidemiology. Int J Epidemiol 44: 1800-13.

[23] Dawber TR, Moore FE, Mann GV. Coronary heart disease in the Framingham study. Am J Public Health Nations Health 1957; 47(4 Pt 2): 4-24.
[http://dx.doi.org/10.2105/AJPH.47.4_Pt_2.4] [PMID: 13411327]

[24] Kannel WB, Dawber TR, Kagan A, Revotskie N, Stokes J III. Factors of risk in the development of coronary heart disease--six year follow-up experience. The Framingham Study. Ann Intern Med 1961; 55: 33-50.
[http://dx.doi.org/10.7326/0003-4819-55-1-33] [PMID: 13751193]

[25] Doyle JT, Dawber TR, Kannel WB, Heslin AS, Kahn HA. Cigarette smoking and coronary heart disease. Combined experience of the Albany and Framingham studies. N Engl J Med 1962; 266: 796-801.
[http://dx.doi.org/10.1056/NEJM196204192661602] [PMID: 13887664]

[26] Kannel WB, Castelli WP, Gordon T, McNamara PM. Serum cholesterol, lipoproteins, and the risk of coronary heart disease. The Framingham study. Ann Intern Med 1971; 74(1): 1-12.
[http://dx.doi.org/10.7326/0003-4819-74-1-1] [PMID: 5539274]

[27] Anderson KM, Castelli WP, Levy D. Cholesterol and mortality. 30 years of follow-up from the Framingham study. JAMA 1987; 257(16): 2176-80.
[http://dx.doi.org/10.1001/jama.1987.03390160062027] [PMID: 3560398]

[28] Kannel WB, McGee DL. Diabetes and cardiovascular disease. The Framingham study. JAMA 1979; 241(19): 2035-8.
[http://dx.doi.org/10.1001/jama.1979.03290450033020] [PMID: 430798]

[29] Bostom AG, Cupples LA, Jenner JL, *et al.* Elevated plasma lipoprotein(a) and coronary heart disease in men aged 55 years and younger. A prospective study. JAMA 1996; 276(7): 544-8.

[http://dx.doi.org/10.1001/jama.1996.03540070040028] [PMID: 8709403]

[30]   Kannel WB, Sorlie P. Some health benefits of physical activity. The Framingham Study. Arch Intern Med 1979; 139(8): 857-61.
[http://dx.doi.org/10.1001/archinte.1979.03630450011006] [PMID: 464698]

[31]   Posner BM, Cupples LA, Franz MM, Gagnon DR. Diet and heart disease risk factors in adult American men and women: the Framingham Offspring-Spouse nutrition studies. Int J Epidemiol 1993; 22(6): 1014-25.
[http://dx.doi.org/10.1093/ije/22.6.1014] [PMID: 8144282]

[32]   Truett J, Cornfield J, Kannel W. A multivariate analysis of the risk of coronary heart disease in Framingham. J Chronic Dis 1967; 20(7): 511-24.
[http://dx.doi.org/10.1016/0021-9681(67)90082-3] [PMID: 6028270]

[33]   Cornfield J, Gordon T, Smith W. Quantal response curves for experimentally uncontrolled variables. Bull Int Stat Inst 1961; p. 28.

[34]   Walker SH, Duncan DB. Estimation of the probability of an event as a function of several independent variables. Biometrika 1967; 54(1): 167-79.
[http://dx.doi.org/10.1093/biomet/54.1-2.167] [PMID: 6049533]

[35]   Kannel WB, McGee D, Gordon T. A general cardiovascular risk profile: the Framingham Study. Am J Cardiol 1976; 38(1): 46-51.
[http://dx.doi.org/10.1016/0002-9149(76)90061-8] [PMID: 132862]

[36]   Gordon T, Kannel WB. Multiple risk functions for predicting coronary heart disease: the concept, accuracy, and application. Am Heart J 1982; 103(6): 1031-9.
[http://dx.doi.org/10.1016/0002-8703(82)90567-1] [PMID: 7044082]

[37]   D'Agostino RB, Lee ML, Belanger AJ, Cupples LA, Anderson K, Kannel WB. Relation of pooled logistic regression to time dependent Cox regression analysis: the Framingham Heart Study. Stat Med 1990; 9(12): 1501-15.
[http://dx.doi.org/10.1002/sim.4780091214] [PMID: 2281238]

[38]   Anderson KM, Wilson PW, Odell PM, Kannel WB. An updated coronary risk profile. A statement for health professionals. Circulation 1991; 83(1): 356-62.
[http://dx.doi.org/10.1161/01.CIR.83.1.356] [PMID: 1984895]

[39]   Wilson PW, D'Agostino RB, Levy D, Belanger AM, Silbershatz H, Kannel WB. Prediction of coronary heart disease using risk factor categories. Circulation 1998; 97(18): 1837-47.
[http://dx.doi.org/10.1161/01.CIR.97.18.1837] [PMID: 9603539]

[40]   D'Agostino RB Sr, Vasan RS, Pencina MJ, *et al.* General cardiovascular risk profile for use in primary care: the Framingham Heart Study. Circulation 2008; 117(6): 743-53.
[http://dx.doi.org/10.1161/CIRCULATIONAHA.107.699579] [PMID: 18212285]

[41]   D'Agostino RB Sr, Pencina MJ, Massaro JM, Coady S. Cardiovascular Disease Risk Assessment: Insights from Framingham. Glob Heart 2013; 8(1): 11-23.
[http://dx.doi.org/10.1016/j.gheart.2013.01.001] [PMID: 23750335]

[42]   Dogan MV, Grumbach IM, Michaelson JJ, Philibert RA. Integrated genetic and epigenetic prediction of coronary heart disease in the Framingham Heart Study. PLoS One 2018; 13(1)e0190549
[http://dx.doi.org/10.1371/journal.pone.0190549] [PMID: 29293675]

[43]   Assmann G, Cullen P, Schulte H. Simple scoring scheme for calculating the risk of acute coronary events based on the 10-year follow-up of the prospective cardiovascular Münster (PROCAM) study. Circulation 2002; 105(3): 310-5.
[http://dx.doi.org/10.1161/hc0302.102575] [PMID: 11804985]

[44]   Prevention of Cardiovascular Disease Guidelines for assessment and management of cardiovascular risk. Geneva: WHO 2007.

[45] Conroy RM, Pyörälä K, Fitzgerald AP, *et al.* Estimation of ten-year risk of fatal cardiovascular disease in Europe: the SCORE project. Eur Heart J 2003; 24(11): 987-1003.
[http://dx.doi.org/10.1016/S0195-668X(03)00114-3] [PMID: 12788299]

[46] Hippisley-Cox J, Coupland C, Vinogradova Y, Robson J, May M, Brindle P. Derivation and validation of QRISK, a new cardiovascular disease risk score for the United Kingdom: prospective open cohort study. BMJ 2007; 335(7611): 136.
[http://dx.doi.org/10.1136/bmj.39261.471806.55] [PMID: 17615182]

[47] Chia YC. Review of tools of cardiovascular disease risk stratification: interpretation, customisation and application in clinical practice. Singapore Med J 2011; 52(2): 116-23.
[PMID: 21373738]

[48] Ko M, Kim MT, Nam JJ. Assessing risk factors of coronary heart disease and its risk prediction among Korean adults: the 2001 Korea National Health and Nutrition Examination Survey. Int J Cardiol 2006; 110(2): 184-90.
[http://dx.doi.org/10.1016/j.ijcard.2005.07.030] [PMID: 16412525]

[49] Ng KK, Chia YC. Utility of Framingham model in predicting coronary heart disease risk in Malaysia, a developing country. Atherosclerosis 2008; 9: 92.
[http://dx.doi.org/10.1016/S1567-5688(08)70367-2]

[50] Empana JP, Ducimetière P, Arveiler D, *et al.* Are the Framingham and PROCAM coronary heart disease risk functions applicable to different European populations? The PRIME Study. Eur Heart J 2003; 24(21): 1903-11.
[http://dx.doi.org/10.1016/j.ehj.2003.09.002] [PMID: 14585248]

[51] Laurier D, Nguyen PC, Cazelles B, Segond P. Estimation of CHD risk in a French working population using a modified Framingham model. J Clin Epidemiol 1994; 47(12): 1353-64.
[http://dx.doi.org/10.1016/0895-4356(94)90079-5] [PMID: 7730844]

[52] Menotti A, Lanti M, Puddu PE, Kromhout D. Coronary heart disease incidence in northern and southern European populations: a reanalysis of the seven countries study for a European coronary risk chart. Heart 2000; 84(3): 238-44.
[http://dx.doi.org/10.1136/heart.84.3.238] [PMID: 10956281]

[53] Brindle P, Emberson J, Lampe F, *et al.* Predictive accuracy of the Framingham coronary risk score in British men: prospective cohort study. BMJ 2003; 327(7426): 1267.
[http://dx.doi.org/10.1136/bmj.327.7426.1267] [PMID: 14644971]

[54] Liu J, Hong Y, D'Agostino RB Sr, *et al.* Predictive value for the Chinese population of the Framingham CHD risk assessment tool compared with the Chinese Multi-Provincial Cohort Study. JAMA 2004; 291(21): 2591-9.
[http://dx.doi.org/10.1001/jama.291.21.2591] [PMID: 15173150]

[55] Ramachandran S, French JM, Vanderpump MP, Croft P, Neary RH. Using the Framingham model to predict heart disease in the United Kingdom: retrospective study. BMJ 2000; 320(7236): 676-7.
[http://dx.doi.org/10.1136/bmj.320.7236.676] [PMID: 10710574]

[56] Ramsay LE, Haq IU, Jackson PR, Yeo WW, Pickin DM, Payne JN. Targeting lipid-lowering drug therapy for primary prevention of coronary disease: an updated Sheffield table. Lancet 1996; 348(9024): 387-8.
[http://dx.doi.org/10.1016/S0140-6736(96)05516-X] [PMID: 8709740]

[57] Yusuf S, Sleight P, Pogue J, Bosch J, Davies R, Dagenais G. Effects of an angiotensin-convertin--enzyme inhibitor, ramipril, on cardiovascular events in high-risk patients. N Engl J Med 2000; 342(3): 145-53.
[http://dx.doi.org/10.1056/NEJM200001203420301] [PMID: 10639539]

[58] Effects of ramipril on cardiovascular and microvascular outcomes in people with diabetes mellitus: results of the HOPE study and MICRO-HOPE substudy. Lancet 2000; 355(9200): 253-9.

[http://dx.doi.org/10.1016/S0140-6736(99)12323-7] [PMID: 10675071]

[59] Hansson L, Lindholm LH, Niskanen L, *et al.* Effect of angiotensin-converting-enzyme inhibition compared with conventional therapy on cardiovascular morbidity and mortality in hypertension: the Captopril Prevention Project (CAPPP) randomised trial. Lancet 1999; 353(9153): 611-6.
[http://dx.doi.org/10.1016/S0140-6736(98)05012-0] [PMID: 10030325]

[60] Estacio RO, Jeffers BW, Hiatt WR, Biggerstaff SL, Gifford N, Schrier RW. The effect of nisoldipine as compared with enalapril on cardiovascular outcomes in patients with non-insulin-dependent diabetes and hypertension. N Engl J Med 1998; 338(10): 645-52.
[http://dx.doi.org/10.1056/NEJM199803053381003] [PMID: 9486993]

[61] Zinman B, Wanner C, Lachin JM, *et al.* Empagliflozin, cardiovascular outcomes, and mortality in type 2 diabetes. N Engl J Med 2015; 373(22): 2117-28.
[http://dx.doi.org/10.1056/NEJMoa1504720] [PMID: 26378978]

[62] Anderson SG, Hutchings DC, Woodward M, *et al.* Phosphodiesterase type-5 inhibitor use in type 2 diabetes is associated with a reduction in all-cause mortality. Heart 2016; 102(21): 1750-6.
[http://dx.doi.org/10.1136/heartjnl-2015-309223] [PMID: 27465053]

[63] Andersson DP, Trolle Lagerros Y, Grotta A, Bellocco R, Lehtihet M, Holzmann MJ. Association between treatment for erectile dysfunction and death or cardiovascular outcomes after myocardial infarction. Heart 2017; 103(16): 1264-70.
[http://dx.doi.org/10.1136/heartjnl-2016-310746] [PMID: 28280146]

[64] Hill AB. The environment and disease: association or causation? Proc R Soc Med 1965; 58: 295-300.
[PMID: 14283879]

[65] Schade DS, Helitzer D, Eaton P. Evidence that Low Density Lipoprotein Is the Primary Cause of Atherosclerotic Cardiovascular Disease: A Bradford-Hill Approach. World J Cardiovasc Dis 2017; 7: 271-84.
[http://dx.doi.org/10.4236/wjcd.2017.79025]

[66] Mulder R, Singh AB, Hamilton A, *et al.* The limitations of using randomised controlled trials as a basis for developing treatment guidelines. Evid Based Ment Health 2018; 21(1): 4-6.
[http://dx.doi.org/10.1136/eb-2017-102701] [PMID: 28710065]

[67] Craig P, Dieppe P, Macintyre S, Michie S, Nazareth I, Petticrew M. Developing and evaluating complex interventions: the new Medical Research Council guidance. BMJ 2008; 337: a1655.
[http://dx.doi.org/10.1136/bmj.a1655] [PMID: 18824488]

[68] Moher D, Hopewell S, Schulz KF, *et al.* CONSORT 2010 explanation and elaboration: updated guidelines for reporting parallel group randomised trials. BMJ 2010; 340: c869.
[http://dx.doi.org/10.1136/bmj.c869] [PMID: 20332511]

[69] Moher D, Schulz KF, Simera I, Altman DG. Guidance for developers of health research reporting guidelines. PLoS Med 2010; 7(2)e1000217
[http://dx.doi.org/10.1371/journal.pmed.1000217] [PMID: 20169112]

[70] Welch VA, Norheim OF, Jull J, Cookson R, Sommerfelt H, Tugwell P. CONSORT-Equity 2017 extension and elaboration for better reporting of health equity in randomised trials. BMJ 2017; 359: j5085.
[http://dx.doi.org/10.1136/bmj.j5085] [PMID: 29170161]

[71] Byrne BE, Rooshenas L, Lambert H, Blazeby JM. Evidence into practice: protocol for a new mixed-methods approach to explore the relationship between trials evidence and clinical practice through systematic identification and analysis of articles citing randomised controlled trials. BMJ Open 2018; 8(11)e023215
[http://dx.doi.org/10.1136/bmjopen-2018-023215] [PMID: 30413510]

[72] Black DM. Gut-acting drugs for lowering cholesterol. Curr Atheroscler Rep 2002; 4(1): 71-5.
[http://dx.doi.org/10.1007/s11883-002-0065-8] [PMID: 11772426]

[73]   Insull W Jr, Toth P, Mullican W, *et al.* Effectiveness of colesevelam hydrochloride in decreasing LDL cholesterol in patients with primary hypercholesterolemia: a 24-week randomized controlled trial. Mayo Clin Proc 2001; 76(10): 971-82.
[http://dx.doi.org/10.4065/76.10.971] [PMID: 11605698]

[74]   The Lipid Research Clinics Coronary Primary Prevention Trial results. I. Reduction in incidence of coronary heart disease. JAMA 1984; 251(3): 351-64.
[http://dx.doi.org/10.1001/jama.1984.03340270029025] [PMID: 6361299]

[75]   Siperstein MD, Guest MJ. Studies on the site of the feedback control of cholesterol synthesis. J Clin Invest 1960; 39: 642-52.
[http://dx.doi.org/10.1172/JCI104079] [PMID: 14447167]

[76]   Burg JS, Espenshade PJ. Regulation of HMG-CoA reductase in mammals and yeast. Prog Lipid Res 2011; 50(4): 403-10.
[http://dx.doi.org/10.1016/j.plipres.2011.07.002] [PMID: 21801748]

[77]   Endo A. The origin of the statins. 2004. Atheroscler Suppl 2004; 5(3): 125-30.
[http://dx.doi.org/10.1016/j.atherosclerosissup.2004.08.033] [PMID: 15531285]

[78]   Pedersen TR. The success story of LDL cholesterol lowering. Circ Res 2016; 118(4): 721-31.
[http://dx.doi.org/10.1161/CIRCRESAHA.115.306297] [PMID: 26892969]

[79]   Sacks FM, Pfeffer MA, Moye LA, *et al.* The effect of pravastatin on coronary events after myocardial infarction in patients with average cholesterol levels. Cholesterol and Recurrent Events Trial investigators. N Engl J Med 1996; 335(14): 1001-9.
[http://dx.doi.org/10.1056/NEJM199610033351401] [PMID: 8801446]

[80]   The effect of aggressive lowering of low-density lipoprotein cholesterol levels and low-dose anticoagulation on obstructive changes in saphenous-vein coronary-artery bypass grafts. N Engl J Med 1997; 336(3): 153-62.
[http://dx.doi.org/10.1056/NEJM199701163360301] [PMID: 8992351]

[81]   Downs JR, Clearfield M, Weis S, *et al.* Primary prevention of acute coronary events with lovastatin in men and women with average cholesterol levels: results of AFCAPS/TexCAPS. Air Force/Texas Coronary Atherosclerosis Prevention Study. JAMA 1998; 279(20): 1615-22.
[http://dx.doi.org/10.1001/jama.279.20.1615] [PMID: 9613910]

[82]   Prevention of cardiovascular events and death with pravastatin in patients with coronary heart disease and a broad range of initial cholesterol levels. N Engl J Med 1998; 339(19): 1349-57.
[http://dx.doi.org/10.1056/NEJM199811053391902] [PMID: 9841303]

[83]   GISSI Prevenzione Investigators (Gruppo Italiano per lo Studio della Sopravivenza nell'Infarto Miocardico). Results of the low dose (20 mg) pravastatin GISSI Prevenzione trial in 4271 patients with recent myocardial infarction; do stopped trials contribute to overall knowledge? Ital Heart J 2000; 1: 810-20.

[84]   Schwartz GG, Olsson AG, Ezekowitz MD, *et al.* Effects of atorvastatin on early recurrent ischemic events in acute coronary syndromes: the MIRACL study: a randomized controlled trial. JAMA 2001; 285(13): 1711-8.
[http://dx.doi.org/10.1001/jama.285.13.1711] [PMID: 11277825]

[85]   MRC/BHF Heart Protection Study of cholesterol lowering with simvastatin in 20,536 high-risk individuals: a randomised placebo-controlled trial. Lancet 2002; 360(9326): 7-22.
[http://dx.doi.org/10.1016/S0140-6736(02)09327-3] [PMID: 12114036]

[86]   Serruys PW, de Feyter P, Macaya C, *et al.* Fluvastatin for prevention of cardiac events following successful first percutaneous coronary intervention: a randomized controlled trial. JAMA 2002; 287(24): 3215-22.
[http://dx.doi.org/10.1001/jama.287.24.3215] [PMID: 12076217]

[87]   Athyros VG, Papageorgiou AA, Mercouris BR, *et al.* Treatment with atorvastatin to the National

Cholesterol Educational Program goal versus 'usual' care in secondary coronary heart disease prevention. The GREek Atorvastatin and Coronary-heart-disease Evaluation (GREACE) study. Curr Med Res Opin 2002; 18(4): 220-8.
[http://dx.doi.org/10.1185/030079902125000787] [PMID: 12201623]

[88]   Shepherd J, Blauw GJ, Murphy MB, *et al.* Pravastatin in elderly individuals at risk of vascular disease (PROSPER): a randomised controlled trial. Lancet 2002; 360(9346): 1623-30.
[http://dx.doi.org/10.1016/S0140-6736(02)11600-X] [PMID: 12457784]

[89]   Major outcomes in moderately hypercholesterolemic, hypertensive patients randomized to pravastatin vs usual care: The Antihypertensive and Lipid-Lowering Treatment to Prevent Heart Attack Trial (ALLHAT-LLT). JAMA 2002; 288(23): 2998-3007.
[http://dx.doi.org/10.1001/jama.288.23.2998] [PMID: 12479764]

[90]   Sever PS, Dahlöf B, Poulter NR, *et al.* Prevention of coronary and stroke events with atorvastatin in hypertensive patients who have average or lower-than-average cholesterol concentrations, in the Anglo-Scandinavian Cardiac Outcomes Trial--Lipid Lowering Arm (ASCOT-LLA): a multicentre randomised controlled trial. Lancet 2003; 361(9364): 1149-58.
[http://dx.doi.org/10.1016/S0140-6736(03)12948-0] [PMID: 12686036]

[91]   Holdaas H, Fellström B, Jardine AG, *et al.* Effect of fluvastatin on cardiac outcomes in renal transplant recipients: a multicentre, randomised, placebo-controlled trial. Lancet 2003; 361(9374): 2024-31.
[http://dx.doi.org/10.1016/S0140-6736(03)13638-0] [PMID: 12814712]

[92]   Colhoun HM, Betteridge DJ, Durrington PN, *et al.* Primary prevention of cardiovascular disease with atorvastatin in type 2 diabetes in the Collaborative Atorvastatin Diabetes Study (CARDS): multicentre randomised placebo-controlled trial. Lancet 2004; 364(9435): 685-96.
[http://dx.doi.org/10.1016/S0140-6736(04)16895-5] [PMID: 15325833]

[93]   Koren MJ, Hunninghake DB. Clinical outcomes in managed-care patients with coronary heart disease treated aggressively in lipid-lowering disease management clinics: the alliance study. J Am Coll Cardiol 2004; 44(9): 1772-9.
[http://dx.doi.org/10.1016/j.jacc.2004.07.053] [PMID: 15519006]

[94]   Cannon CP, Braunwald E, McCabe CH, *et al.* Intensive versus moderate lipid lowering with statins after acute coronary syndromes. N Engl J Med 2004; 350(15): 1495-504.
[http://dx.doi.org/10.1056/NEJMoa040583] [PMID: 15007110]

[95]   de Lemos JA, Blazing MA, Wiviott SD, *et al.* Early intensive vs a delayed conservative simvastatin strategy in patients with acute coronary syndromes: phase Z of the A to Z trial. JAMA 2004; 292(11): 1307-16.
[http://dx.doi.org/10.1001/jama.292.11.1307] [PMID: 15337732]

[96]   LaRosa JC, Grundy SM, Waters DD, *et al.* Intensive lipid lowering with atorvastatin in patients with stable coronary disease. N Engl J Med 2005; 352(14): 1425-35.
[http://dx.doi.org/10.1056/NEJMoa050461] [PMID: 15755765]

[97]   Wanner C, Krane V, März W, *et al.* Atorvastatin in patients with type 2 diabetes mellitus undergoing hemodialysis. N Engl J Med 2005; 353(3): 238-48.
[http://dx.doi.org/10.1056/NEJMoa043545] [PMID: 16034009]

[98]   Pedersen TR, Faergeman O, Kastelein JJ, *et al.* High-dose atorvastatin vs usual-dose simvastatin for secondary prevention after myocardial infarction: the IDEAL study: a randomized controlled trial. JAMA 2005; 294(19): 2437-45.
[http://dx.doi.org/10.1001/jama.294.19.2437] [PMID: 16287954]

[99]   Nakamura H, Arakawa K, Itakura H, *et al.* Primary prevention of cardiovascular disease with pravastatin in Japan (MEGA Study): a prospective randomised controlled trial. Lancet 2006; 368(9542): 1155-63.
[http://dx.doi.org/10.1016/S0140-6736(06)69472-5] [PMID: 17011942]

[100]   Amarenco P, Bogousslavsky J, Callahan A III, *et al.* High-dose atorvastatin after stroke or transient

ischemic attack. N Engl J Med 2006; 355(6): 549-59.
[http://dx.doi.org/10.1056/NEJMoa061894] [PMID: 16899775]

[101] Kjekshus J, Apetrei E, Barrios V, *et al.* Rosuvastatin in older patients with systolic heart failure. N Engl J Med 2007; 357(22): 2248-61.
[http://dx.doi.org/10.1056/NEJMoa0706201] [PMID: 17984166]

[102] Tavazzi L, Maggioni AP, Marchioli R, *et al.* Effect of rosuvastatin in patients with chronic heart failure (the GISSI-HF trial): a randomised, double-blind, placebo-controlled trial. Lancet 2008; 372(9645): 1231-9.
[http://dx.doi.org/10.1016/S0140-6736(08)61240-4] [PMID: 18757089]

[103] Ridker PM, Danielson E, Fonseca FAH, *et al.* Rosuvastatin to prevent vascular events in men and women with elevated C-reactive protein. N Engl J Med 2008; 359(21): 2195-207.
[http://dx.doi.org/10.1056/NEJMoa0807646] [PMID: 18997196]

[104] Fellström BC, Jardine AG, Schmieder RE, *et al.* Rosuvastatin and cardiovascular events in patients undergoing hemodialysis. N Engl J Med 2009; 360(14): 1395-407.
[http://dx.doi.org/10.1056/NEJMoa0810177] [PMID: 19332456]

[105] Armitage J, Bowman L, Wallendszus K, *et al.* Intensive lowering of LDL cholesterol with 80 mg versus 20 mg simvastatin daily in 12,064 survivors of myocardial infarction: a double-blind randomised trial. Lancet 2010; 376(9753): 1658-69.
[http://dx.doi.org/10.1016/S0140-6736(10)60310-8] [PMID: 21067805]

[106] Baigent C, Landray MJ, Reith C, *et al.* The effects of lowering LDL cholesterol with simvastatin plus ezetimibe in patients with chronic kidney disease (Study of Heart and Renal Protection): a randomised placebo-controlled trial. Lancet 2011; 377(9784): 2181-92.
[http://dx.doi.org/10.1016/S0140-6736(11)60739-3] [PMID: 21663949]

[107] Yusuf S, Bosch J, Dagenais G, *et al.* Cholesterol Lowering in Intermediate-Risk Persons without Cardiovascular Disease. N Engl J Med 2016; 374(21): 2021-31.
[http://dx.doi.org/10.1056/NEJMoa1600176] [PMID: 27040132]

[108] Sabatine MS, Giugliano RP, Keech AC, *et al.* Evolocumab and clinical outcomes in patients with cardiovascular disease. N Engl J Med 2017; 376(18): 1713-22.
[http://dx.doi.org/10.1056/NEJMoa1615664] [PMID: 28304224]

[109] Schwartz GG, Steg PG, Szarek M, *et al.* ODYSSEY OUTCOMES Committees and Investigators. 2018. https://www.nejm.org/doi/pdf/ 10.1056/NEJMoa1801174

[110] Knatterud GL, Rosenberg Y, Campeau L, *et al.* Long-term effects on clinical outcomes of aggressive lowering of low-density lipoprotein cholesterol levels and low-dose anticoagulation in the post coronary artery bypass graft trial. Circulation 2000; 102(2): 157-65.
[http://dx.doi.org/10.1161/01.CIR.102.2.157] [PMID: 10889125]

[111] Knopp RH, d'Emden M, Smilde JG, Pocock SJ. Efficacy and safety of atorvastatin in the prevention of cardiovascular end points in subjects with type 2 diabetes: the Atorvastatin Study for Prevention of Coronary Heart Disease Endpoints in non-insulin-dependent diabetes mellitus (ASPEN). Diabetes Care 2006; 29(7): 1478-85.
[http://dx.doi.org/10.2337/dc05-2415] [PMID: 16801565]

[112] Iqbal J, Al Qarni A, Hawwari A. Regulation of intestinal cholesterol absorption: A disease perspective. Adv Biol Chem 2017; 7: 60-75.
[http://dx.doi.org/10.4236/abc.2017.71004]

[113] Altmann SW, Davis HR Jr, Zhu LJ, *et al.* Niemann-Pick C1 Like 1 protein is critical for intestinal cholesterol absorption. Science 2004; 303(5661): 1201-4.
[http://dx.doi.org/10.1126/science.1093131] [PMID: 14976318]

[114] Brown MS, Anderson RG, Goldstein JL. Recycling receptors: the round-trip itinerary of migrant membrane proteins. Cell 1983; 32(3): 663-7.

[http://dx.doi.org/10.1016/0092-8674(83)90052-1] [PMID: 6299572]

[115] Horton JD, Cohen JC, Hobbs HH. PCSK9: a convertase that coordinates LDL catabolism. J Lipid Res 2009; 50 (Suppl.): S172-7.
[http://dx.doi.org/10.1194/jlr.R800091-JLR200] [PMID: 19020338]

[116] Sabatine MS, Giugliano RP, Wiviott SD, *et al.* Efficacy and safety of evolocumab in reducing lipids and cardiovascular events. N Engl J Med 2015; 372(16): 1500-9.
[http://dx.doi.org/10.1056/NEJMoa1500858] [PMID: 25773607]

[117] Robinson JG, Farnier M, Krempf M, *et al.* Efficacy and safety of alirocumab in reducing lipids and cardiovascular events. N Engl J Med 2015; 372(16): 1489-99.
[http://dx.doi.org/10.1056/NEJMoa1501031] [PMID: 25773378]

[118] Nicholls SJ, Puri R, Anderson T, *et al.* Effect of evolocumab on progression of coronary disease in statin-treated patients: the GLAGOV randomized clinical trial. JAMA 2016; 316(22): 2373-84.
[http://dx.doi.org/10.1001/jama.2016.16951] [PMID: 27846344]

[119] Jarcho JA, Keaney JF Jr. Proof that lower is better – LDL cholesterol and IMPROVE-IT. N Engl J Med 2015; 372(25): 2448-50.
[http://dx.doi.org/10.1056/NEJMe1507041] [PMID: 26039520]

[120] Bruckert E, Labreuche J, Deplanque D, Touboul PJ, Amarenco P. Fibrates effect on cardiovascular risk is greater in patients with high triglyceride levels or atherogenic dyslipidemia profile: a systematic review and meta-analysis. J Cardiovasc Pharmacol 2011; 57(2): 267-72.
[http://dx.doi.org/10.1097/FJC.0b013e318202709f] [PMID: 21052016]

[121] Shipman KE, Strange RC, Ramachandran S. Use of fibrates in the metabolic syndrome: A review. World J Diabetes 2016; 7(5): 74-88.
[http://dx.doi.org/10.4239/wjd.v7.i5.74] [PMID: 26981181]

[122] Frick MH, Elo O, Haapa K, *et al.* Helsinki Heart Study: primary-prevention trial with gemfibrozil in middle-aged men with dyslipidemia. Safety of treatment, changes in risk factors, and incidence of coronary heart disease. N Engl J Med 1987; 317(20): 1237-45.
[http://dx.doi.org/10.1056/NEJM198711123172001] [PMID: 3313041]

[123] Rubins HB, Robins SJ, Collins D, *et al.* Gemfibrozil for the secondary prevention of coronary heart disease in men with low levels of high-density lipoprotein cholesterol. N Engl J Med 1999; 341(6): 410-8.
[http://dx.doi.org/10.1056/NEJM199908053410604] [PMID: 10438259]

[124] Secondary prevention by raising HDL cholesterol and reducing triglycerides in patients with coronary artery disease. Circulation 2000; 102(1): 21-7.
[http://dx.doi.org/10.1161/01.CIR.102.1.21] [PMID: 10880410]

[125] Keech A, Simes RJ, Barter P, *et al.* Effects of long-term fenofibrate therapy on cardiovascular events in 9795 people with type 2 diabetes mellitus (the FIELD study): randomised controlled trial. Lancet 2005; 366(9500): 1849-61.
[http://dx.doi.org/10.1016/S0140-6736(05)67667-2] [PMID: 16310551]

[126] Ginsberg HN, Elam MB, Lovato LC, *et al.* Effects of combination lipid therapy in type 2 diabetes mellitus. N Engl J Med 2010; 362(17): 1563-74.
[http://dx.doi.org/10.1056/NEJMoa1001282] [PMID: 20228404]

[127] Jun M, Foote C, Lv J, *et al.* Effects of fibrates on cardiovascular outcomes: a systematic review and meta-analysis. Lancet 2010; 375(9729): 1875-84.
[http://dx.doi.org/10.1016/S0140-6736(10)60656-3] [PMID: 20462635]

[128] Rohatgi A, Khera A, Berry JD, *et al.* HDL cholesterol efflux capacity and incident cardiovascular events. N Engl J Med 2014; 371(25): 2383-93.
[http://dx.doi.org/10.1056/NEJMoa1409065] [PMID: 25404125]

[129] Niacin in patients with low HDL cholesterol levels receiving intensive statin therapy. N Engl J Med

2011; 365: 2255-2267.32.

[130]   Barter PJ, Caulfield M, Eriksson M, *et al.* Effects of torcetrapib in patients at high risk for coronary events. N Engl J Med 2007; 357(21): 2109-22.
[http://dx.doi.org/10.1056/NEJMoa0706628] [PMID: 17984165]

[131]   Bowman L, Hopewell JC, Chen F, *et al.* Effects of Anacetrapib in Patients with Atherosclerotic Vascular Disease. N Engl J Med 2017; 377(13): 1217-27.
[http://dx.doi.org/10.1056/NEJMoa1706444] [PMID: 28847206]

[132]   Lipid modification: cardiovascular risk assessment and the modification of blood lipids for the primary and secondary prevention of cardiovascular disease 2014.http://www.nice.org.uk/guidance/CG181

[133]   Ridker PM, Cushman M, Stampfer MJ, Tracy RP, Hennekens CH. Inflammation, aspirin, and the risk of cardiovascular disease in apparently healthy men. N Engl J Med 1997; 336(14): 973-9.
[http://dx.doi.org/10.1056/NEJM199704033361401] [PMID: 9077376]

[134]   Ridker PM, Hennekens CH, Buring JE, Rifai N. C-reactive protein and other markers of inflammation in the prediction of cardiovascular disease in women. N Engl J Med 2000; 342(12): 836-43.
[http://dx.doi.org/10.1056/NEJM200003233421202] [PMID: 10733371]

[135]   Ridker PM, Rifai N, Clearfield M, *et al.* Measurement of C-reactive protein for the targeting of statin therapy in the primary prevention of acute coronary events. N Engl J Med 2001; 344(26): 1959-65.
[http://dx.doi.org/10.1056/NEJM200106283442601] [PMID: 11430324]

[136]   Nissen SE, Tuzcu EM, Schoenhagen P, *et al.* Statin therapy, LDL cholesterol, C-reactive protein, and coronary artery disease. N Engl J Med 2005; 352(1): 29-38.
[http://dx.doi.org/10.1056/NEJMoa042000] [PMID: 15635110]

[137]   Ridker PM, Everett BM, Thuren T, *et al.* Antiinflammatory therapy with canakinumab for atherosclerotic disease. N Engl J Med 2017; 377(12): 1119-31.
[http://dx.doi.org/10.1056/NEJMoa1707914] [PMID: 28845751]

[138]   Chhabra N. Endothelial dysfunction – A predictor of atherosclerosis. Internet Journal of Medical Update 2009; 4: 33-41.

[139]   Baratchi S, Khoshmanesh K, Woodman OL, Potocnik S, Peter K, McIntyre P. Molecular cells of blood flow in endothelial cells. Trends Mol Med 2017; 23(9): 850-68.
[http://dx.doi.org/10.1016/j.molmed.2017.07.007] [PMID: 28811171]

[140]   Peiffer V, Sherwin SJ, Weinberg PD. Does low and oscillatory wall shear stress correlate spatially with early atherosclerosis? A systematic review. Cardiovasc Res 2013; 99(2): 242-50.
[http://dx.doi.org/10.1093/cvr/cvt044] [PMID: 23459102]

[141]   Zhou J, Li YS, Chien S. Shear stress-initiated signaling and its regulation of endothelial function. Arterioscler Thromb Vasc Biol 2014; 34(10): 2191-8.
[http://dx.doi.org/10.1161/ATVBAHA.114.303422] [PMID: 24876354]

[142]   Srikanth S, Deedwania P. Management of Dyslipidemia in Patients with Hypertension, Diabetes, and Metabolic Syndrome. Curr Hypertens Rep 2016; 18(10): 76.
[http://dx.doi.org/10.1007/s11906-016-0683-0] [PMID: 27730495]

[143]   Gupta N, Herati A, Gilbert BR. Penile Doppler ultrasound predicting cardiovascular disease in men with erectile dysfunction. Curr Urol Rep 2015; 16(3): 16.
[http://dx.doi.org/10.1007/s11934-015-0482-1] [PMID: 25677231]

[144]   Corona G, Fagioli G, Mannucci E, *et al.* Penile doppler ultrasound in patients with erectile dysfunction (ED): role of peak systolic velocity measured in the flaccid state in predicting arteriogenic ED and silent coronary artery disease. J Sex Med 2008; 5(11): 2623-34.
[http://dx.doi.org/10.1111/j.1743-6109.2008.00982.x] [PMID: 18783349]

[145]   Westholm C, Johnson J, Sahlen A, Winter R, Jernberg T. Peak systolic velocity using color-coded tissue Doppler imaging, a strong and independent predictor of outcome in acute coronary syndrome

patients. Cardiovasc Ultrasound 2013; 11: 9.
[http://dx.doi.org/10.1186/1476-7120-11-9] [PMID: 23547949]

[146]   Joint British Societies' consensus recommendations for the prevention of cardiovascular disease (JBS3). Heart 2014; 100 (Suppl. 2): ii1-ii67.
[http://dx.doi.org/10.1136/heartjnl-2014-305693] [PMID: 24667225]

[147]   Hackett G, Jones PW, Strange RC, Ramachandran S. Statin, testosterone and phosphodiesterase 5-inhibitor treatments and age related mortality in diabetes. World J Diabetes 2017; 8(3): 104-11.
[http://dx.doi.org/10.4239/wjd.v8.i3.104] [PMID: 28344753]

[148]   Ramachandran S, Hackett GI, Strange RC. Hypogonadism in men with diabetes: Should testosterone replacement therapy be based on evidence based testosterone levels and lifetime risk reduction? Edorium J Biochem 2017; 2: 1-3.
[http://dx.doi.org/10.5348/B01-2017-4-ED-4]

CHAPTER 2

The Role of SGLT2i in the Prevention and Treatment of Heart Failure

Hasan AlTurki[1], Ahmed AlTurki[2], Mark Sherman[3], Abhinav Sharma[2] and Thao Huynh[2,*]

[1] *Department of Medicine, University of British Columbia, Vancouver, Canada*

[2] *Division of Cardiology, McGill University Health Center, Montreal, Canada*

[3] *Division of Endocrinology, McGill University Health Center, Montreal, Canada*

Abstract: Diabetes mellitus (DM) is an important independent risk factor for incident heart failure (HF). DM is also a prominent prognostic factor for major cardiovascular (CV) adverse events in patients with established HF with reduced (HFrEF) or preserved ejection fraction (HFpEF). Sodium-glucose cotransporter 2 inhibitors (SGLT2i) are recently approved drugs for DM treatment. SGLT2i lead to natriuresis and glycosuria with subsequent reductions in blood glucose, intravascular volume, and blood pressure. SGLT2i demonstrated a remarkable relative risk reduction in hospitalization for heart failure in large CV outcome trials of patients with DM. In addition, there was a more modest but also a relevant reduction in CV mortality with empagliflozin. SGLT2i reduce recurrent myocardial infarctions in patients with prior myocardial infarction. SGLT2i were subsequently evaluated in patients with HFrEF, including those without DM. Dapagliflozin was associated with reductions in the primary composite endpoint of worsening heart failure or CV death and each component separately. Considering their remarkable CV benefits and nephroprotection, SGLT2i represent invaluable therapy for the primary and secondary prevention of heart diseases in patients with DM or HFrEF. Ongoing trials may confirm the potential impact of SGTL2i in patients with HFpEF and acutely decompensating HF.

Keywords: Diabetes Mellitus, Heart Failure, SGLT2 Inhibitors.

INTRODUCTION

Diabetes Mellitus (DM) is a common disease associated with debilitating microvascular and macrovascular consequences [1, 2]. Macrovascular diseases can lead to acute coronary syndromes, heart failure (HF), and cardiovascular (CV) death, which is the most common cause of death in this population [3 - 5].

* **Corresponding author Thao Huynh:** Division of Cardiology, McGill University Health Center, Montreal, Canada;
Tel: 514-934-1934 Ext-44649 ; Fax: 514-934-8569;
E-mail: thao.huynhthanh@mail.mcgill.ca

The mainstay of DM management is optimal glycemic control [1, 2].

In 2008, the American Food and Drug Administration (FDA) mandated a compulsory assessment of long-term CV outcomes in all trials evaluating novel anti-diabetic agents [6]. Similar requirements were also set forth by the European Medicines Agency [7]. Both recommendations were in response to a meta-analysis by Nissen and colleagues, which showed 43% and 64% increased odds of myocardial infarction and CV death, respectively, associated with rosiglitazone [8]. Subsequently, rosiglitazone was banned or severely restricted globally. In the later ten years following the above recommendation, 22 randomized controlled trials (RCTS) were completed or ongoing to assess CV outcomes in anti-diabetic agents [9]. Almost all novel anti-diabetic agents were non-inferior to placebo for CV safety [10 - 14] except for one notable exception with increased risk of heart failure (HF) hospitalizations (HHF) associated with saxagliptin [15]. Glucagon-like peptide 1 agonists show excellent glycemic control and weight loss [12]. In 2016, the LEADER trial showed a reduction in the major adverse cardiovascular outcome (MACE), including CV death with liraglutide [16]. Sodium-glucose cotransporter-2 inhibitors (SGLT2i) emerged with promising CV benefits in several safety trials [17 - 19]. In this chapter, we will review the impact of SGLT2i in the primary and secondary prevention of CV diseases with an emphasis on HF.

HEART FAILURE

HF is a complex clinical condition characterized by the heart's inability to provide adequate forward flow or filling without pulmonary congestion [20 - 22]. HF has been declared a global pandemic affecting over 26 million people worldwide [23]. HF is classified into two main categories. HF with preserved left ventricle's ejection fraction and HF with reduced left ventricle's ejection fraction [21]. The importance of HF resides in two essential facts. First, HF is common with an annual incidence of 1% and a lifetime risk of 20% [24, 25]. Second, HF is generally associated with poor outcomes [26]. The Initiation Management Predischarge Process for Assessment of Carvedilol Therapy for Heart Failure (IMPACT-HF) study reported six-month mortality and repeated HHF approximating 5% and 23%, respectively [27].

The Canadian Enhanced Feedback for Effective Cardiac Treatment (EFFECT) study demonstrated 30-day and 1-year heart failure readmissions of 4.9% and 16.1%, as well as mortality of 7.1% and 25.5%, respectively, in 1,570 patients with HFrEF [28]. During the last two decades, angiotensin pathway inhibitors, beta-blockers, and mineralocorticoid receptor antagonists (so-called triple therapies) have markedly improved heart failure outcomes [29]. However, despite the triple therapies, the residual risks of HF-related hospitalization and mortality remain high and innovative approaches are needed.

Patients with DM have more than twice the risk of developing HF than individuals without DM [30]. DM-induced cardiomyopathy has been postulated as HF in the absence of coronary artery disease and hypertension in patients with DM [31]. The potential causal factors of DM cardiomyopathy include oxidative stress, inflammation, apoptosis, and microvascular coronary artery disease. In the Framingham Heart Study, DM independently increased the risk of HF up to two-fold in men and five-fold in women compared with age-matched controls (adjusted for age, hypertension, dyslipidemia, and coronary artery disease) [32, 33]. The prevalence of DM in HF patients is three to four-fold higher than the general population [34]. Moreover, DM is independently associated with increased risks of death and HHF in individuals with HF [35, 36]. HF was responsible for a substantial mortality burden of patients with DM in the TECOS trial [37].

Since elevated HbA1c level is associated with an increased incidence of HF [38], one may postulate that intensive glycemic control would reduce CV, and specifically HF-related outcomes. Unexpectedly, trials designed to evaluate the above hypothesis showed the contrary. The ADVANCE trial (Action in Diabetes and Vascular Disease: Preterax and Diamicron MR Controlled Evaluation) demonstrated that intensive glucose control, aiming for HbA1c 6.5% or better, failed to reduce macrovascular events or total mortality [39]. The ACCORD trial (Action to Control CV Risk in Diabetes), showed that intensive glycemic control (HbA1c of 6% and less) increased mortality by 22% compared to patients in the standard treatment arm [40]. Castagno *et al* completed a meta-analysis of eight RCTs evaluating the reduction in HF by an intensive glucose-lowering regimen compared to standard treatment in 37,229 patients [41]. The mean difference in the HbA1C level between the standard treatment and an intensive regimen was 0.9% (follow-up ranging from two to ten years) [41]. Overall, the risk of HF-related events was similar between the intensive and standard treatment arms (odds ratio (OR)1.20; 95% confidence interval (CI): 0.96-1.48) [41].

MECHANISMS OF ACTION OF SGLT2 AND SGTL2I

In this section, we will examine the potential mechanisms by which SGLT2i may be beneficial in the prevention and treatment of HF. We summarize the mechanisms by which SGLT2i exert its cardioprotective effects in Fig. (**1**).

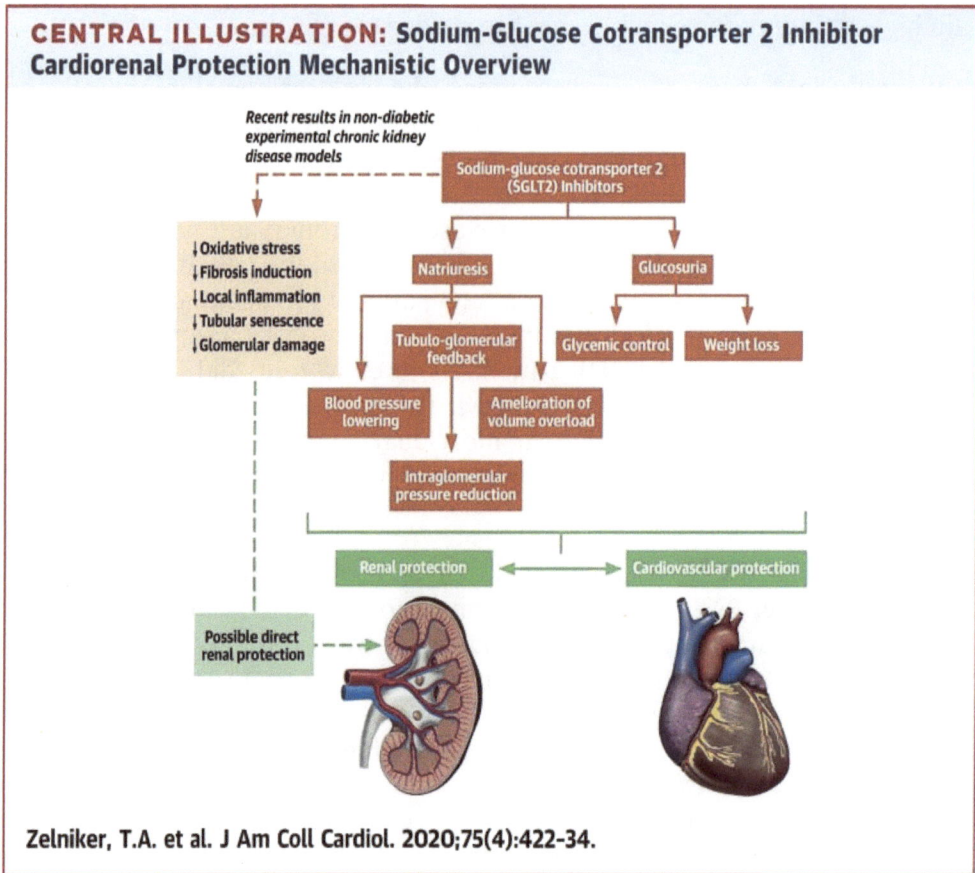

CENTRAL ILLUSTRATION: Sodium-Glucose Cotransporter 2 Inhibitor Cardiorenal Protection Mechanistic Overview

Zelniker, T.A. et al. J Am Coll Cardiol. 2020;75(4):422-34.

Fig. (1). Mechanisms of Cardio-Renal Protection of Sodium-Glucose Cotransporter 2 Inhibitors[54]. (Reproduced with permission).

Glucose Homeostasis

SGLTs are responsible for tissue glucose translocation, with SGLT2 being specific to the kidney and pancreas [42]. SGLT2 is a high-capacity, low-affinity glucose transporter located on the epithelial cells lining the S1 and S2 segments of the proximal convoluted tubules in the kidneys. It is responsible for about 90% of filtered glucose reabsorption [43]. Sodium-glucose cotransporter-1 (SGLT1) is a low-capacity and high-affinity glucose transport, located in the S3 segment of the proximal convoluted tubules, as well as the enterocytes of the small intestine [44]. SGLT1 is responsible for the reabsorption of the remaining 10% of filtered glucose [45]. In the pancreas, SGLT2 is part of an alpha cell glucose uptake system [46]. SGLT2i may directly block glucose transport into alpha cells, leading to an increase in glucagon secretion [47]. One particular concern of

SGLT2i in the pancreas is an increased risk of pancreatitis (based on case reports), but a meta-analysis of thirty-five trials of SGLT2i did not show increased risks in pancreatitis or pancreatic cancer [48].

The active transport of glucose *via* SGLT2 is linked to Na+ transport maintained by its active extrusion *via* the Na+/K+ ATPase of the basolateral membrane into the intracellular fluid [43]. Under normal conditions, glucose is freely filtered into the urine at the glomerulus (180 g/day) and reabsorbed in the proximal tubule by SGLT2 (90%) and SGLT1 (10%) [43, 45]. The plasma glucose concentration above which urinary glucose excretion occurs is approximately 180–200 mg/dl (10.0-11.1 mmol/L), and in patients with DM, this threshold can increase up to 300 mg/dl (16.7 mmol/L) because of the increased activity of SGLT2 [49].

SGLT2i reduce HbA1c by about 0.5%– 0.7% [50]. SGLT2i exert its benefits though several mechanisms: **1)** by blocking the reuptake of glucose in the proximal tubule, thereby promoting urinary glucose excretion, **2)** due to glycosuria-induced associated caloric losses, SGLT2i can induce mild weight loss of 0.5-1 kg [18], and **3)** SGLT2i promotes urinary excretion of sodium (natriuresis) [51]. SGLT2i shift the renal tubular threshold for glycosuria to 50 mg/dl (2.8 mmol/L), reduce the reabsorption of filtered glucose (30–50%), and increase glycosuria, decreasing glycemia and HbA1c levels independent of insulinemia [52]. The insulin-independent mechanism allows feedback reductions in insulin secretion and the risk of hypoglycemia. The glycosuria with SGLT2i is dose-dependent and without tachyphylaxis [53].

Cardiovascular Effects of SGLT2i

There are several potential pathways by which SGLT2i can exert its CV benefits: reduction of sarcoplasmic calcium leak with resulting improved cardiac contractility, decreased reactive sympathetic system hyperactivation associated with HF, improved oxygen delivery, lower inflammation and oxidative stress and improvement of endothelial function [54]. Inhibition of the sodium-hydrogen exchanger lowers myocardial cytoplasmic sodium and calcium levels while increasing mitochondrial calcium levels which [55] reduces cardiac injury, hypertrophy, fibrosis, remodeling, and left ventricular systolic dysfunction [53, 54]. SGLT2i also attenuate the upregulation of the sodium-hydrogen exchanger, which can occur in patients with HF [56]. There is also evidence that SGLT2i may improve obesity-mediated cardiac dysfunction by maintaining redox homeostasis through the regulation of Sestrin2-mediated AMPK-mTOR signaling [57]. Another potential mechanism is the inhibition of SGLT1. Inhibition of cardiac SGLT1 decreases the myocardial sodium and glucose uptake and reduces the generation of reactive oxygen species due to hyperglycemia [58].

Canagliflozin has the highest potential to inhibit SGLT1 due to its non-specific inhibition of SGLT 1 and 2. However, inhibition of SGLT1 occurs to much lesser degrees than SGLT2. Therefore, it remains unclear whether the inhibition of SGLT1 has any clinical consequence.

Another potential mechanism of the beneficial effect of SGLT2i in HF may also be the inhibition of the sodium-hydrogen exchanger in the renal tubules rather than only on glucose reabsorption [59]. The sodium-hydrogen exchanger is responsible for most of the sodium reuptake after filtration, and its activity is markedly increased in patients with HF, in whom it may be responsible for their resistance to diuretics and to endogenous natriuretic peptides. The natriuretic effect of SGLT2i contributes to intravascular volume contraction and improves intrarenal hemodynamics *via* tubulo-glomerular feedback. This natriuresis can reduce approximately five mmHg of systolic blood pressure and 30%–50% in albuminuria.

Nephroprotective Effects of SGLT2I

SGLT2i exerts its nephroprotective effects by both hemodynamic and non-hemodynamic mechanisms [54]. SGLT2i lowers intraglomerular pressure by decreasing blood pressure. By reducing the glucose reabsorption, SGLT2i decreases the energy demand on the kidney tubular cells resulting in more erythropoietin production, which in turn can attenuate the hypoxic injury of these cells [54]. SGLT2i augment uric acid secretion by stimulating uric transporter 1 with increased glucose concentrations in the distal tubule [54]. By decreasing uricemia, SGLT2i can prevent the inflammation, oxidative stress, and activation of renin-angiotensin pathways on the kidneys and cardiovascular system. The nephroprotective effects of SGLT2i appear to be independent of their actions on glucose homeostasis [54].

CV OUTCOMES IN PATIENTS WITH T2DM

To date, there are five major randomized controlled trials (RCTs) examining the CV effects of different SGLT2i in various populations [17 - 19, 60, 61]. In this section, we will be discussing the results of these trials, as well as their subgroup analyses for patients with T2DM, Chronic Kidney Disease (CKD), and established HF (Table **2**). We summarize the baseline characteristics of these trials in Table **1**. The Empagliflozin CV Outcome Event Trial in Type 2 Diabetes Mellitus Patients - Removing Excess Glucose (EMPA-REG OUTCOME) trial was the first large RCT to show reductions in CV outcomes with an SGLT2i in patients with T2DM [18]. There were 7,020 patients with T2DM with an estimated glomerular filtration (eGFR) of greater than 30 ml/min, and established CV disease, randomized to either empagliflozin (10mg or 25mg) or placebo.

Table 1. Study and baseline patient characteristics of CV outcome trials assessing SGLT2i.

Trials	EMPA-REG OUTCOME	CANVAS	DECLARE-TIMI 58	CREDENCE	DAPA-HF
Drug	Empagliflozin	Canagliflozin	Dapagliflozin	Canagliflozin	Dapagliflozin
Primary outcomes	MACE	MACE	MACE and HHF or CV death	Doubling of serum Cr, or ESRD, or CV/renal death	CV death, HHF or urgent HF visit
Dose	10mg or 20mg	100mg or 300mg	10mg	100mg	10mg
Inclusion Criteria	-T2DM with HbA1c 7% to 10% (9 if drug naïve) -Established CVD -eGFR>30 ml/min -Age >18 years -BMI <45	-T2DM with HbA1c 7% - 10.5% -Established CVD or high CV risk	-T2DM -Age>40 years -CrCl>60 ml/min -Established CV disease or multiple risk factors	-T2DM with HbA1c 6.5-12 - eGFR 30-90 ml/min -ACR 300 to 5000mg/g -ACEi/ARB -Age>30 years	-Age>18 years -Symptomatic HFrEF with NYHA II-IV -LVEF<40% - NT pro BNP>600pg/ml if no HHF in last 12 months, otherwise >400pg/ml -Standard HF therapy -eGFR>30 ml/min
Main Exclusion Criteria	-Liver disease -Planned cardiac surgery or PCI within 3 months -Bariatric surgery within 2 years -Systemic steroids within 6 weeks -ACS, CVA within 2 months	-T1DM -Prior DKA -Pancreas or beta cell transplant -Severe hypoglycemia within 6 months	-T1DM -Chronic cystitis -Recurrent UTIs -Radiation therapy to lower abdomen or pelvis	-T1DM -DKA -Primary renal glucosuria -Renal disease on immunosuppressive therapy -Liver disease -NYHA IV HF -Blood potassium >5.5mEq/L	-T1DM -Hypotension (symptomatic or SBP<95) -Acute HF within 4 weeks -ACS, CVA, CRT, PCI or CABG within 3 months -HF due to restrictive cardiomyopathy, active myocarditis, constrictive pericarditis, HOCM or primary uncorrected valve disease

(Table 1) cont.....

Trials	EMPA-REG OUTCOME	CANVAS	DECLARE-TIMI 58	CREDENCE	DAPA-HF
Total Patients (% female)	7,020 (29%)	10,142 (35.8%)	17,160 (37.4%)	4,401 (33.9%)	4,744 (24%)
Mean Age (years)	63 ±8.7	63.3 ±-8.3	63.9 ±-6.8	63.0 ±-9.2	66±11
Median follow-up (years)	3.1	2.4	4.2	2.6	1.5
Prior CV disease	100%	65.6%	40.7%	50.4%	56%
Prior HF	10%	14.4%	10.0%	14.8%	100%
T2DM	100%	100%	100%	100%	41.8%
eGFR<60 ml/min	26%	20.1%	7.4%	59.8%	40.7%
Albuminuria	40%	29.8%	30.3%	99.3%	Not reported

Abbreviations: MACE: Major adverse cardiovascular events, HHF: Hospitalization for heart failure, CV: Cardiovascular, Cr: Creatinine, ESRD: End stage renal disease, T2DM: Type 2 diabetes mellitus, HbA1c: Glycosylated hemoglobin, CVD: Cardiovascular disease, eGFR: Estimated glomerular filtration rate, BMI: Body mass index, CrCl: Creatinine clearance, ACR: Albumin to creatinine ratio, ACEi: Angiotensin converting enzyme inhibitor, ARB: Angiotensin receptor blocker, HFrEF: Heart failure with reduced ejection fraction, NYHA: New York heart association, LVEF: Left ventricular ejection fraction, NT pro BNP: N terminal prohormone of brain natriuretic peptide, HF: Heart failure, ACS: Acute coronary syndrome, CVA: Cerebrovascular accident, T1DM: Type 1 diabetes mellitus, DKA: Diabetic ketoacidosis, UTI: Urinary tract infection, CRT: Cardiac resynchronization therapy, PCI: Percutaneous coronary intervention, CABG: Coronary artery bypass graft, HOCM: Hypertrophic obstructive cardiomyopathy.

Empagliflozin was associated with a reduction in the primary outcome (composite of death from CV causes, and non-fatal myocardial infarction) 10.5% *versus* 12.1% in placebo (hazard ratio (HR) 0.86, confidence intervals (CI) 0.74 to 0.99, p<0.001 for non-inferiority and p<0.04 for superiority). Empagliflozin was also associated with marked reductions in CV deaths (3.7% *versus* 5.9%; HR: 0.62, CI: 0.49 to 0.77, p<0.001), all-cause mortality (5.7% *versus* 8.3%;HR: 0.68, CI: 0.57 to 0.82, p<0.001), and hospitalization for heart failure (HHF) (2.7% *versus* 4.1%, HR: 0.65, CI: 0.5 to 0.85, p=0.002). These benefits were independent of empagliflozin dose, baseline renal function, presence of HF, and HbA1c. Of note, 65% of patients in this study had a prior myocardial infarction (MI) or stroke. The benefits of empagliflozin were consistent across all subgroups, stratified by the Thrombolysis in Myocardial infarction (TIMI) risk score [62]. Similarly, in the patients without HF at baseline (90%), empagliflozin provided consistent benefits across all subgroups, stratified for 5-year risk for incident HF (Health ABC HF Risk score) [63]. Interestingly, while hypoglycemia in the placebo group was associated with an increase in HHF, the CV benefits in the empagliflozin group persisted independent of hypoglycemic events. Finally, although 25 mg of empagliflozin was more effective in decreasing HbA1c than the 10 mg dose, the CV benefits were similar between the two doses.

Table 2. Main Results of the SGLT2i Outcome Trials.

Trials	EMPA-REG OUTCOME	CANVAS	DECLARE-TIMI 58	CREDENCE	DAPA-HF
Primary outcomes	MACE	MACE	MACE and HHF or CV death	Doubling of serum Cr, or ESRD, or CV/renal death	CV death, HHF or urgent HF visit
Primary results, HR (95% CI)	0.86 (0.74-0.99)	0.86 (0.75-0.97)	0.93 (0.84-1.03)	0.70 (0.59-0.82)	0.74 (0.65-0.85)
HHF, HR (95% CI)	0.65 (0.50-0.85)	0.67 (0.52-0.87)	0.73 (0.61-0.88)	0.61 (0.47-0.80)	0.70 (0.59 to 0.83)
CV death, HR (95% CI)	0.62 (0.49-0.77)	0.87 (0.72-1.06)	0.98 (0.82-1.17)	0.78 (0.61-1.00)	0.82 (0.69 to 0.98)
All-cause mortality, HR (95% CI)	0.68 (0.57-0.82)	0.87 (0.74-1.01)	0.93 (0.82-1.04)	0.83 (0.68-1.02)	0.83 (0.71 to 0.97)
Progression of renal disease*, HR (95% CI)	0.54 (0.40-0.75)	0.60 (0.47-0.77)	0.53 (0.43-0.66)	0.66 (0.53-0.81)	0.71 (0.44 to 1.16)

*EMPA-REG OUTCOME: Doubling of serum creatinine with eGFR less than 45ml/min, initiation of RRT or renal death. CANVAS: 40% reduction in eGFR, RRT or renal death. DECLARE-TIMI 58: Over 40% decrease in eGFR to less than 60ml/min, ESRD, or renal death. CREDENCE: Doubling of serum creatinine, ESRD, or renal death. DAPA-HF: Over 50% decline in eGFR, ESRD, RRT, or renal death Abbreviations: MACE: Major adverse cardiovascular events, HHF: Hospitalization for heart failure, CV: Cardiovascular, Cr: Creatinine, ESRD: End stage renal disease, HF: Heart failure, HR: Hazard ration, CI: Confidence interval, eGFR: Estimated glomerular filtration rate, RRT: Renal replacement therapy.

The Canagliflozin CV Assessment Study (CANVAS) Program was the second large-scale RCT demonstrating a benefit in CV outcomes with SGLT2i (canagliflozin) in patients with T2DM [19]. This study enrolled 10,142 patients with T2DM, an eGFR greater than 30ml/min, and with either established CV disease or at high CV risk (more than two CV risk factors or older than 50 years old). These patients were randomized to either canagliflozin (100 mg daily or 300 mg daily) or placebo. Canagliflozin was associated with a reduction in the primary outcome (CV death, MI, or stroke) of 2.69% compared to 3.15% placebo. The HR was 0.86, 95% CI: 0.75-0.97, p=0.02 for superiority and p<0.001 for non-inferiority. The CV benefits were observed in patients with and without baseline CV disease independent of baseline renal function [64].

The Dapagliflozin Effect on CV Events (DECLARE) – Thrombolysis in Myocardial Infarction (TIMI)-58 trial was the third RCT to examine CV outcomes with an SGLT2i, specifically dapagliflozin, in patients with T2DM [17]. This trial included 17,160 patients with T2DM, and notably with a creatinine clearance (CrCl) greater than 60 ml/min, differentiating it from previous trials. At baseline, 59% of these patients did not have pre-existing atherosclerotic CV disease. Dapagliflozin was non-inferior to placebo in reduction of major cardiovascular events (MACE) (8.8% compared to 9.4%, HR 0.93, 95% CI 0.84-1.03, p<0.001 for non-inferiority and p = 0.17 for superiority). Dapagliflozin was associated with 24% reduction in HF hospitalization (2.5% compared to 3.3%, p=0.005).

Zelniker *et al* completed a meta-analysis of the above three studies (totaling 34,322 patients) [65]. SGLT2i was associated with reduced risk of CV death, non-fatal MI or stroke (HR: 0·89, CI: 0·83–0·96, p=0·0014), in addition to a lowered risk of CV death or HHF (HR: 0·77, CI: 0·71–0·84, p<0·0001), and HHF alone (HR: 0·69, CI: 0·61–0·79, p<0·0001). Furthermore, patients with existing HF (10-15% of the patients) appeared to derive a greater benefit from SGLT2i, as did those with mild to moderate renal dysfunction.

In summary, there were three large-scale CV outcome trials EMPA-REG OUTCOME (empagliflozin), CANVAS (canagliflozin), and DECLARE-TIMI 58 (dapagliflozin) which showed a reduction of MACE with SGLT2i in patients with T2DM [17 - 19]. Notably, SGLT2i reduced the risk of HHF in all three trials, regardless of HF status at baseline or presence of atherosclerotic CV disease, making SGLT2i the first class of anti-diabetic medications associated with reductions in HHF. These encouraging results subsequently prompted investigators to examine the benefits of SGLT2 inhibitors in other populations.

RENAL OUTCOMES IN PATIENTS WITH T2DM AND CHRONIC KIDNEY DISEASE (CKD)

CKD is one of the main risk factors for CV death and HHF, particularly in patients with underlying HF [66 - 68]. The CREDENCE trial is the only large RCT to date, which examined the use of a SGLT2i (canagliflozin) in patients with concomitant T2DM and CKD [61]. The trial enrolled 4,401 patients with T2DM and renal disease (eGFR 30-90 ml/min), already on angiotensin pathway inhibitors, to receive either 100mg of canagliflozin daily or placebo. The trial was stopped prematurely due to marked benefit with canagliflozin in reducing the primary composite outcome of progression to end-stage renal disease (ESRD), doubling of serum creatinine and renal or CV death compared to placebo (HR: 0.70, 95% CI: 0.59-0.82, p<0.00001). Additionally, canagliflozin was also beneficial in decreasing several secondary outcomes, *i.e.* CV death, MI, stroke, HHF, and UA. All of these benefits were independent of baseline HbA1c [61].

We observed similar benefits for patients with CKD and macroalbuminuria in subgroup analyses of previous SGLT2i trials. The EMPA-REG OUTCOMES, CANVAS, and DECLARE-TIMI 58 trials reported reductions in risk of composite renal outcomes, defined as progression to ESRD, renal death, kidney failure (40% reduction in eGFR or doubling of serum creatinine) [69 - 71]. In patients with T2DM and CKD, there was also evidence supporting CV benefit with SGLT2i. In CREDENCE, canagliflozin was associated with a reduction in MACE (HR: 0.80, 95% CI: 0.67–0.95) and HHF (HR: 0.61, 95% CI: 0.47–0.80) [61]. In EMPA-REG, empagliflozin decreased CV death (HR 0.76, 95% CI 0.59-0.99), HHF (HR 0.61, 95% CI 0.72-0.92), and all-cause hospitalization (HR 0.81, 95% CI 0.72-0.92) in patients with CKD (baseline eGFR<60 ml/min) regardless of the empagliflozin dose [71]. In CANVAS, 20% of patients had a baseline eGFR 30- 60 ml/min; 72% of whom had prior CV disease [19]. Canagliflozin diminished MACE's risk by 30% (95% CI 0.55-0.90) compared to placebo [69]. The nephroprotection coupled with reduction in risks of CV outcomes and HF with SGLT2i in patients with CKD is promising. For this reason, SLGT2i represent a compelling choice as the ideal anti-diabetic agents in patients with CKD.

HEART FAILURE

To date, the DAPA-HF trial is the only fully published RCT examining the use of an SGLT2i, dapagliflozin, in patients with stable heart failure with reduced ejection fraction (HFrEF) and New York Heart Association (NYHA) class II-IV [60]. The study randomized 4,744 patients to either dapagliflozin 10 mg daily or placebo. Compared to placebo, dapagliflozin was associated with a 26% reduction in risk of CV death, HHF, or urgent HF visits (95% CI 0.65-0.85, p<0.001). This was primarily driven by a reduction in HHF (HR 0.70, 95%CI 0.59-0.83) and CV death (HR 0.82, 95% CI 0.69-0.98). These benefits were consistent among all subgroups of patients, regardless of age, diabetes status, or baseline health status (as measured by the Kansas City Cardiomyopathy Score) [72 - 74].

Subgroup analyses of prior CV outcome trials (EMPA-REG, CANVAS, and DECLARE-TIMI 58) also supported the advantages of SGLT2i in patients with HF [75 - 77]. Compared to placebo, empagliflozin resulted in less HHF or CV death (5.7% *vs* 8.5%, respectively), (HR: 0.66, 95% CI: 0.55-0.79, p<0.001). Interestingly, this benefit was consistent in patients with HF and without baseline HF [75]. Empagliflozin also decreased HHF or HF-related deaths compared to placebo (2.8% *vs* 4.5%; HR 0.61, 95% CI 0.82-0.96, p = 0.003). Similar findings were also observed in the CANVAS program, in which 14.4% of patients had baseline HF [19]. Canagliflozin was associated with a reduction in CV death or HHF (HR: 0.78, 95% CI: 0.67-0.91), as well as fatal or hospitalized HF (HR: 0.70, 95% CI: 0.55-0.89) and HHF alone (HR 0.67, 95% CI 0.52-0.87) compared to placebo [76]. Of note, the reductions in CV death or HHF were more remarkable in patients with baseline HF (HR: 0.61, 95% CI 0.46-0.80) than those without baseline HF (HR 0.87, 95% CI 0.72-2.06, p interaction = 0.021). In DECLARE-TIMI 58, 7.7% of patients had HFrEF. In these patients, dapagliflozin reduced CV death or HHF (HR: 0.62, CI: 0.45-0.86), HHF (HR: 0.64, CI: 0.43-0.95), CV death (HR: 0.55, CI: 0.34-0.90), and all-cause mortality (HR: 0.59, CI: 0.40-0.88) [77]. Dapagliflozin did not reduce CV death and all-cause mortality in those without HFrEF [77].

Brain natriuretic peptide (BNP) and N-terminal prohormone of BNP (NT-proBNP) are biomarkers primarily released by the heart's ventricles in response to myocyte stretch and increased ventricular pressure [78]. These biomarkers are used in the diagnosis and prognostication of HF. The DEFINE HF trial was the first trial to investigate the effects of an SGLT2i, dapagliflozin, on NT-proBNP levels [79]. When adjusted for baseline NT-proBNP, baseline DM status, age, and baseline eGFR, there was no difference in the proportion of patients with the primary endpoint with dapagliflozin (20% reduction in NT-proBNP at six weeks) compared to placebo (34.4% *vs* 33.3%, adjusted OR: 1.1, CI: 0.6-1.9, p=0.74). However, dapagliflozin was associated with a more than 20% reduction in NT-proBNP at 12 weeks (44% compared to 29.4%, adjusted OR 1.9, 95% CI 1.1-3.3). At 12-month, canagliflozin was associated with reduced NT-proBNP, while NT-proBNP was elevated in patients on placebo [80].

SGLT2i may also improve the quality of life in patients with chronic and stable HF. In a subgroup analysis of the DAPA-HF trial, dapagliflozin was associated with a 2.3-point increase in the summary KCCQ score [73]. Similarly, in DEFINE-HF, patients in the dapagliflozin arm showed more considerable improvement in the summary KCCQ score compared to placebo (42.9% compared to 32.5%, adjusted OR: 1.73, 95% CI: 0.98-3.05) [79].

PERIPHERAL ARTERIAL DISEASE

Concerns were raised concerning the potential worsening of peripheral arterial disease (PAD) and increased risk of major lower limb amputation (MALE) with SGLT2i. The CANVAS investigators noted a two-fold increase in the risk of MALE with canagliflozin compared to placebo (HR: 1.97, 95% CI: 1.41–2.75) [81]. This report prompted the FDA to issue a black box warning of MALE with canagliflozin and motivates our detailed evaluation of the risk of MALE with

SGLT2i.

In the EMPA-REG trial, 20% of patients had PAD at enrollment. In these patients, empagliflozin reduced CV death by 43% (HR 0.57, 95% CI 0.37-0.88), all-cause mortality by 38% (HR 0.62, 95% CI 0.44-0.88), CV death, MI or stroke by 16% (HR 0.84, 95% CI 0.62-1.14), CV death, MI, stroke, or unstable angina by 7% (HR 0.93, 95% CI 0.70-1.24), HHF by 44% (HR 0.56, 95% CI 0.35-0.92), and incident or worsening nephropathy by 46% (HR 0.54, 95% CI 0.41-0.71) compared to placebo [62]. These benefits were consistent with findings in patients without PAD (p for interaction for all endpoints > 0.05). The incidences of MALE were similar between the empagliflozin and placebo arms and between patients with and without PAD.

In the DECLARE-TIMI trial, 1,205 patients had PAD at enrollment. Patients with PAD had more MALE (20.3% compared to 2.1%) and more MACE and renal events [17]. The presence of PAD did not modify the impact of dapagliflozin on the incidence of MALE. Limb events were similar in the dapagliflozin and placebo groups including major adverse limb events (1.4% *vs* 1.2%), amputation (1.4% *vs* 1.3%), urgent revascularization (0.5% *vs* 0.6%) and elective revascularization (1.6% *vs* 1.5%).

In the CREDENCE trial, approximately 5% of the patients in both treatment arms had a prior amputation. The rate of MALE was similar in both treatment groups: 12.3 *versus* 11.2 per 1,000 patient-years (HR: 1.11; 95% CI: 0.79-1.56). In summary, there was no convincing increase in the risk of MALE with empagliflozin and dapagliflozin, or with subsequent clinical trial of canagliflozin [61], suggesting that this complication may not be an actual drug-related complication but more likely due to the underlying PAD often associated with DM [82].

ACUTE HEART FAILURE

Acute HF is a leading cause of hospitalization and carries a high risk of mortality. In contrast to therapies for chronic HF, there are currently no lifesaving medical therapies [29, 83]. Up to 20% of patients hospitalized with acute HF have residual volume overload at discharge despite loop diuretics [84]. Residual volume overload was associated with increased readmission and mortality risks, particularly in patients with underlying renal disease and those who responded poorly to diuretics [85]. Due to the natriuretic and glycosuric effect of SGLT2i, it has been hypothesized that this class of medications may be useful in acute decompensated HF.

The EMPA-RESPONSE-AHF was a pilot study, and the first RCT to date, examining SGLT2i (empagliflozin) in patients presenting with acute decompensated HF [86]. Eighty patients with acute HF were randomized to 10mg of empagliflozin daily or placebo for 30 days. All patients received standard diuretics. Of note, about 30% of the enrolled patients had pre-existing T2DM. There were no differences in the primary outcome between the two groups (composite of visual analogue dyspnea score, diuretic response, change in NT-proBNP, and length of hospital stay). On the other hand, compared to placebo, empagliflozin reduced the secondary composite outcome of in-hospital worsening HF, re-hospitalization for HF or death within 60 days (10% compared to 33%, p = 0.01).

The safety results were encouraging in this trial with similar rates of adverse events between the two treatment groups. There was no difference in diuretic response, as defined by the weight/furosemide dose, dyspnea severity, and NT-proBNP levels across both groups (empagliflozin *vs.* placebo) [86]. Nevertheless, empagliflozin induced greater cumulative urine output (difference 3,449 mL, 95% confidence interval 578–6320 mL, p <0.01, n =28) after four days and higher net fluid loss (−2163 mL *vs.* −1007 mL, p <0.01, n =53) after one day. Overall, these findings supported a beneficial diuresis with SGLT2i in acutely decompensating HF. This pilot study may pave the way for larger outcome trials of SGLT2i in patients with acute decompensated HF.

REAL-WORLD DATA

The majority of patients enrolled in the above RCTs were mainly from the United States and Europe [17 - 19, 61, 62]. Furthermore, these RCTs focused mainly on CV and kidney outcomes and did not evaluate stroke. To remediate the limited external validity of the above RCTs, the CVD-REAL investigators examined further the safety and benefits of SGLT2i in a large observational study of six countries: South Korea, Japan, Singapore, Australia, Israel, and Canada [6]. Compared to other types of anti-diabetic medications (including insulin), SGLT2i was associated with a lower risk of death (HR: 0.51; 95% confidence interval ; 95%CI: 0.37 to 0.70; p < 0.001), HHF (HR: 0.64; 95% CI: 0.50 to 0.82; p ¼ 0.001), death or HHF (HR: 0.60; 95% CI: 0.47 to 0.76; p < 0.001), MI (HR: 0.81; 95% CI: 0.74 to 0.88; p < 0.001), and stroke (HR: 0.68; 95% CI: 0.55 to 0.84; p < 0.001). The benefits of SGLT2i were consistent across both countries and patient subgroups, and across individuals with and without CV disease.

CURRENT SGLT2I USES

Up to now, there are four FDA approved SGLT-2 inhibitors: empagliflozin, dapagliflozin, canagliflozin, and ertugliflozin. Other SGLT2i are currently in use in Asia: ipragliflozin, tofogliflozin and luseogliflozin [6]. The various SGLT2 inhibitors express varying levels of selectivity for SGLT2 over SGLT1: 2500-fold for empagliflozin, 2235-fold for ertugliflozin, 1200-fold for dapagliflozin and 200 fold for canagliflozin [87 - 90].

We summarize the current American, European and Canadian guidelines in Table **3**. The 2018 American Diabetes Association (ADA) and European Association for the Study of Diabetes (EASD) consensus guidance support SGLT2i as a second-line anti-diabetic medication in patients with DM and concomitant atherosclerotic CV disease. Given metformin's low cost and favorable safety profile, it remains the first agent of choice [91]. In their 2019 updates, the ADA and EASD went a step further and suggested SGLT2i to reduce MACE, HHF, CV death, or CKD progression in patients with DM, independent of HbA1c target [92]. Specifically, they recommended SGLT2i in patients with HFrEF, CKD, or albuminuria, regardless of CV risk status.

Table 3. Current guideline recommendations for SGLT2i.

American College of Cardiology 2018	• Consider SGLT2i in patients with T2DM and ASCVD and when patient and clinician priorities include:
	  • -Reducing MACE and CV death
	  • -Preventing HHF
	  • - BP control
	  • -Orally administered therapies

American Diabetes Association and European Association for the Study of Diabetes 2019	• -Consider SGLT2i in patients with T2DM at high risk, to reduce MACE, HHF, CV death or CKD progression, independent of baseline HbA1c.
	  • -Benefit is greatest in patients with HFrEF (EF<45%) or CKD (eGFR 30 to 60 ml/min or UACR over 30mg/g, particularly over 300mg/g).
	  • -SGLT2i recommended in patients with T2DM and HF (particularly HFrEF) to reduce HHF, MACE and CV death.
	  • -SGLT2i recommended in patients with T2DM and CKD to reduce progression of CKD, HHF, MACE, and CV death.
	  • -Careful shared decision making for patients with foot ulcers or at high risk for amputation prior to SGLT2i initiation.

European Society of Cardiology 2019	• -SGLT2i to lower risk of HHF in patients with DM (recommendation Ia)
	  • -Empagliflozin, Canagliflozin or Dapagliflozin in patients with T2DM and CVD (or at high risk) to reduce CV events (recommendation Ia)
	  • -Empagliflozin in patients with T2DM and CVD to reduce risk of death (recommendation Ia)
	  • -SGLT2i in patients with T2DM and CKD to reduce progression of diabetic kidney disease (recommendation Ia)
	  • -SGLT2i or GLP1-RA as first line treatment in drug naïve patients with T2DM and with ASCVD or with high CV risk (second line for patients already on metformin) (recommendation Ia)

(Table 3) cont.....

Canadian CV Society and Canadian Heart Failure Society 2020	• -SGLT2i for patients with T2DM and ASCVD to reduce risk of HHF and death (Strong Recommendation, High-Quality Evidence) • -SGLT2i for patients over 50 with T2DM and risk factors for ASCVD to reduce risk of HHF (Strong Recommendation, High-Quality Evidence) • -SGLT2i for patients over 50 with T2DM and macroalbuminuric renal disease to reduce risk of HHF and progression of renal disease (Strong Recommendation, High-Quality Evidence) • -SGLT2i in patients with T2DM and mild to moderate HFrEF to improve symptoms and quality of life and to reduce risk of hospitalization and CV mortality (Strong Recommendation, High-Quality Evidence) • --SGLT2i in patients without T2DM and mild to moderate HFrEF to improve symptoms and quality of life and reduce risk of hospitalization and CV mortality (Conditional Recommendation, High-Quality Evidence)

Abbreviations: SGLT2i: Sodium glucose cotransporter 2 inhibitor, T2DM: Type 2 diabetes mellitus, ASCVD: Atherosclerotic cardiovascular disease, MACE: Major adverse cardiovascular events, CV: cardiovascular, HHF: Hospitalization for heart failure, BP: Blood pressure, CKD: Chronic kidney disease, HbA1c: Glycosylated hemoglobin, HFrEF: Heart failure with reduced ejection fraction, EF: Ejection fraction, eGFR: Estimated glomerular filtration rate, UACR: Urine albumin to creatinine ratio, HF: Heart failure, DM: Diabetes mellitus, GLP-RA: Glucagon-like peptide 1 receptor agonist Recommendation 1a denotes a strong recommendation where the benefits outweigh the risks for most patients, supported by high quality evidence Reproduced with permission from Elsevier. Reproduced with permission from Elsevier.

The American College of Cardiology expert consensus decision pathway suggested using SGLT2i when priorities include reducing MACE and CV death, preventing HHF, lowering BP, or using oral agents [93]. In 2019, the European Society of Cardiology (ESC) collaborated with the European Association for the Study of Diabetes for guidelines on diabetes, pre-diabetes, and CV diseases [94]. These experts included new class Ia recommendations for SGLT2i to reduce CV events, and specifically for empagliflozin to decrease the mortality risk in patients with T2DM and CVD (or those at high CV risk), as well as to reduce HHF in patients with T2DM, and to slow the progression of kidney disease in patients with CKD. Of note, they no longer recommended metformin as first-line therapy for all patients. Moreover, they recommended SGLT2i or glucagon-like peptide-1 receptor agonist monotherapy as first-line anti-diabetic medication in specific subgroups of patients with T2DM (drug naïve, atherosclerotic CVD, or high CV risk).

The CCS/HF heart failure guidelines 2020 issued several new recommendations concerning SGLT2i [95]. They recommended SGLT2i in the following subgroups of patients: T2DM and atherosclerotic CVD, T2DM over 50 years, and with risk factors for atherosclerotic CVD, T2DM over the age of 30 years with macroalbuminuria, T2DM and HFrEF, and mild to moderate HFrEF in persons without T2DM.

CURRENT USE OF SGLT2 INHIBITORS IN CLINICAL PRACTICE

While there is mounting evidence to support the CV and renal benefits of SGLT2i, in the United States, only 5% of eligible patients received SGLT2i [96, 97]. Similar care gaps were noted with other HF therapies. For example, in 2017, only 15% of eligible patients were treated with an angiotensin receptor neprilysin inhibitor (ARNI) [98]. In the DAPA-HF trial, only 10% of patients received ARNI, and in EMPA-RESPONSE-AHF only 5% of patients were treated with ARNI [60]. Therefore, the benefits and side effects of SGLT2i used in combination with an ARNI could not be reliably ascertained [99].

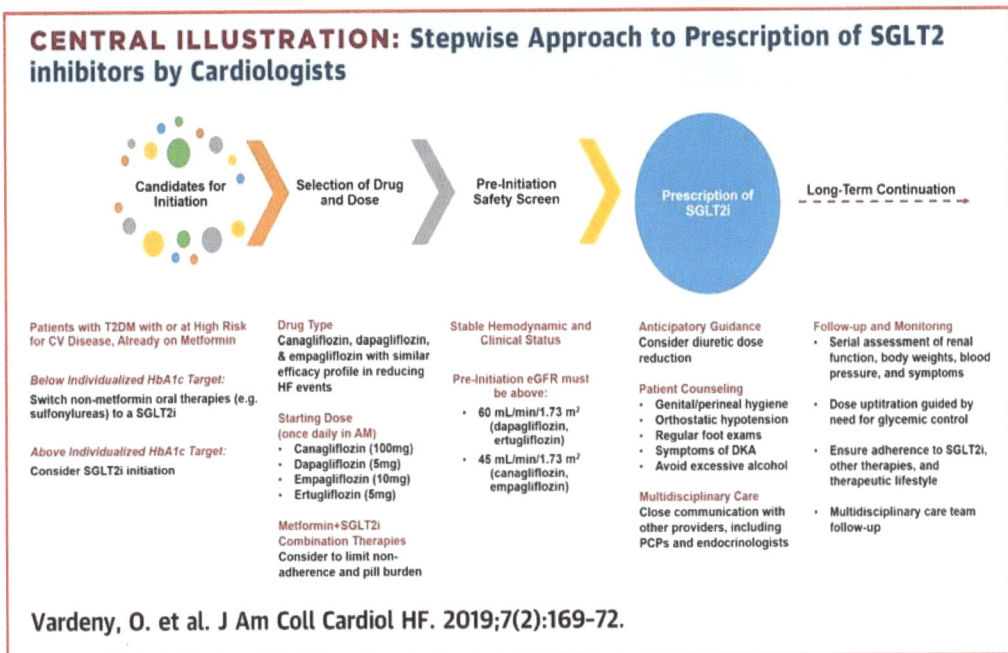

CENTRAL ILLUSTRATION: Stepwise Approach to Prescription of SGLT2 inhibitors by Cardiologists

Candidates for Initiation → Selection of Drug and Dose → Pre-Initiation Safety Screen → Prescription of SGLT2i → Long-Term Continuation

Candidates for Initiation

Patients with T2DM with or at High Risk for CV Disease, Already on Metformin

Below Individualized HbA1c Target:
Switch non-metformin oral therapies (e.g. sulfonylureas) to a SGLT2i

Above Individualized HbA1c Target:
Consider SGLT2i initiation

Selection of Drug and Dose

Drug Type
Canagliflozin, dapagliflozin, & empagliflozin with similar efficacy profile in reducing HF events

Starting Dose
(once daily in AM)
· Canagliflozin (100mg)
· Dapagliflozin (5mg)
· Empagliflozin (10mg)
· Ertugliflozin (5mg)

Metformin+SGLT2i Combination Therapies
Consider to limit non-adherence and pill burden

Pre-Initiation Safety Screen

Stable Hemodynamic and Clinical Status

Pre-Initiation eGFR must be above:
· 60 mL/min/1.73 m² (dapagliflozin, ertugliflozin)
· 45 mL/min/1.73 m² (canagliflozin, empagliflozin)

Prescription of SGLT2i

Anticipatory Guidance
Consider diuretic dose reduction

Patient Counseling
· Genital/perineal hygiene
· Orthostatic hypotension
· Regular foot exams
· Symptoms of DKA
· Avoid excessive alcohol

Multidisciplinary Care
Close communication with other providers, including PCPs and endocrinologists

Long-Term Continuation

Follow-up and Monitoring
· Serial assessment of renal function, body weights, blood pressure, and symptoms
· Dose uptitration guided by need for glycemic control
· Ensure adherence to SGLT2i, other therapies, and therapeutic lifestyle
· Multidisciplinary care team follow-up

Vardeny, O. et al. J Am Coll Cardiol HF. 2019;7(2):169-72.

Fig. (2). Practical considerations with Sodium-Glucose Cotransporter 2 Inhibitors[100]. (Reproduced with permission).

PRACTICAL CONSIDERATIONS WITH SGLT2I PRESCRIPTION

The CV benefit of SGLT2i is most likely a class effect with consistent benefits shown with empagliflozin, canagliflozin and dapagliflozin [17 - 19]. CV outcome trials with ertugliflozin have not yet been reported (VERTIS CV Trial NCT01986881). All four SGLT2i are available in once-daily dosing regimens and are available in FDA-approved combinations with metformin. We summarized the practical considerations for SGLT2i's use in Fig. (2). The starting dose for empagliflozin is 10mg, for canagliflozin is 100 mg, for dapagliflozin is 5 mg, and for ertugliflozin is 5mg. The higher doses were 25 mg, 300 mg, 10 mg, and 15 mg, respectively for these medications. Given the lack of incremental benefit of higher doses on CV outcomes, SGLT-2 inhibitors' dose should be up-titrated mainly in accordance with glycemic control, renal function and tolerability [100].

SGLT2i are not approved for patients with T1DM in North America. In patients with T2DM already on sulfonylurea and/or insulin, initiation of SGLT-2 inhibitors should be with precautions since these combinations may induce hypoglycemia [101]. In these circumstances, one may consider reducing the dose of the other hypoglycemic agents such as sulfonylureas or insulin, as well as reinforcing glucose monitoring to minimise the risk of hypoglycemia. In patients with optimal glycosylated hemoglobin, reducing or discontinuing anti-diabetic agents such as sulfonylureas may be considered before initiation of SGLT2i.

Patients with T2DM on SGLT2i can rarely present with euglycemic ketoacidosis. This can occur due to SGLT2i's hypoinsulinemia's effect (through reduction in blood glucose levels) and increase of secretion of glucagon [102]. Reduction of insulin levels result in increase of lipolysis and production of free fatty acids, which are then converted to ketones by hepatic beta-oxidation. Both reduction in insulin levels and an increase in glucagon levels result in an increase in fatty acid transport into the liver *via* activation of carnitine palmitoyltransferase-I (CPT-I) [103]. All of these metabolic disturbances will increase beta-oxidation and ketone production [103]. Consequently, it is crucial to educate patients of "sick day" rules. Specifically, patients should be instructed to hold these drugs when suffering from volume depletion, infection, trauma, and around the time of an elective surgery [101]. Excessive alcohol intake and ketogenic diets should also be avoided. Clinicians should have a high index of suspicion for euglycemic ketoacidosis in these patients and should measure serum anion gap during acute illness [100].

As SGLT2i are diuretic medications, it is essential to hold or avoid initiating them in volume-depleted patients. In euvolemic patients already on a loop diuretic, a reduction in the loop diuretic dose may be considered [101]. Patients should also be advised about possible orthostatic hypotension with SGLT2i [100].

SGLT2i are safe for use in patients with an eGFR of ≥30 ml/min. It should be noted that the FDA approves empagliflozin only in patients with an eGFR of ≥45 ml/min, and ertugliflozin in patients with an eGFR of ≥60 ml/min. Patients should have their renal function verified at baseline and regularly monitored while on an SGLT2i [100]. It is common for patients to experience a transient drop of up to 20% of their eGFR after initiation of an SGLT2 inhibitor. This temporary decline in eGFR generally resolves within the first three months of treatment. In patients who experience a larger than expected drop in their eGFR, readjustment of diuretics or other nephrotoxic medications should be considered [101].The FDA has issued a black box warning of the risk for MALE for canagliflozin. This risk appears to be the highest in those with PAD or prior amputation [104]. SGLT2i should be used cautiously in patients with PAD, prior amputation, or active arterial ulcers.In this subgroup of patients, SGLT2i should be initiated after a thorough risk/benefit discussion with the patient. Additionally, patients should be counseled on maintaining proper foot care to minimize the risk of diabetic foot ulcer [100].

Genital mycotic infections are the most common adverse events associated with SGLT2i and occur more commonly in patients with previous genital infections, women, and uncircumcised men [105]. In the occurrence of a fungal genital infection, the SGLT2i can be continued and the mycosis generally resolves with a single 150 mg dose of fluconazole. Finally, the FDA has issued a class-wide warning related to twelve cases of Fournier's gangrene with SGLT2i [106]. Although this infection is rare, it is dangerous, life-threatening, and potentially disfiguring. Patients should be advised about the importance of good genital hygiene.

FUTURE DIRECTIONS AND ONGOING TRIALS

Several RCTs are underway to evaluate SGLT2i in patients across the spectrum of HF. These RCTs will be vital in bridging the existing knowledge gaps. In particular, these trials will determine the potential impact of SGLT2i in patients with HFrEF, HFpEF, and acutely decompensating HF with or without DM. In this section, we will review the designs and potential impacts of these patients.

The Empagliflozin outcome trial in people with chronic HFrEF (EMPEROR-Reduced) randomized 3,600 subjects with HFrEF and elevated natriuretic peptide levels to empagliflozin 10 mg daily *vs.* placebo (NCT03057977). This RCT is similar in design to the DAPA-HF trial. It will confirm the potential class effect of SGLT2i in reducing HF events in patients with HFrEF independent of baseline DM status. The primary outcome will be the time-to-first event of the combined endpoint of death and hospitalization for heart failure. This trial will also evaluate the effects of empagliflozin on renal function, CV death, all-cause mortality, and recurrent hospitalization events at an estimated mean follow-up of 38 months. By enrolling only patients with elevated natriuretic peptide levels, the trial aims to include mainly high-risk patients with an expected annual event rate of at least 15% [107]. On the date of 30 July 2020, EMPEROR-Reduced met its primary endpoint, demonstrating superiority with empagliflozin (10 mg) compared to placebo in reducing the risk for the composite of cardiovascular death or hospitalization due to heart failure, when added to standard of care. The full results of this RCT will be presented at the European Society of Cardiology 2020.

The Empagliflozin Outcome Trial in People with Chronic Heart Failure with Preserved Ejection Fraction (EMPEROR-Preserved) is randomizing 5,750 patients with HFpEF, with and without T2DM, to empagliflozin 10 mg/day or placebo (NCT03057951). The primary outcome will be the time-to-first event (mean follow-up expected to be 38 months) of the combined endpoint of CV death or hospitalization for heart failure. The trial will also evaluate the effects of empagliflozin on biomarkers of renal function, CV death, all-cause mortality, and recurrent hospitalization events. EMPEROR-Preserved will determine whether empagliflozin would benefit patients with HFpEF (for which there are currently few therapeutic options) [108]. Similarly, the Dapagliflozin Evaluation to Improve the Lives of Patients with Preserved Ejection Fraction Heart Failure (DELIVER) trial is enrolling 4,700 patients with HFpEF ((LVEF >40% and evidence of structural heart disease)) to dapagliflozin 10 mg *versus* placebo, (NCT03619213). The primary outcome is the time to the first occurrence of any of the components of the composite of CV death, HHF, or urgent HF visit.

There are ongoing trials to evaluate the effects of SGLT2i on quality of life and exercise capacity in patients with HF. The Dapagliflozin Effect on Exercise Capacity Using a 6-minute Walk Test in Patients With Heart Failure With Reduced Ejection Fraction (DETERMINE-Reduced) (NCT03877237) is randomizing 313 patients with HFrEF (EF of 40% and less) to receive either dapagliflozin or placebo, with the primary outcome defined as a change in KCCQ score (total symptom score and physical limitation score), and 6-minute walk distance. DETERMINE-Preserved (NCT03877224) will evaluate the same primary outcome in 504 patients with HFpEF.

CONCLUSIONS

SGLT2i are innovating therapies of DM and HF. Through several mechanisms such as glycosuria and natriuresis, SGLT2i reduce CV adverse events, including HF outcomes in patients with DM, and improve CV outcomes in patients with HFrEF with and without DM. The results of trials in progress of SGLT2i in HFpEF and acute HF are eagerly anticipated. These trials will revolutionize further the management of patients with HF, regardless of their DM status. If proven beneficial, SGTL2i will be particularly useful for patients with HFpEF in whom there is currently no disease-modifying therapy.

CONSENT FOR PUBLICATION

Not applicable.

CONFLICTS OF INTEREST

Dr Thao Huynh received research grants and consulting honoraria from Boehringer-Ingelheim and Astra-Zeneca.

Dr. Mark Sherman received speaker and consulting honoraria from Akcea, Astra-Zeneca, Gilead, Janssen, Novo-Nordisk, and Sanofi.

Dr Abhinav Sharma received support Roche Diagnostics, Boeringer-Ingelheim, AstraZeneca, Novartis, and Takeda.

ACKNOWLEDEGEMENTS

Dr. Abhinav Sharma is supported by the Fonds de Recherche Santé Quebec (FRSQ) Junior 1 clinician scholars program, Alberta Innovates Health Solution, European Society of Cardiology young investigator grant.

REFERENCES

[1]   Punthakee Z, Goldenberg R, Katz P. Definition, classification and diagnosis of diabetes, prediabetes and metabolic syndrome. Can J Diabetes 2018; 42 (Suppl. 1): S10-5.
[http://dx.doi.org/10.1016/j.jcjd.2017.10.003] [PMID: 29650080]

[2]   Stratton IM, Adler AI, Neil HAW, *et al.* Association of glycaemia with macrovascular and microvascular complications of type 2 diabetes (UKPDS 35): prospective observational study. BMJ 2000; 321(7258): 405-12.
[http://dx.doi.org/10.1136/bmj.321.7258.405] [PMID: 10938048]

[3]   Baena-Díez JM, Peñafiel J, Subirana I, *et al.* Risk of cause-specific death in individuals with diabetes: A competing risks analysis. Diabetes Care 2016; 39(11): 1987-95.
[http://dx.doi.org/10.2337/dc16-0614] [PMID: 27493134]

[4]   Rawshani A, Rawshani A, Franzén S, *et al.* Mortality and cardiovascular disease in type 1 and type 2 diabetes. N Engl J Med 2017; 376(15): 1407-18.
[http://dx.doi.org/10.1056/NEJMoa1608664] [PMID: 28402770]

[5]   Garber AJ, Abrahamson MJ, Barzilay JI, *et al.* AACE comprehensive diabetes management algorithm 2013. Endocr Pract 2013; 19(2): 327-36.
[http://dx.doi.org/10.4158/endp.19.2.a38267720403k242] [PMID: 23598536]

[6]   Kosiborod M, Lam CSP, Kohsaka S, *et al.* Cardiovascular events associated with SGLT-2 inhibitors *versus* other glucose-lowering drugs: The CVD-REAL 2 study. J Am Coll Cardiol 2018; 71(23): 2628-39.
[http://dx.doi.org/10.1016/j.jacc.2018.03.009] [PMID: 29540325]

[7]   Nathan DM, Buse JB, Davidson MB, *et al.* Medical management of hyperglycemia in type 2 diabetes: A consensus algorithm for the initiation and adjustment of therapy A consensus statement of the American Diabetes Association and the European Association for the Study of Diabetes 2009; 32: 193-203.

[8]   Nissen SE, Wolski K. Effect of rosiglitazone on the risk of myocardial infarction and death from cardiovascular causes. N Engl J Med 2007; 356(24): 2457-71.
[http://dx.doi.org/10.1056/NEJMoa072761] [PMID: 17517853]

[9]   Cefalu WT, Kaul S, Gerstein HC, *et al.* Cardiovascular outcomes trials in type 2 diabetes: Where do we go from here? Reflections from a *diabetes care* editors' expert forum. Diabetes Care 2018; 41(1):

14-31.
[http://dx.doi.org/10.2337/dci17-0057] [PMID: 29263194]

[10]   Green JB, Bethel MA, Armstrong PW, *et al.* Effect of sitagliptin on cardiovascular outcomes in type 2 diabetes. N Engl J Med 2015; 373(3): 232-42.
[http://dx.doi.org/10.1056/NEJMoa1501352] [PMID: 26052984]

[11]   White WB, Cannon CP, Heller SR, *et al.* Alogliptin after acute coronary syndrome in patients with type 2 diabetes. N Engl J Med 2013; 369(14): 1327-35.
[http://dx.doi.org/10.1056/NEJMoa1305889] [PMID: 23992602]

[12]   Pfeffer MA, Claggett B, Diaz R, *et al.* Lixisenatide in patients with type 2 diabetes and acute coronary syndrome. N Engl J Med 2015; 373(23): 2247-57.
[http://dx.doi.org/10.1056/NEJMoa1509225] [PMID: 26630143]

[13]   Marso SP, Bain SC, Consoli A, *et al.* Semaglutide and cardiovascular outcomes in patients with type 2 diabetes. N Engl J Med 2016; 375(19): 1834-44.
[http://dx.doi.org/10.1056/NEJMoa1607141] [PMID: 27633186]

[14]   Holman RR, Bethel MA, Mentz RJ, *et al.* Effects of once-weekly exenatide on cardiovascular outcomes in type 2 diabetes. N Engl J Med 2017; 377(13): 1228-39.
[http://dx.doi.org/10.1056/NEJMoa1612917] [PMID: 28910237]

[15]   Scirica BM, Bhatt DL, Braunwald E, *et al.* Saxagliptin and cardiovascular outcomes in patients with type 2 diabetes mellitus. N Engl J Med 2013; 369(14): 1317-26.
[http://dx.doi.org/10.1056/NEJMoa1307684] [PMID: 23992601]

[16]   Marso SP, Daniels GH, Brown-Frandsen K, *et al.* Liraglutide and cardiovascular outcomes in type 2 diabetes. N Engl J Med 2016; 375(4): 311-22.
[http://dx.doi.org/10.1056/NEJMoa1603827] [PMID: 27295427]

[17]   Wiviott SD, Raz I, Bonaca MP, *et al.* Dapagliflozin and cardiovascular outcomes in type 2 diabetes. N Engl J Med 2019; 380(4): 347-57.
[http://dx.doi.org/10.1056/NEJMoa1812389] [PMID: 30415602]

[18]   Zinman B, Wanner C, Lachin JM, *et al.* Empagliflozin, cardiovascular outcomes, and mortality in type 2 diabetes. N Engl J Med 2015; 373(22): 2117-28.
[http://dx.doi.org/10.1056/NEJMoa1504720] [PMID: 26378978]

[19]   Neal B, Perkovic V, Mahaffey KW, *et al.* Canagliflozin and cardiovascular and renal events in type 2 diabetes. N Engl J Med 2017; 377(7): 644-57.
[http://dx.doi.org/10.1056/NEJMoa1611925] [PMID: 28605608]

[20]   Parmley WW. Pathophysiology of congestive heart failure. Am J Cardiol 1985; 56(2): 7A-11A.
[http://dx.doi.org/10.1016/0002-9149(85)91199-3] [PMID: 4014051]

[21]   Drazner MH, Velez-Martinez M, Ayers CR, *et al.* Relationship of right- to left-sided ventricular filling pressures in advanced heart failure: insights from the ESCAPE trial. Circ Heart Fail 2013; 6(2): 264-70.
[http://dx.doi.org/10.1161/CIRCHEARTFAILURE.112.000204] [PMID: 23392790]

[22]   Yancy CW, Jessup M, Bozkurt B, *et al.* 2017 ACC/AHA/HFSA Focused Update of the 2013 ACCF/AHA Guideline for the Management of Heart Failure A Report of the American College of Cardiology/American Heart Association Task Force on Clinical Practice Guidelines and the Heart Failure Society of America 2017; 70: 776-803.

[23]   Ponikowski P, Anker SD, AlHabib KF, *et al.* Heart failure: preventing disease and death worldwide. ESC Heart Fail 2014; 1(1): 4-25.
[http://dx.doi.org/10.1002/ehf2.12005] [PMID: 28834669]

[24]   Savarese G, Lund LH. Global public health burden of heart failure. Card Fail Rev 2017; 3(1): 7-11.
[http://dx.doi.org/10.15420/cfr.2016:25:2] [PMID: 28785469]

[25]   Lloyd-Jones DM, Larson MG, Leip EP, *et al.* Lifetime risk for developing congestive heart failure: the framingham heart study. Circulation 2002; 106(24): 3068-72.
[http://dx.doi.org/10.1161/01.CIR.0000039105.49749.6F] [PMID: 12473553]

[26]   Solomon SD, Anavekar N, Skali H, *et al.* Influence of ejection fraction on cardiovascular outcomes in a broad spectrum of heart failure patients. Circulation 2005; 112(24): 3738-44.
[http://dx.doi.org/10.1161/CIRCULATIONAHA.105.561423] [PMID: 16330684]

[27]   Gattis WA, O'Connor CM, Gallup DS, Hasselblad V, Gheorghiade M. Predischarge initiation of carvedilol in patients hospitalized for decompensated heart failure: results of the Initiation Management Predischarge: Process for Assessment of Carvedilol Therapy in Heart Failure (IMPACT-HF) trial. J Am Coll Cardiol 2004; 43(9): 1534-41.
[http://dx.doi.org/10.1016/j.jacc.2003.12.040] [PMID: 15120808]

[28]   Tu JV, Donovan LR, Lee DS, *et al.* Effectiveness of public report cards for improving the quality of cardiac care: the EFFECT study: a randomized trial. JAMA 2009; 302(21): 2330-7.
[http://dx.doi.org/10.1001/jama.2009.1731] [PMID: 19923205]

[29]   Ponikowski P, Voors AA, Anker SD, *et al.* 2016 ESC Guidelines for the diagnosis and treatment of acute and chronic heart failure: The Task Force for the diagnosis and treatment of acute and chronic heart failure of the European Society of Cardiology (ESC)Developed with the special contribution of the Heart Failure Association (HFA) of the ESC. Eur Heart J 2016; 37(27): 2129-200.
[http://dx.doi.org/10.1093/eurheartj/ehw128] [PMID: 27206819]

[30]   Kenny HC, Abel ED. Heart failure in type 2 diabetes mellitus. Circ Res 2019; 124(1): 121-41.
[http://dx.doi.org/10.1161/CIRCRESAHA.118.311371] [PMID: 30605420]

[31]   Jia G, Hill MA, Sowers JR. Diabetic cardiomyopathy: An update of mechanisms contributing to this clinical entity. Circ Res 2018; 122(4): 624-38.
[http://dx.doi.org/10.1161/CIRCRESAHA.117.311586] [PMID: 29449364]

[32]   Kannel WB, Hjortland M, Castelli WP. Role of diabetes in congestive heart failure: the Framingham study. Am J Cardiol 1974; 34(1): 29-34.
[http://dx.doi.org/10.1016/0002-9149(74)90089-7] [PMID: 4835750]

[33]   Kannel WB, McGee DL. Diabetes and cardiovascular disease. The Framingham study. JAMA 1979; 241(19): 2035-8.
[http://dx.doi.org/10.1001/jama.1979.03290450033020] [PMID: 430798]

[34]   Echouffo-Tcheugui JB, Xu H, DeVore AD, *et al.* Temporal trends and factors associated with diabetes mellitus among patients hospitalized with heart failure: Findings from Get With The Guidelines-Heart Failure registry. Am Heart J 2016; 182: 9-20.
[http://dx.doi.org/10.1016/j.ahj.2016.07.025] [PMID: 27914505]

[35]   Echouffo-Tcheugui JB, Masoudi FA, Bao H, Spatz ES, Fonarow GC. Diabetes mellitus and outcomes of cardiac resynchronization with implantable cardioverter-defibrillator therapy in older patients with heart failure. Circ Arrhythm Electrophysiol 2016; 9(8)e004132
[http://dx.doi.org/10.1161/CIRCEP.116.004132] [PMID: 27489243]

[36]   Ziaeian B, Hernandez AF, DeVore AD, *et al.* Long-term outcomes for heart failure patients with and without diabetes: From the Get With The Guidelines-Heart Failure Registry. Am Heart J 2019; 211: 1-10.
[http://dx.doi.org/10.1016/j.ahj.2019.01.006] [PMID: 30818060]

[37]   Sharma A, Green JB, Dunning A, *et al.* Causes of death in a contemporary cohort of patients with type 2 diabetes and atherosclerotic cardiovascular disease: Insights from the TECOS trial. Diabetes Care 2017; 40(12): 1763-70.
[http://dx.doi.org/10.2337/dc17-1091] [PMID: 28986504]

[38]   Erqou S, Lee C-TC, Suffoletto M, *et al.* Association between glycated haemoglobin and the risk of congestive heart failure in diabetes mellitus: systematic review and meta-analysis. Eur J Heart Fail

2013; 15(2): 185-93.
[http://dx.doi.org/10.1093/eurjhf/hfs156] [PMID: 23099356]

[39]   Patel A, MacMahon S, Chalmers J, *et al.* Intensive blood glucose control and vascular outcomes in patients with type 2 diabetes. N Engl J Med 2008; 358(24): 2560-72.
[http://dx.doi.org/10.1056/NEJMoa0802987] [PMID: 18539916]

[40]   Gerstein HC, Miller ME, Byington RP, *et al.* Effects of intensive glucose lowering in type 2 diabetes. N Engl J Med 2008; 358(24): 2545-59.
[http://dx.doi.org/10.1056/NEJMoa0802743] [PMID: 18539917]

[41]   Castagno D, Baird-Gunning J, Jhund PS, *et al.* Intensive glycemic control has no impact on the risk of heart failure in type 2 diabetic patients: evidence from a 37,229 patient meta-analysis. Am Heart J 2011; 162(5): 938-948.e2.
[http://dx.doi.org/10.1016/j.ahj.2011.07.030] [PMID: 22093212]

[42]   Thomas MC, Cherney DZI. The actions of SGLT2 inhibitors on metabolism, renal function and blood pressure. Diabetologia 2018; 61(10): 2098-107.
[http://dx.doi.org/10.1007/s00125-018-4669-0] [PMID: 30132034]

[43]   Vallon V, Platt KA, Cunard R, *et al.* SGLT2 mediates glucose reabsorption in the early proximal tubule. J Am Soc Nephrol 2011; 22(1): 104-12.
[http://dx.doi.org/10.1681/ASN.2010030246] [PMID: 20616166]

[44]   Gorboulev V, Schürmann A, Vallon V, *et al.* Na(+)-D-glucose cotransporter SGLT1 is pivotal for intestinal glucose absorption and glucose-dependent incretin secretion. Diabetes 2012; 61(1): 187-96.
[http://dx.doi.org/10.2337/db11-1029] [PMID: 22124465]

[45]   Ghezzi C, Loo DDF, Wright EM. Physiology of renal glucose handling *via* SGLT1, SGLT2 and GLUT2. Diabetologia 2018; 61(10): 2087-97.
[http://dx.doi.org/10.1007/s00125-018-4656-5] [PMID: 30132032]

[46]   Bonner C, Kerr-Conte J, Gmyr V, *et al.* Inhibition of the glucose transporter SGLT2 with dapagliflozin in pancreatic alpha cells triggers glucagon secretion. Nat Med 2015; 21(5): 512-7.
[http://dx.doi.org/10.1038/nm.3828] [PMID: 25894829]

[47]   Goldenberg RM, Verma S, Perkins BA, Gilbert JD, Zinman B. Can the combination of incretin agents and sodium-glucose cotransporter 2 (SGLT2) inhibitors reconcile the yin and yang of glucagon? Can J Diabetes 2017; 41(1): 6-9.
[http://dx.doi.org/10.1016/j.jcjd.2016.08.001] [PMID: 27838228]

[48]   Tang H, Yang K, Li X, Song Y, Han J. Pancreatic safety of sodium-glucose cotransporter 2 inhibitors in patients with type 2 diabetes mellitus: A systematic review and meta-analysis. Pharmacoepidemiol Drug Saf 2020; 29(2): 161-72.
[http://dx.doi.org/10.1002/pds.4943] [PMID: 32017292]

[49]   Gerich JE. Role of the kidney in normal glucose homeostasis and in the hyperglycaemia of diabetes mellitus: therapeutic implications. Diabet Med 2010; 27(2): 136-42.
[http://dx.doi.org/10.1111/j.1464-5491.2009.02894.x] [PMID: 20546255]

[50]   Zurek AM, Yendapally R, Urteaga EM. A review of the efficacy and safety of sodium-glucose cotransporter 2 inhibitors: a focus on diabetic ketoacidosis. Diabetes Spectr 2017; 30(2): 137-42.
[http://dx.doi.org/10.2337/ds16-0030] [PMID: 28588380]

[51]   Kalra S. Sodium glucose co-transporter-2 (SGLT2) inhibitors: a review of their basic and clinical pharmacology. Diabetes Ther 2014; 5(2): 355-66.
[http://dx.doi.org/10.1007/s13300-014-0089-4] [PMID: 25424969]

[52]   Chao EC. SGLT-2 inhibitors: A new Mechanism for glycemic control Clinical diabetes : A publication of the American Diabetes Association 2014; 32: 4-11.

[53]   Thomson SC, Vallon V. Renal effects of sodium-glucose co-transporter inhibitors. Am J Cardiol 2019; 124 (Suppl. 1): S28-35.

[http://dx.doi.org/10.1016/j.amjcard.2019.10.027] [PMID: 31741437]

[54]   Zelniker TA, Braunwald E. Mechanisms of cardiorenal effects of sodium-glucose cotransporter 2 inhibitors: JACC state-of-the-art review. J Am Coll Cardiol 2020; 75(4): 422-34.
[http://dx.doi.org/10.1016/j.jacc.2019.11.031] [PMID: 32000955]

[55]   Baartscheer A, Schumacher CA, Wüst RCI, *et al.* Empagliflozin decreases myocardial cytoplasmic Na$^+$ through inhibition of the cardiac Na$^+$/H$^+$ exchanger in rats and rabbits. Diabetologia 2017; 60(3): 568-73.
[http://dx.doi.org/10.1007/s00125-016-4134-x] [PMID: 27752710]

[56]   Ye Y, Jia X, Bajaj M, Birnbaum Y. Dapagliflozin Attenuates Na$^+$/H$^+$ Exchanger-1 in Cardiofibroblasts via AMPK Activation. Cardiovasc Drugs Ther 2018; 32(6): 553-8.
[http://dx.doi.org/10.1007/s10557-018-6837-3] [PMID: 30367338]

[57]   Sun X, Han F, Lu Q, *et al.* Empagliflozin ameliorates obesity-related cardiac dysfunction by regulating sestrin2-mediated ampk-mTOR signaling and redox homeostasis in high-fat diet-induced obese mice. Diabetes 2020; 69(6): 1292-305.
[PMID: 32234722]

[58]   Bell RM, Yellon DM. SGLT2 inhibitors: hypotheses on the mechanism of cardiovascular protection. Lancet Diabetes Endocrinol 2018; 6(6): 435-7.
[http://dx.doi.org/10.1016/S2213-8587(17)30314-5] [PMID: 29030201]

[59]   Packer M, Anker SD, Butler J, Filippatos G, Zannad F. Effects of Sodium-Glucose Cotransporter 2 Inhibitors for the Treatment of Patients With Heart Failure: Proposal of a Novel Mechanism of Action. JAMA Cardiol 2017; 2(9): 1025-9.
[http://dx.doi.org/10.1001/jamacardio.2017.2275] [PMID: 28768320]

[60]   McMurray JJV, Solomon SD, Inzucchi SE, *et al.* Dapagliflozin in Patients with Heart Failure and Reduced Ejection Fraction. N Engl J Med 2019; 381(21): 1995-2008.
[http://dx.doi.org/10.1056/NEJMoa1911303] [PMID: 31535829]

[61]   Perkovic V, Jardine MJ, Neal B, *et al.* Canagliflozin and Renal Outcomes in Type 2 Diabetes and Nephropathy. N Engl J Med 2019; 380(24): 2295-306.
[http://dx.doi.org/10.1056/NEJMoa1811744] [PMID: 30990260]

[62]   Fitchett D, Inzucchi SE, Cannon CP, *et al.* Empagliflozin Reduced Mortality and Hospitalization for Heart Failure Across the Spectrum of Cardiovascular Risk in the EMPA-REG OUTCOME Trial. Circulation 2019; 139(11): 1384-95.
[http://dx.doi.org/10.1161/CIRCULATIONAHA.118.037778] [PMID: 30586757]

[63]   Fitchett D, Butler J, van de Borne P, *et al.* Effects of empagliflozin on risk for cardiovascular death and heart failure hospitalization across the spectrum of heart failure risk in the EMPA-REG OUTCOME® trial. Eur Heart J 2018; 39(5): 363-70.
[http://dx.doi.org/10.1093/eurheartj/ehx511] [PMID: 29020355]

[64]   Mahaffey KW, Neal B, Perkovic V, *et al.* Canagliflozin for Primary and Secondary Prevention of Cardiovascular Events: Results From the CANVAS Program (Canagliflozin Cardiovascular Assessment Study). Circulation 2018; 137(4): 323-34.
[http://dx.doi.org/10.1161/CIRCULATIONAHA.117.032038] [PMID: 29133604]

[65]   Zelniker TA, Wiviott SD, Raz I, *et al.* SGLT2 inhibitors for primary and secondary prevention of cardiovascular and renal outcomes in type 2 diabetes: a systematic review and meta-analysis of cardiovascular outcome trials. Lancet 2019; 393(10166): 31-9.
[http://dx.doi.org/10.1016/S0140-6736(18)32590-X] [PMID: 30424892]

[66]   Aguilar D. Heart Failure, Diabetes Mellitus, and Chronic Kidney Disease: A Clinical Conundrum. Circ Heart Fail 2016; 9(7)e003316
[http://dx.doi.org/10.1161/CIRCHEARTFAILURE.116.003316] [PMID: 27413031]

[67]   Smith DH, Thorp ML, Gurwitz JH, *et al.* Chronic kidney disease and outcomes in heart failure with

preserved versus reduced ejection fraction: the Cardiovascular Research Network PRESERVE Study. Circ Cardiovasc Qual Outcomes 2013; 6(3): 333-42.
[http://dx.doi.org/10.1161/CIRCOUTCOMES.113.000221] [PMID: 23685625]

[68]   Patel PA, Liang L, Khazanie P, *et al.* Antihyperglycemic Medication Use Among Medicare Beneficiaries With Heart Failure, Diabetes Mellitus, and Chronic Kidney Disease. Circ Heart Fail 2016; 9(7)e002638
[http://dx.doi.org/10.1161/CIRCHEARTFAILURE.115.002638] [PMID: 27413035]

[69]   Neuen BL, Cherney DZ, Jardine MJ, Perkovic V. Sodium-glucose cotransporter inhibitors in type 2 diabetes: thinking beyond glucose lowering. CMAJ 2019; 191(41): E1128-35.
[http://dx.doi.org/10.1503/cmaj.190047] [PMID: 31615819]

[70]   Mosenzon O, Wiviott SD, Cahn A, *et al.* Effects of dapagliflozin on development and progression of kidney disease in patients with type 2 diabetes: an analysis from the DECLARE-TIMI 58 randomised trial. Lancet Diabetes Endocrinol 2019; 7(8): 606-17.
[http://dx.doi.org/10.1016/S2213-8587(19)30180-9] [PMID: 31196815]

[71]   Wanner C, Inzucchi SE, Lachin JM, *et al.* Empagliflozin and Progression of Kidney Disease in Type 2 Diabetes. N Engl J Med 2016; 375(4): 323-34.
[http://dx.doi.org/10.1056/NEJMoa1515920] [PMID: 27299675]

[72]   Martinez FA, Serenelli M, Nicolau JC, *et al.* Efficacy and Safety of Dapagliflozin in Heart Failure With Reduced Ejection Fraction According to Age: Insights From DAPA-HF. Circulation 2020; 141(2): 100-11.
[http://dx.doi.org/10.1161/CIRCULATIONAHA.119.044133] [PMID: 31736328]

[73]   Kosiborod MN, Jhund PS, Docherty KF, *et al.* Effects of Dapagliflozin on Symptoms, Function, and Quality of Life in Patients With Heart Failure and Reduced Ejection Fraction: Results From the DAPA-HF Trial. Circulation 2020; 141(2): 90-9.
[http://dx.doi.org/10.1161/CIRCULATIONAHA.119.044138] [PMID: 31736335]

[74]   Petrie MC, Verma S, Docherty KF, *et al.* Effect of Dapagliflozin on Worsening Heart Failure and Cardiovascular Death in Patients With Heart Failure With and Without Diabetes. JAMA 2020; 323: 1353-68.
[http://dx.doi.org/10.1001/jama.2020.1906] [PMID: 32219386]

[75]   Fitchett D, Zinman B, Wanner C, *et al.* Heart failure outcomes with empagliflozin in patients with type 2 diabetes at high cardiovascular risk: results of the EMPA-REG OUTCOME® trial. Eur Heart J 2016; 37(19): 1526-34.
[http://dx.doi.org/10.1093/eurheartj/ehv728] [PMID: 26819227]

[76]   Rådholm K, Figtree G, Perkovic V, *et al.* Canagliflozin and Heart Failure in Type 2 Diabetes Mellitus: Results From the CANVAS Program. Circulation 2018; 138(5): 458-68.
[http://dx.doi.org/10.1161/CIRCULATIONAHA.118.034222] [PMID: 29526832]

[77]   Kato ET, Silverman MG, Mosenzon O, *et al.* Effect of Dapagliflozin on Heart Failure and Mortality in Type 2 Diabetes Mellitus. Circulation 2019; 139(22): 2528-36.
[http://dx.doi.org/10.1161/CIRCULATIONAHA.119.040130] [PMID: 30882238]

[78]   Calzetta L, Orlandi A, Page C, *et al.* Brain natriuretic peptide: Much more than a biomarker. Int J Cardiol 2016; 221: 1031-8.
[http://dx.doi.org/10.1016/j.ijcard.2016.07.109] [PMID: 27447810]

[79]   Nassif ME, Windsor SL, Tang F, *et al.* Dapagliflozin Effects on Biomarkers, Symptoms, and Functional Status in Patients With Heart Failure With Reduced Ejection Fraction: The DEFINE-HF Trial. Circulation 2019; 140(18): 1463-76.
[http://dx.doi.org/10.1161/CIRCULATIONAHA.119.042929] [PMID: 31524498]

[80]   Januzzi JL Jr, Butler J, Jarolim P, *et al.* Effects of Canagliflozin on Cardiovascular Biomarkers in Older Adults With Type 2 Diabetes. J Am Coll Cardiol 2017; 70(6): 704-12.
[http://dx.doi.org/10.1016/j.jacc.2017.06.016] [PMID: 28619659]

[81]   Matthews DR, Li Q, Perkovic V, *et al.* Effects of canagliflozin on amputation risk in type 2 diabetes: the CANVAS Program. Diabetologia 2019; 62(6): 926-38.
       [http://dx.doi.org/10.1007/s00125-019-4839-8] [PMID: 30868176]

[82]   Scheen AJ. Does lower limb amputation concern all SGLT2 inhibitors? Nat Rev Endocrinol 2018; 14(6): 326-8.
       [http://dx.doi.org/10.1038/s41574-018-0001-9] [PMID: 29626204]

[83]   Chioncel O, Collins SP, Ambrosy AP, *et al.* Improving Postdischarge Outcomes in Acute Heart Failure. Am J Ther 2018; 25(4): e475-86.
       [http://dx.doi.org/10.1097/MJT.0000000000000791] [PMID: 29985826]

[84]   Chioncel O, Mebazaa A, Harjola VP, *et al.* Clinical phenotypes and outcome of patients hospitalized for acute heart failure: the ESC Heart Failure Long-Term Registry. Eur J Heart Fail 2017; 19(10): 1242-54.
       [http://dx.doi.org/10.1002/ejhf.890] [PMID: 28463462]

[85]   Rubio-Gracia J, Demissei BG, Ter Maaten JM, *et al.* Prevalence, predictors and clinical outcome of residual congestion in acute decompensated heart failure. Int J Cardiol 2018; 258: 185-91.
       [http://dx.doi.org/10.1016/j.ijcard.2018.01.067] [PMID: 29544928]

[86]   Damman K, Beusekamp JC, Boorsma EM, *et al.* double-blind, placebo-controlled, multicentre pilot study on the effects of empagliflozin on clinical outcomes in patients with acute decompensated heart failure (EMPA-RESPONSE-AHF) European Journal of Heart Failure

[87]   Anker SD, Butler J. Empagliflozin, calcium, and SGLT1/2 receptor affinity: another piece of the puzzle. ESC Heart Fail 2018; 5(4): 549-51.
       [http://dx.doi.org/10.1002/ehf2.12345] [PMID: 30024112]

[88]   Washburn WN. Evolution of sodium glucose co-transporter 2 inhibitors as anti-diabetic agents. Expert Opin Ther Pat 2009; 19(11): 1485-99.
       [http://dx.doi.org/10.1517/13543770903337828] [PMID: 19852718]

[89]   Grempler R, Thomas L, Eckhardt M, *et al.* Empagliflozin, a novel selective sodium glucose cotransporter-2 (SGLT-2) inhibitor: characterisation and comparison with other SGLT-2 inhibitors. Diabetes Obes Metab 2012; 14(1): 83-90.
       [http://dx.doi.org/10.1111/j.1463-1326.2011.01517.x] [PMID: 21985634]

[90]   Mascitti V, Maurer TS, Robinson RP, *et al.* Discovery of a clinical candidate from the structurally unique dioxa-bicyclo[3.2.1]octane class of sodium-dependent glucose cotransporter 2 inhibitors. J Med Chem 2011; 54(8): 2952-60.
       [http://dx.doi.org/10.1021/jm200049r] [PMID: 21449606]

[91]   Davies MJ, D'Alessio DA, Fradkin J, *et al.* Management of Hyperglycemia in Type 2 Diabetes, 2018. A Consensus Report by the American Diabetes Association (ADA) and the European Association for the Study of Diabetes (EASD). Diabetes Care 2018; 41(12): 2669-701.
       [http://dx.doi.org/10.2337/dci18-0033] [PMID: 30291106]

[92]   Buse JB, Wexler DJ, Tsapas A, *et al.* Update to: Management of Hyperglycemia in Type 2 Diabetes, 2018. A Consensus Report by the American Diabetes Association (ADA) and the European Association for the Study of Diabetes (EASD). Diabetes Care 2019; 2019dci190066
       [PMID: 31857443]

[93]   Das SR, Everett BM, Birtcher KK, *et al.* 2018 ACC Expert Consensus Decision Pathway on Novel Therapies for Cardiovascular Risk Reduction in Patients With Type 2 Diabetes and Atherosclerotic Cardiovascular Disease A Report of the American College of Cardiology Task Force on Expert Consensus Decision Pathways 2018; 72: 3200-23.

[94]   Grant PJ, Cosentino F. The 2019 ESC Guidelines on diabetes, pre-diabetes, and cardiovascular diseases developed in collaboration with the EASD: New features and the 'Ten Commandments' of the 2019 Guidelines are discussed by Professor Peter J. Grant and Professor Francesco Cosentino, the

Task Force chairmen. Eur Heart J 2019; 40(39): 3215-7.
[http://dx.doi.org/10.1093/eurheartj/ehz687] [PMID: 31608951]

[95] O'Meara E, McDonald M, Chan M, *et al.* CCS/CHFS Heart Failure Guidelines: Clinical Trial Update on Functional Mitral Regurgitation, SGLT2 Inhibitors, ARNI in HFpEF, and Tafamidis in Amyloidosis. Can J Cardiol 2020; 36(2): 159-69.
[http://dx.doi.org/10.1016/j.cjca.2019.11.036] [PMID: 32036861]

[96] Vaduganathan M, Sathiyakumar V, Singh A, *et al.* Prescriber Patterns of SGLT2i After Expansions of U.S. Food and Drug Administration Labeling. J Am Coll Cardiol 2018; 72(25): 3370-2.
[http://dx.doi.org/10.1016/j.jacc.2018.08.2202] [PMID: 30409566]

[97] Arnold SV, Inzucchi SE, Tang F, *et al.* Real-world use and modeled impact of glucose-lowering therapies evaluated in recent cardiovascular outcomes trials: An NCDR® Research to Practice project. Eur J Prev Cardiol 2017; 24(15): 1637-45.
[http://dx.doi.org/10.1177/2047487317729252] [PMID: 28870145]

[98] Greene SJ, Butler J, Albert NM, *et al.* Medical Therapy for Heart Failure With Reduced Ejection Fraction: The CHAMP-HF Registry. J Am Coll Cardiol 2018; 72(4): 351-66.
[http://dx.doi.org/10.1016/j.jacc.2018.04.070] [PMID: 30025570]

[99] Fang JC. Heart-Failure Therapy - New Drugs but Old Habits? N Engl J Med 2019; 381(21): 2063-4.
[http://dx.doi.org/10.1056/NEJMe1912180] [PMID: 31535828]

[100] Vardeny O, Vaduganathan M. Practical Guide to Prescribing Sodium-Glucose Cotransporter 2 Inhibitors for Cardiologists. JACC Heart Fail 2019; 7(2): 169-72.
[http://dx.doi.org/10.1016/j.jchf.2018.11.013] [PMID: 30704605]

[101] van Baar MJB, van Ruiten CC, Muskiet MHA, van Bloemendaal L, IJzerman RG, van Raalte DH. SGLT2 Inhibitors in Combination Therapy: From Mechanisms to Clinical Considerations in Type 2 Diabetes Management. Diabetes Care 2018; 41(8): 1543-56.
[http://dx.doi.org/10.2337/dc18-0588] [PMID: 30030256]

[102] Kibbey RG. SGLT-2 inhibition and glucagon: Cause for alarm? Trends Endocrinol Metab 2015; 26(7): 337-8.
[http://dx.doi.org/10.1016/j.tem.2015.05.011] [PMID: 26059706]

[103] Ogawa W, Sakaguchi K. Euglycemic diabetic ketoacidosis induced by SGLT2 inhibitors: possible mechanism and contributing factors. J Diabetes Investig 2016; 7(2): 135-8.
[http://dx.doi.org/10.1111/jdi.12401] [PMID: 27042263]

[104] Chatterjee S, Bandyopadhyay D, Ghosh RK, *et al.* SGLT-2 Inhibitors and Peripheral Artery Disease: A Statistical Hoax or Reality? Curr Probl Cardiol 2019; 44(7): 207-22.
[http://dx.doi.org/10.1016/j.cpcardiol.2018.06.004] [PMID: 30195639]

[105] Sarafidis PA, Ortiz A. The risk for urinary tract infections with sodium-glucose cotransporter 2 inhibitors: no longer a cause of concern? Clin Kidney J 2019; 13(1): 24-6.
[http://dx.doi.org/10.1093/ckj/sfz170] [PMID: 32082549]

[106] Bersoff-Matcha SJ, Chamberlain C, Cao C, Kortepeter C, Chong WH. Fournier Gangrene Associated With Sodium-Glucose Cotransporter-2 Inhibitors: A Review of Spontaneous Postmarketing Cases. Ann Intern Med 2019; 170(11): 764-9.
[http://dx.doi.org/10.7326/M19-0085] [PMID: 31060053]

[107] Packer M, Butler J, Filippatos GS, *et al.* Evaluation of the effect of sodium-glucose co-transporter 2 inhibition with empagliflozin on morbidity and mortality of patients with chronic heart failure and a reduced ejection fraction: rationale for and design of the EMPEROR-Reduced trial. Eur J Heart Fail 2019; 21(10): 1270-8.
[http://dx.doi.org/10.1002/ejhf.1536] [PMID: 31584231]

[108]   Anker SD, Butler J, Filippatos GS, *et al.* Evaluation of the effects of sodium-glucose co-transporter 2 inhibition with empagliflozin on morbidity and mortality in patients with chronic heart failure and a preserved ejection fraction: rationale for and design of the EMPEROR-Preserved Trial. Eur J Heart Fail 2019; 21(10): 1279-87.
[http://dx.doi.org/10.1002/ejhf.1596] [PMID: 31523904]

CHAPTER 3

Natural Products and Semi-Synthetic Compounds as Antithrombotics: A Review of the Last Ten Years (2009-2019)

Angelo Piato[1,*] and **Cedric Stephan Graebin**[2,*]

[1] *Departamento de Farmacologia, Instituto de Ciências Básicas da Saúde, Universidade Federal do Rio Grande do Sul, Porto Alegre, Brasil*

[2] *Departamento de Química Orgânica, Instituto de Química, Universidade Federal Rural do Rio de Janeiro, Seropédica, Brasil*

Abstract: Pathologies associated with hypercoagulable states, including myocardial infarction, deep vein thrombosis, and pulmonary embolism, are one of the most important causes of morbidity and mortality worldwide. Despite the approval of several new synthetic (including orally active) antithrombotic agents in recent years for treating such diseases, mainly direct thrombin, and factor Xa inhibitors, concerns still exist for side-effects, especially bleeding. There is still a therapeutic demand for safe and effective anticoagulant agents that present fewer side effects than the currently available drugs. Natural products and semi-synthetic molecules, as well as molecules inspired by natural scaffolds, have been an important source of drugs in the past decades. This chapter covers reports published in the last ten years concerning natural (or semi-synthetic) products that have been reported as *in vitro* and/or *in vivo* antithrombotic agents.

Keywords: Antithrombotics, Anticoagulants, Antiplatelets, Drug Discovery, Fibrinogen, Factor Xa, Medicinal Chemistry, Natural Products, Platelet Aggregation, Semi-Synthesis, Thrombin.

INTRODUCTION

Cardiovascular diseases (CVDs) (or circulatory diseases) is a collective term for a group of diseases and disorders of the heart and blood vessels, such as coronary heart disease, cerebrovascular disease, peripheral arterial disease, rheumatic heart disease, congenital heart disease, deep vein thrombosis and pulmonary embolism [1].

* **Address correspondence to Angelo Piato:** Departamento de Farmacologia, Instituto de Ciências Básicas da Saúde, Universidade Federal do Rio Grande do Sul, Porto Alegre, Brasil; Tel: +55 (51) 3308-3121; E-mail: angelopiato@ufrgs.br, **Cedric S. Graebin:** Departamento de Química Orgânica, Instituto de Química, Universidade Federal Rural do Rio de Janeiro, Seropédica, Brasil; Tel: +55 (21) 2682-1872; E-mail: cedric@ufrrj.br

According to data from the World Health Organization (WHO), CVDs are the major cause of death globally, both in developed and developing countries. In 2016, an estimated number of 17.9 million people (31% of all global deaths) died from CVDs, being 85% of these deaths due to heart attacks and strokes. The annual mortality of CVDs is expected to reach approximately 23.6 million deaths by 2030 [1 - 4]. The WHO also estimates that at least 75% of the CVD-related deaths occur in low and middle-income countries, mostly due to the lack of preventive care and access to effective and equitable health care services [5, 6]. Also, the economic burden of CVDs in low and middle-income countries is significant; some studies affirm that CVDs and the burden they bring to patients can be a cause of poverty itself [7]. In the past few years, the number of CVD deaths in high-income countries has declined but there is evidence pointing that this long-term decline is either staggering or reversing [8].

Natural products, with their chemical diversity and remarkable and complex structures, have been a significant source of therapeutic agents used to treat several diseases throughout the last centuries. Furthermore, semi-synthetic (*i.e.* compounds that were obtained from organic synthetic methods employing a natural product as starting material) and fully synthetic molecules whose pharmacophoric group is directly inspired from a natural source have also been an important source of new drugs [9 - 11]. Although it seemed that, in the past few years, natural products were being pushed aside in favor of fully synthetic drug candidates [12], it can be said that they are expendable experiencing a return of sorts as useful sources of hit and lead compounds [13-15]. In addition to that, the growing interest in natural products from marine sources [16] is revealing new and interesting bioactive molecules that are structurally diverse from ground-based natural products [17, 18].

Nonetheless, this "going out/in favor" trend regarding the use of natural products as drug candidates was not reflected in the scientific literature. Our search in the SCOPUS database [†] , looking for articles reporting the antithrombotic activity of natural products (search key:*TITLE-ABS-KEY ("natural products" OR alkaloid OR flavonoid OR terpene OR saponin OR polysaccharide) AND (antithrombotic OR antiplatelet OR anticoagulant OR thrombin OR "factor Xa" OR platelet)* in the last 20 years has returned a steady growing trend (Fig. **1**) which indicates that, despite the perceived lack of therapeutic applicability for natural products in the pharmaceutical industry in the past, the global community of researchers investigating the antithrombotic activity of natural products kept and continues to investigate these molecules and their biological properties.

Publications of "natural products" and antithrombotics per year, 1999-2019

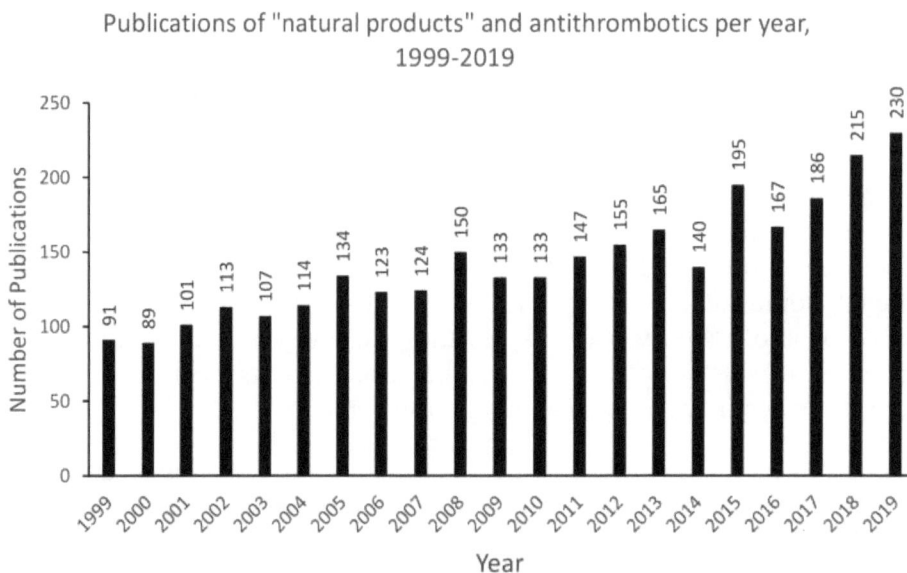

Fig. (1). The plot of the number of published articles regarding the antithrombotic activity of natural products during 1999-2019. Search terms: ("natural products" OR alkaloid OR flavonoid OR terpene OR saponin OR polysaccharide) AND (antithrombotic OR antiplatelet OR anticoagulant OR thrombin OR "factor Xa" OR platelet) Source: SCOPUS.

Despite the recent approval of several new synthetic (including orally active) anticoagulant agents in recent years for treating such diseases, mainly direct thrombin, and factor Xa (fXa) inhibitors (Fig. **2**), concerns still exist for side-effects, in particular the bleeding associated with their use [19 - 22]. Therefore, there is still a therapeutic demand for safe and effective antithrombotic agents that present fewer side effects than the currently available drugs.

In the past few years, several reports discussing the antithrombotic activity of natural (and semi-synthetic) products from several sources (plants, microorganisms, and marine organisms) have been published [23 - 27]. This chapter aims to cover these reports published in the last ten years concerning natural (or semi-synthetic) products that have been reported as *in vitro* and/or *in vivo* anticoagulants. Since one of the aims of this chapter is to highlight the molecular diversity of the natural products reported, we decided to focus our literature survey on isolated products. Reports concerning whole-extract activities without any indication of the active compound (or compounds) were, consequently, excluded. In order to have a more comprehensive discussion of the chemical entities reported, we decided to separate our findings into four categories: a) natural products from marine sources; b) natural products from microorganisms; natural products from plant-based sources and d) semi-synthetic molecules.

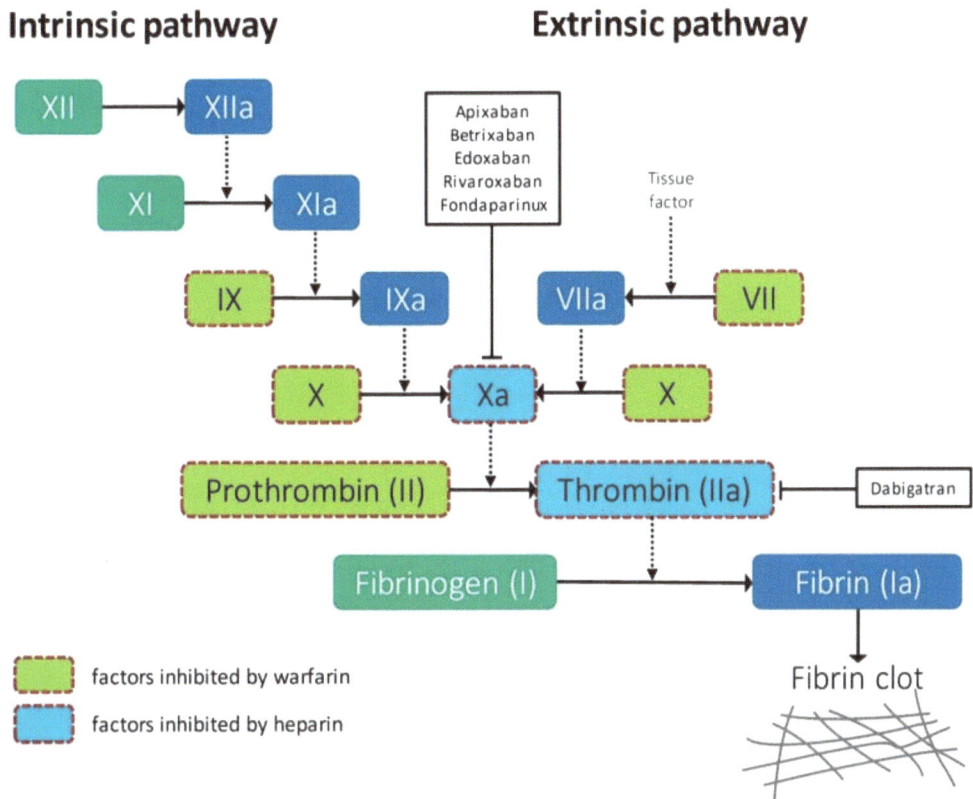

Fig. (2). The coagulation cascade and the currently available anticoagulant drugs, indicating their known mechanisms of action.

NATURAL PRODUCTS WITH ANTITHROMBOTIC ACTIVITY

Antithrombotic Molecules Obtained from Marine-based Sources

Organisms present in the marine ecosystem have received special attention in the last decades as a potential source mainly due to their bioactive substances [28]. These organisms produce a wide repertoire of substances with biological activities, for example, antibacterial, anticancer, antivirus, fungicidal, anti-inflammatory, analgesic, antihypertensive, antidepressant, and more [28 - 35]. Although many studies review and/or assess the effects of extracts [28, 30, 31, 36 - 43], here our focus is to describe a compendium of studies (Table **1**) about isolated compounds particularly with activity in the hemostasis cascade, a complex process that involves platelet aggregation and coagulation phenomena.

Table 1. Anticoagulant molecules from marine sources

Structure	Source Organism	Biological Assays and/or Mechanism of Action	Ref.
1	*Canistrocarpus cervicornis*	Inhibition of plasma or fibrinogen coagulation induced by thrombin at 1-100 μM; inhibited platelet aggregation induced by ADP and collagen. At 80 and 100 μM, the compound inhibited 100% of the platelet aggregation induced by ADP or collagen. IC_{50}: 35 μM when induced by ADP or collagen.	[47]
2: R = H **3**: R = Br	*Plocamium brasiliense*	Inhibition of proteolysis and protection from hemorrhage induced by snakebite venom in 30% *in vivo*, although compound **2** inhibited 100% and 20% of the hemorrhagic and proteolytic activities (15 μg mL^{-1}).	[44]

(Table 1) cont.....

Structure	Source organism	Biological assays and/or mechanism of action	Ref.
Pachydictyol A **4** Isopachydictyol A **5** Dichotomanol	*Dictyota menstrualis*	Compounds **4** and **5** (0.18 mM – 0.7 mM) inhibited aggregation induced by collagen (IC_{50}: 0.12 mM) or thrombin (IC_{50}: 0.25 mM). Compound **6** (0.18 mM–1.38 mM) inhibited platelet aggregation in platelet-rich plasma (PRP) induced by ADP or collagen. IC_{50}: 0.31 mM and 1.06 mM, respectively.	[45]
Clavatadine A **7**	*Suberea clavata*	Selective and irreversible inhibitor of factor XIa at 1.3 μM.	[48]
Fascaplysin **8**	*Fascaplysinopsis sp.*	Decreased platelet aggregation (10 μM); decreased formation of platelet-leukocyte aggregates (PLA) (10 μM); increased *in vivo* tail bleeding time and reduced thrombus formation (5 mg kg^{-1}).	[51]

Structure	Source organism	Biological assays and/or mechanism of action	Ref.
NH$_2$-Asn-Met-Glu-Lys-Gly-Ser-Ser-Ser-Val-Val-Ser-Ser-Arg-Met-Lyz-Gln-COOH (VITPOR AI) **9**	*Porphyra yezoensis* (Nori) pepsin hydrolysate.	fXII inhibitor (IC$_{50}$: 70.24 µM). The authors also performed molecular modeling studies with the peptide docked with fXII.	[52]
	Bohadschia argus Compounds isolated from deaminative depolymerization of the fucosylated glycosaminoglycan found in sea cucumber	The oligosaccharides **11** and **12** increased APTT (47.4 and 334.3 µg mL^{-1}) and **12** presented anti-FXase activity (IC$_{50}$: 597 ng mL^{-1}). Compound **10** was inactive in those assays.	[53]
"1000RS" (**13**), a sulfated galactan mainly composed of 4-linked Galp and 3-O-sulfated Galp units	*Microcosmus exasperatus*	Inhibition of the intrinsic coagulation pathway, prolongation of the activated partial thromboplastin time (aPTT) at manner (1.7–39.2 g mL^{-1}).	[54]

From algae, there are some studies showing the effects of different molecules on the coagulation process [39, 44 - 46]. Andrade Moura *et al.* [47] reported that **1**, a dolastane diterpene found in the marine brown algae *Canistrocarpus cervicornis* inhibited either plasma or fibrinogen coagulation induced by thrombin and increased the time for coagulation in a concentration-dependent manner.

Da Silva *et al.* [44] extracted two monoterpenes (**2** and **3**) from the seaweed *Plocamium brasiliense*. These compounds inhibited the coagulant activity induced by *Bothrops jararaca* venom. The authors suggested that these monoterpenes could be useful for treating the effects induced by the venom snake.

In another study [45], the diterpenes pachydictyol A (**4**), isopachydictyol A (**5**) and dichotomanol (**6**), isolated from the marine algae *Dictyota menstrualis*, inhibited platelet aggregation induced by collagen. Compounds **4** and **5** also inhibited platelet aggregation induced by adenosine diphosphate (ADP) and **6** inhibited thrombin-induced platelet aggregation.

Beyond algae, compounds from other marine organisms have been studied as blood hemostasis modulators.

Buchanan *et al.* [48] analyzed the effects of Clavatadine A (**7**), a molecule obtained from an extract of the marine sponge *Suberea clavata* in high-throughput screening, on factor XIa, a plasma protease related to blood coagulation [49].

Fascaplysin (**8**), a marine pigment with known antimicrobial and kinase inhibitory activities isolated from the Fijian sea sponge *Fascaplysinopsis sp.* [50], was reported as presenting *in vitro* and *in vivo* anticoagulant and antithrombotic properties, being able to reduce platelet aggregation, inhibit the formation of platelet-leukocyte aggregates (PLA), increasing tail bleeding time and reducing thrombus formation in experimental models [51].

Syed, Venkatraman and Mehta studied the peptide VITPOR AI (**9**), isolated from the pepsin hydrolysate of the seaweed *Porphyra yezoensis*. The authors determined that the peptide – already known for its anticoagulant properties – was an *in vitro* factor XII (fXII) inhibitor and performed several computer-guided assays to determine how the peptide binds to this receptor [52].

In a study with the tropical sea cucumber *Bohadschia argus*, commonly found in seafood markets in China, the authors isolated oligosaccharides (**10-12**) from depolymerized fucosylated glycosaminoglycan and these molecules presented anti-fXase activity [53], potentially inducing the inhibition of thrombus formation.

Restrepo-Espinosa *et al.* [54] evaluated the effects of sulfated galactan 1000RS (**13**) from the tunic of the ascidian *Microcosmus exasperatus* on the intrinsic coagulation pathway. The compound can inhibit the intrinsic coagulation pathway, although it was less effective than heparin.

Antithrombotics from microorganisms

Microorganisms have been a very important source of new drugs in the past decades. From the pivotal discovery of the antibacterial Penicillin G to more recent examples such as the immunosuppressant drug tacrolimus and the cholesterol-lowering agent lovastatin, secondary metabolites found in a diverse range of bacteria, fungi, and other microorganisms have been successfully used to treat several diseases [10, 55]. Although there is not any approved antithrombotic drug originating from microbial sources, a small number of reports concerning the antithrombotic activity of these classes of natural products have been published in the past years. These findings are described below and summarized in Table **2** .

Table 2. Anticoagulant molecules from microorganisms.

Structure	Source Organism	Biological Assays and/or Mechanism of Action	Ref.
Indothiazinone **14**	Cultures of Myxobac-terial strain 706	Inhibition of platelet integrin αIIbβ3-dependent cell adhesion, platelet spreading, and talin-induced integrin activation at 200 μM.	[56]

(Table 2) cont.....

Structure	Source Organism	Biological Assays and/or Mechanism of Action	Ref.
FGFC1 **15**	*Stachybotrys longispora* FG216	Fibrinolytic activity at 0.1-0.4 mmol L^{-1}; stimulate the generation of plasmin activity *in vitro* and dissolve pulmonary thrombus of Wistar rats at 10 mg kg^{-1}.	[58]
16: Anabaenopeptin B (R_1 = H; R_2 = NHC(NH)NH$_2$) **17**: Anabaenopeptin F (R_1 = Me; R_2 = NHC(NH)NH$_2$) **18**: Anabaenopeptin C (R_1 = H; R_2 = NH$_2$)	*Planktothrix rubescens*	Inhibition of Thrombin Activatable Fibrinolysis Inhibitor (TAFIa). IC_{50}: 1.5, 1.5, and 1.9 nM for compounds **16**, **17**, and **18**, respectively.	[59]

(Table 2) cont.....

Structure	Source Organism	Biological Assays and/or Mechanism of Action	Ref.
Micropeptin MZ859 **19**	*Microcystis sp.*	Thrombin was moderately inhibited by **19** with an IC_{50} of 52.9 µM. Other micropeptins tested in the same protease inhibition assays were not active.	[60]
Micropeptin MM978 **20**	*Microcystis sp.*	Thrombin inhibition (IC_{50}: 52.9 µM). Other compounds reported in the publication were inactive.	[61]

(Table 2) cont.....

Structure	Source Organism	Biological Assays and/or Mechanism of Action	Ref.
Aeruginosin TR642 **21**	*Microcystis sp.*	Compound **21** had trypsin and thrombin inhibitory properties (IC_{50} of 3.80 and 0.85 µM, respectively). Another compound reported by the authors was inactive as a thrombin inhibitor.	[62]
Aeruginosin K-139 **22** Micropeptin K-139 **23** Microviridin B **24**	*Microcystis aeruginosa* K-134	**22**: thrombin EC_{50}: 0.66 µM; fVII-sTF EC_{50}: 166 µM; **23**: thrombin EC_{50}: 26.94 µM; fVII-sTF EC_{50}: 10.62 µM; **24**: thrombin EC_{50}: 4.58 µM; fVII-sTF EC_{50}: inactive.	[63]

Yang *et al.* [56] studied the antiplatelet effects of indothiazinone (**14**). This alkaloid was initially identified and isolated from myxobacterial strains [57] and presented antiplatelet effects by inhibiting integrin αIIbβ3 activation [56].

In a study by Wang *et al.* [58], an isoindolone derivative FGFC1 (**15**) from marine fungus *Stachybotrys longispora* presented fibrinolytic activity *in vitro* (stimulating the generation of plasmin activity) as well as *in vivo* (degrading pulmonary thrombus of rats).

Schreuder *et al.* [59] studied three anabaenopeptins B, F, and C (**16-18**), isolated from the cyanobacteria *Planktothrix rubescens*, as an inhibitor of thrombin activatable fibrinolysis (TAFIa). TAFIa is a carboxypeptidase that stabilizes fibrin clots, removing C-terminal arginines and lysines from partially degraded fibrin. The inhibition of TAFIa promotes the degradation of fibrin clots and may help to prevent thrombosis. The three anabaenopeptins were able to inhibit TAFIa and, therefore, are potential agents for the prevention of thrombosis.

Zafrir and Carmeli [60] studied the effects of micropeptins MZ845, MZ859, MZ939A, MZ925, MZ939B, MZ1019, and MZ771 from a hydrophilic extract of the cyanobacterium *Microcystis sp.* as serine protease inhibitors. Only micropeptin MZ859 (**19**) presented moderate effects inhibiting thrombin. In another study using the same approach, micropeptin MM978 (**20**) was able to inhibit thrombin [61].

In recent work, Hasan-Amer and Carmeli evaluated the effects of aeruginosin TR642 (**21**), also from *Microcystis sp.* This compound was active as a trypsin and thrombin inhibitor [62].

Anas *et al.* also investigated a *Microcystis* species, *Microcystis aeruginosa* K-134. The peptide Aeruginosin K-134 (**22**), and the macrocyclic peptides Micropeptin K-134 (**23**) and Microviridin B (**24**) presented thrombin inhibitory activities. Compounds **22** and **23** were also factor VIIa soluble Tissue Factor (fVIIa-sTF) inhibitors, being **23** more active than **22** [63].

Antithrombotics from Plant-based Sources

Several plant-based natural products were reported, in the past ten years, as presenting anticoagulant properties. The products reported and their biological activities are summarized in Table **3**, below.

Using activity-guided isolation coupled with mass spectrometry techniques, Gao *et al.* [64] were able to isolate two monoterpenoid glycosides, **25** and **26**, from Hawthorn (*Crataegus pinnatifida*) leaves. These compounds presented antico-agulant activity in *in vitro* and in an *in vivo* zebrafish thrombosis model. Other products (a monoterpenoid and a flavanone) were also active, but less than the two glycosides. The authors also investigated, using molecular docking techniques, the interaction of these compounds with ADP receptors $P2Y_1$ and $P2Y_{12}$. The same research group [65] isolated **27**, a sesquiterpene, also from Hawthorn leaves. This product exerted an inhibitory effect in ADP-induced platelet aggregation in *in vitro* models, as well as antithrombotic activity in an *in vivo* caudal zebrafish model. The authors also used molecular docking assays to investigate its interaction with $P2Y_{12}$.

Table 3. Anticoagulants from plant-based sources

Compound	Source Organism	Biological Assays and/or Mechanism of Action	Ref.
25 **26**	Hawthorn (*Crataegus pinnatifida*) leaf extract (activity-guided isolation)	Platelet aggregation inhibition induced by ADP; *In* vitro increased $FeCl_3$-induced thrombosis time (zebrafish model) at 150 and 250 µg mL^{-1}. In silico docking assays (P2Y1 and P2Y12).	[64]
27	*Crataegus pinnatifida* seeds; compound tested after purification and characterization	Inhibited ADP-induced platelet aggregation at 1 mg mL^{-1}.	[65]
28	*Crataegus pinnatifida* leaves; compound tested after purification and characterization	Inhibited ADP-induced platelet aggregation (250 µg mL^{-1}) and prolonged $FeCl_3$-induced thrombocyte formation time in zebrafish caudal vessels (50 and 150 µg mL^{-1}). Molecular modeling studies with **23** and P2Y$_{12}$ receptor.	[66]
Berberine **29**	Compound acquired from commercial sources.	Prolonged whole blood clotting time (CT), aPTT, PT and thrombin time (TT) (2.5 µM); Decreased *in vitro* fibrinogen (FIB) concentration (2.5 µM). Prolonged *in vivo* whole blood CT, prolonged aPTT, PT and TT (100 – 200 mg Kg^{-1}).	[67]

(Table 3) cont.....

Compound	Source Organism	Biological Assays and/or Mechanism of Action	Ref.
 Dihydrocaffeic acid **30** Amentoflavone **31**	Processed 'Juan Bai' (*Selaginela tamarascina*) extract and also tested isolated	Compound **30** increased activated partial thrombin time (aPTT), prothrombin time (PT) increased *in vivo* tail bleeding time (171.1 μM); compound **31** inhibited platelet aggregation induced by adenosine diphosphate (ADP) and arachidonic acid (AA) at 40.7 μM.	[68]
 32: Orientin (R1 = Glu, R2 = H) **33:** Isoorientin (R1 = H, R2 = Glu)	*Vaccinium bracteatum.* Compounds were acquired from commercial sources	Prolonged *in vitro* coagulation times (PT, aPTT). Prolonged *in vivo* tail bleeding time; **33** was less active (20 μM) than **32** (5 μM). Inhibition of intrinsic and extrinsic coagulation pathways by inhibiting fXa and thrombin production (HUVEC model). Inhibition of TNF-α induced secretion of plasminogen-activated inhibitor 1 (PAI-1).	[69]

(Table 3) cont.....

Compound	Source Organism	Biological Assays and/or Mechanism of Action	Ref.
Fisetin **34**	Chinese lacquer tree (*Toxicodendron vernicifluum*, formerly *Rhus vernificulia*) heartwood extract (the extract and the isolated natural products were tested)	*In vitro* inhibition of platelet aggregation (IC$_{50}$: 19-44 µM when induced by collagen; 238-331 µM when induced by thrombin and 34-38 µM when induced by ADP). Compound **34** (100 µM) prevented extracellular signal-regulated kinase (ERK)/mitogen activated protein kinase (MAPK) activation. None of these compounds affected p38 activation.	[70]
Butein **35**			
Sulfuretin **36**			

(Table 3) cont.....

Compound	Source Organism	Biological Assays and/or Mechanism of Action	Ref.
 (-)-Epigallocatechin **37**	Green tea (*Camellia sinensis*) leaves and buds extract. The compound was tested isolated from the extract	*In vivo* mice platelet aggregation inhibition. Prolonged bleeding time (BT) and blood clotting time (CT) in mice models (500 mg kg⁻¹). Prolonged aPTT; no effect on PT and FIB levels.	[71]
 Vicenin-2 **38**	Honeybush tea, "vleitee" or "valeitee" (*Cyclopia subternata*) Vicenin-2 was acquired from commercial sources	Prolonged *in vitro* (5 µM) and *ex* vivo (5.9 µg/mouse) aPTT and PT; Prolonged *in vivo* mouse tail bleeding time (11.9 µg/mouse). Inhibits activation and production of thrombin and fXa. Inhibition of TNF-a induced secretion of PAI-1.	[72]
 Scolymoside **39**	*Cyclopia subternata*. Scolymoside was acquired from commercial sources	Prolonged *in vitro* aPTT and PT (> 5 µM). Prolonged *in vivo* tail bleeding time (> 11.9 µg/mouse). Compound **39** also inhibits the activation and production of thrombin and fXa. Inhibition of thrombin-induced fibrin polymerization and platelet aggregation.	[73]

(Table 3) cont.....

Compound	Source Organism	Biological Assays and/or Mechanism of Action	Ref.
Quercetin-3-O-α-rhamnoside **40**	White mangrove or "Mangueira branca" (*Lagunclaria racemosa* (L.) C.F. Gaerth) leaves. Extracts were tested first and, from the most active extract, these two compounds were identified as the most active.	Thrombin inhibition (chromogenic substrate assay) and prolonged coagulation time (0.5 μmol mL⁻¹).	[74]
Quercetin-3-O-α-arabinoside **41**			[74]

(Table 3) cont.....

Compound	Source Organism	Biological Assays and/or Mechanism of Action	Ref.
Pelargonidin **42**	Acquired from commercial sources	Prolonged *in vitro* aPTT and PT; Inhibition of fXa and thrombin production (5-20 µM). Prolonged *in vivo* bleeding times (5.4 µg/mouse). Inhibition of TNF-a induced secretion of PAI-1.	[75]
Zingerone **43**	Ginger (*Zingiber officinale*). The compound was acquired from commercial sources	Prolonged *in vitro* and *ex vivo* APTT; prolonged *in vivo* tail bleeding time. *Ex vivo* antithrombotic effect in mice arterial and pulmonary thrombosis models. Decreases induction of P-selectin and procaspase-activating compound 1 (PAC-1) induced by ADP or U46619. Non-competitive inhibitor of fXa ($K_i = 4.96$ µM).	[76]
44: Methyl ferulate ($R_1 = OCH_3$) **45**: Methyl 4-hydroxycinnamate ($R_1 = H$)	*Illigera luzonensis* stems and roots. Compounds were isolated before testing.	Inhibition of rabbit platelet aggregation induced by AA (> 0.2 µg mL^{-1}).	[77]

(Table 3) cont.....

Compound	Source Organism	Biological Assays and/or Mechanism of Action	Ref.
COOH H₃CO — OCH₃ OH **Syringic acid** **46**	Compound acquired from commercial sources	Decreased the *in vitro* expression of density-enhanced phosphatase 1 (DEP-1)/protein tyrosine phosphatase 1B (PTP1B)/$\alpha_{IIb}\beta_3$; Inhibits *in vitro* clot retraction and *in vivo* FeCl3-induced vascular occlusion of the carotid artery (> 5-20 μg).	[78]
O OH HO OH OH **Shikimic acid** **47**	Compound acquired from commercial sources.	*Ex vivo* study using blood samples from 22 sedentary patients. The compound lowered PAC-1 expression (> 1 mM); reduction of monocyte-platelet aggregate formation and whole-blood platelet aggregation stimulated by ADP but not by collagen (1-2 mM).	[79]

(Table 3) cont.....

Compound	Source Organism	Biological Assays and/or Mechanism of Action	Ref.
  Geniposide **48**	Gardenia (*Gardenia jasminoides*) extract; geniposide (main constituent) was acquired from commercial sources and tested isolated.	Both geniposide isolated and the extract inhibited *ex vivo* thrombin and collagen-induced platelet aggregation; also inhibited *in vivo* thrombosis induced by arteriovenous shunt in rats (> 50 mg kg^{-1}).	[80]
  Chikusetsusaponin IVa **49**	Fruits of Maté (*Ilex paraguariensis*); the compound was isolated and characterized before testing.	Prolonged TT, aPTT and PT; Inhibits the amidolytic activity of fXa and thrombin over synthetic substrates; inhibits thrombin-induced fibrinogen clotting and thrombin and collagen-induced platelet aggregation. Competitive thrombin inhibitor (K_i = 219.6 μM).	[81]

(Table 3) cont.....

Compound	Source Organism	Biological Assays and/or Mechanism of Action	Ref.
	Acanthopanax sessiliflorus fruit extract. Compounds were tested after purification.	Inhibition of platelet aggregation induced by ADP (IC$_{50}$: 4.2 – 5.6 µM).	[82]

(Table 3) cont.....

Compound	Source Organism	Biological Assays and/or Mechanism of Action	Ref.
 Lancolide A **53** Lancolide D **54**	Magnolia vine (*Schisandra lancifolia*) leaves and stems; compounds were tested after purification.	Inhibition of platelet aggregation induced by PAF (100 μg mL⁻¹). Inactive when using AA, thrombin or collagen as aggregation inducer.	[83]

(Table 3) cont.....

Compound	Source Organism	Biological Assays and/or Mechanism of Action	Ref.
 epi-Sesamin **55**	Wild ginger (*Asarum sieboldii*) roots; the compound was isolated and characterized before testing	Prolonged PT and APTT (> 2 µM); inhibited activity of thrombin and fXa, thrombin-catalyzed fibrin polymerization platelet aggregation; *In vivo* anticoagulant effects in mice (7 µg/mouse); Reduction of TNFa- induced production of PAI-1. Sesamin (an epimer of **41**) was less active in these assays.	[84]
 (-)-Synringaresinol **56**	Stems of 'Choijwal' (*Piper wallichii*); Compounds were isolated and characterized before testing.	*In vitro* PAF-induced platelet aggregation inhibition (0.52 mM); *In vivo* antithrombotic activity (zebrafish model) at 125 µM.	[85]

(Table 3) cont.....

Compound	Source Organism	Biological Assays and/or Mechanism of Action	Ref.
 57 **58:** Licarin A (R$_1$ = OH, R$_2$ = OMe) **59:** Licarin B (R$_1$/R$_2$ = -OCH2CH2O-) (-)-dihydroguaiaretic acid **60**	"Asian Lizard's tail" (*Saururus chinensis*) whole plant extract. Compounds were tested after isolation and purification.	Inhibition of ADP-induced platelet aggregation (0.1 – 0.25 µM).	[86]
 61	*Illigera luzonensis* stems and roots. Compound was isolated before testing.	Inhibition of rabbit platelet aggregation induced by AA (0.5 µg mL^{-1}).	[77]

The sesquiterpene glycoside **28**, isolated by Zhou *et al.* [66] from Hawthorn seeds, also presented *in vitro* anticoagulant properties, inhibiting platelet aggregation induced by ADP.

Berberine (**29**), a quaternary ammonium alkaloid salt found in several plants and used as a natural dye due to its intense yellow color, was investigated by Wang *et al.* [67]. The alkaloid presented moderate anticoagulant activity in several *in vitro* and *in vivo* models.

Investigating the effects of processed 'Juan Bai' (*S. tamariscina*), a plant used in Tradicional Chinese Medicine (TCM), Zhang *et al.* [68] found that dihydrocaffeic acid (**30**), presented in a greater concentration in the extract of the processed plant (when compared with the raw plant extract) presented *in vitro* and *in vivo* anticoagulant effect. Amentoflavone (**31**), also found in the processed plant extract, showed *in vitro* anticoagulant activity inhibiting ADP and Arachidonic Acid (AA)-induced platelet aggregation.

Lee and Bae [69] reported the anticoagulant activity of orientin (**32**) and isoorientin (**33**), two structurally related flavonoid *C*-glycosides. Both presented *in vitro* and *in vivo* anticoagulant activity, being **32** more active than **33**. The authors suggest that their mechanism of action is due to the inhibition of the extrinsic and intrinsic coagulation pathways by the inhibition of thrombin and fXa production.

Fisetin (**34**), butein (**35**) and sulfuretin (**36**), three polyphenols found in the heartwood extract of the Chinese lacquer tree (*Toxicodendron vernicifluum*, formerly *Rhus vernificulia*) were reported by Lee *et al.* [70] as *in vitro* inhibitors of platelet aggregation. Extracellular signal-regulated kinase (ERK) mitogen-activated protein kinase (MAPK) activated by collagen was inhibited by fisetin (**34**), but not by **35** or **36**. Fisetin also had a longer *in vitro* activity and was active in an *in vivo* arterial thrombosis protocol.

Chen *et al.* [71] reported the anticoagulant activity of (-)-epigallocatechin (**37**), a polyphenol found in green tea (*Camellia sinensis*) leaves and bud extracts. The polyphenol presented *in vivo* prolonged bleeding time and aPTT, but no effect on prothrombin time (PT) and fibrinogen levels.

Lee and Bae [72] investigated the anticoagulant properties of vicenin-2 (**38**), a flavonoid *C*-glycoside found in the Honeybush tea (*C. subternata*). The flavonoid showed *in vivo* and *in vitro* anticoagulant activity, inhibiting both intrinsic and extrinsic coagulation pathways. Another flavonoid from the same plant, scolymoside (**39**), had its anticoagulant properties reported by Yoon *et al.* [73], being active in *in vitro* and *in vivo* assays.

Rodrigues *et al.* studied the thrombin inhibitory activity of White Mangrove (*Lagunclaria racemosa*) leaf extracts. They isolated and identified two flavonoid glycosides, Quercetin-3-O-α-rhamnoside (**40**) and the correspondent arabnoside (**41**) as the most active compounds. Both were able to inhibit thrombin and also prolong coagulation time when compared with control and the flavonoid quercetin, indicating that the glycosylation of the flavonoid is important to the inhibitory activities reported [74].

Pelagornidin (**42**), an anthocyanin used as a pigment, was reported by Ku *et al.* [75] as an anticoagulant, prolonging *in vitro* aPTT and PT and inhibiting the production of fXa and thrombin in Human umbilical vein endothelial cells (HUVEC). This anthocyanin also exerted *in vivo* anticoagulant effects in mice (tail bleeding assay).

Zingerone (**43**), a phenolic alkanone found in ginger (*Zingiber officinale*), was reported by Lee *et al.* [76] as both an antiplatelet aggregator and a fXa inhibitor, being also active in an *in vivo* protocols, including arterial and pulmonary thrombosis animal models.

Methyl ferulate (**44**) and methyl-4-hydroxycinnamate (**45**), two benzenoids isolated from *Illigera luzonensis* stems and roots, presented *in vitro* anticoagulant properties, inhibiting rabbit platelet aggregation induced by AA [77].

Syringic acid (**46**), a phenolic compound found in several fruits and vegetables, was investigated by Choi and Kim [78]. The acid was able to inhibit clot formation and attenuated the density-enhanced phosphatase 1 (DEP-1)/protein tyrosine phosphatase 1B (PTP1B)/$\alpha_{IIb}\beta_3$ signaling pathway.

Veach *et al.* [79] performed an *ex vivo* study in sedentary patients to investigate the anticoagulant effects of shikimic acid (**47**), a phenolic metabolite. The acid reduced platelet aggregation induced by ADP and lowered procaspase-activating compound 1 (PAC-1) expression.

Zhang *et al.* [80] studied the *in vivo* effects of geniposide (**48**), an iridoid glycoside found in the extract of Gardenia (*Gardenia jasminoides*). Both the plant extract and **39** presented *in vivo* antithrombotic effect in several mice protocols.

Chikusetsusaponin IVa (**49**), a triterpenic saponin found in the fruits of "Maté" or "Mate" (*Ilex paraguariensis*) had its antithrombotic properties reported by Dahmer *et al.* [81]. The saponin was found to be a weak direct thrombin inhibitor, reducing thrombin- and collagen-induced platelet aggregation and prolonging PT, aPTT, and TT.

Yang *et al.* [82] isolated a triterpenic saponin (**50**) and two lupane-derived triterpenes (**51** and **52**, respectively) from the fruits of *Acanthopanax sessiliflorus*. The three compounds were able to inhibit platelet aggregation induced by ADP.

Lancolides A and D (**53** and **54**, respectively), two nortriterpenoids with very interesting and complex structures, were isolated from the Magnolia vine (*Schisandra lancifolia*) by Shi *et al.* [83]. Both nortriterpenoids showed antithrombotic properties in *in vitro* assays, inhibiting platelet aggregation induced by the platelet aggregation factor (PAF), but not by AA, thrombin or collagen.

Ku *et al.* [84] reported that epi-sesamin (**55**), a lignan found in the roots of wild ginger (*Asarum sieboldii*) presented *in vitro* and *in vivo* anticoagulant properties. Sesamin, its epimer, was either inactive or less active in the protocols employed in this study.

(-)-Syringaresinol (**56**), a lignan found in the stems of 'Choijwal' (*Piper wallichii*), had its anticoagulant properties described by Shi *et al.* [85]. The lignan presented *in vitro* and *in vivo* antithrombotic activity in the caudal zebrafish model. It is worth noticing the structural similarities between this lignan, epi-Sesamin (**55**), and their antithrombotic activities.

Studying the lignans found in the "Asian lizard's tail" (*Saururus chinensis*) whole plant extract, Qu *et al.* [86] reported that four lignans: **57**, licarin A (**58**), licarin B (**59**) and (-)-dihydroguaiaretic acid (**60**), presented *in vitro* anti-platelet aggregation activity.

Huang *et al.* [77] isolated several new and already reported products from *Illigera luzonensis*. A bisaporphine alkaloid (**61**) presented *in vitro* anticoagulant properties, inhibiting rabbit platelet aggregation induced by AA.

Semi-synthetic compounds with antithrombotic activity

As briefly mentioned in this chapter's introduction, there is a considerable number of approved drugs that are obtained by semisynthetic processes [10]. The same can be found concerning antithrombotic agents, with a good number of new natural product analogs with antithrombotic properties being reported in the past ten years. These compounds, a simplified synthetic route leading to them, the natural product that was used as inspiration, and their anticoagulant properties are summarized in Table **4**, below.

Table 4. Semi-synthetic anticoagulant compounds.

Natural Product Used as Inspiration and Source Organism	Compounds and Simplified Synthetic Route	Biological Assays and/or Mechanism of Action	Ref.
 Sargahydroquinoic acid **62** Source: *Sargassum micracanthum*	 Geranyl acetone **63** 5 steps **64**	Inhibition of platelet aggregation induced by ADP, thrombin, and collagen (IC$_{50}$: 55-74 μM).	[87]
 OH **OH** Andrographolide **65** Source: Green chireta (*Andrographis paniculate*)	 Andrographolide **65** 13 steps **66**	Inhibited platelet aggregation induced by TRAP (SLLRNNH$_2$) and Thrombin (0.6 – 1.65 μM), but not by ADP or collagen; Inhibited *ex vivo* platelet aggregation (30 mg kg^{-1}).	[88]
Kirenol (**67**) Source: *Siegesbeckia pubescens* Makino	 Kirenol **67** 2 steps **68** 2 steps 1 step **69** **70**	*In vitro* fXa inhibition (IC$_{50}$: 0.22 – 1.7 μM). Other synthesized derivatives were less active than Kirenol (IC$_{50}$: 2.5 μM).	[89]
Kirenol (**63**). Source: same as above.	 Kirenol **67** 6 steps **71**	*In vitro* fXa inhibition (IC$_{50}$: 87 nM). Other synthesized derivatives were inactive.	[90]

(Table 4) cont.....

Natural Product Used as Inspiration and Source Organism	Compounds and Simplified Synthetic Route	Biological Assays and/or Mechanism of Action	Ref.
Spumigin A **72** Source: *Nodularia spumigena*	(six steps from *L*-proline methyl ester) **73**: R$_1$ = H, R$_2$ = (*R*)-OH **74**: R$_1$ = OH, R$_2$ = (*R/S*)-OH (six steps from *D*-leucine) **75**	*In vitro* thrombin and fXa inhibition (**73**: K$_i$ = 3.8 – 18 μM; **74**: K$_i$ = 0.92 – 3.9 μM; **75**: K$_i$ = 5.2 – 30 μM). Other synthesized derivatives were reported as active.	[91]
Anabaenopeptin B **16** Source: *Planktothrix rubescens* strain Cya3	**76** 4 steps **77**	Thrombin Activable Fibrinolysis Inhibitor (TAFIa) inhibitor (IC$_{50}$: 3 nM).	[92]
Cephaindole A **78** Source: *Cephalanceropsis gracilis*	**79** 2 steps **80**: R$_1$ = H, R$_2$ = NO$_2$ **81**: R$_1$ = NO$_2$, R$_2$ = H **82**: R$_1$/R$_2$ = NO$_2$	Inhibition of platelet aggregation induced by AA (IC$_{50}$: 18.9 – 21.5 μg mL^{-1}). Cephaindole A (**78**) was also active in this assay (IC$_{50}$: 19.34 μg mL^{-1}).	[93]

(Table 4) cont.....

Natural Product Used as Inspiration and Source Organism	Compounds and Simplified Synthetic Route	Biological Assays and/or Mechanism of Action	Ref.
Chlorodysinosin A **83** No sources were given in the original report.	11 steps **84** → **85**	Thrombin inhibitor (IC$_{50}$: 3 nM); ca. 95 times less active as a trypsin inhibitor.	[94]
86 (Glycyrrhizin): R$_1$ = GlcA(β1$\rightarrow$2)GlcA **87** (Glycyrrhetinic acid): R$_1$ = H Source: *Glycyrrhiza glabra*	**87** → **88**	Increased TT, PT and bleeding time. Compound **88** is an allosteric thrombin inhibitor (IC$_{50}$: 110 μM).	[95]
Rosmarinic acid **89**	**90** **91** (one-step synthesis from gallic or caffeic acid)	Inhibition of platelet aggregation induced by thrombin (100 μM); Inhibition of thrombin-stimulated Ca^{2+}- mobilization.	[96]

(Table 4) cont.....

Natural Product Used as Inspiration and Source Organism	Compounds and Simplified Synthetic Route	Biological Assays and/or Mechanism of Action	Ref.
Designed as a "flavonoid analog".	**92**	Inhibition of platelet aggregation induced by U466919 and collagen (IC$_{50}$: 27-31 μM). Not active when thrombin was used as an inducer. Also inhibited U466919-induced P-selectin expression.	[97]

Shin, Oh and Lee [87] obtained, in a 5-step synthetic protocol starting from geranyl acetone (**63**), a farnesyl acetone derivative (**64**) analog to the natural product sargahydroquinoic acid (**62**), isolated from seaweeds *Sargassum micracanthum* and *S. yezoense*. This farnesyl acetone was able to inhibit platelet aggregation induced by ADP, collagen, and thrombin.

Using the natural product androgapholide (**65**) as starting material, Liu *et al*. [88] synthesized, in a 13-step convergent synthetic route after a few rounds of pharmacological evaluation and optimizations, an analog (**66**) that presented *in vitro* anticoagulant properties, inhibiting platelet aggregation induced by the peptide TRAP (SLLRNNH$_2$) and thrombin, but not by ADP or collagen. The compound obtained in the synthesis was also identified as a Protease-activated Receptor-1 (PAR-1) antagonist.

Kirenol (**67**), a diterpenoid isolated from *Siegesbeckia pubescens*, was used as a starting material for the synthesis of derivatives (**68-70**) by Wang *et al*. [89]. Some of the synthesized derivatives, alongside with **67**, were *in vitro* fXa inhibitors. The diterpenoid was also used in the 6-step synthesis of a ring-expanded derivative (**71**), which was also found to be an *in vitro* fXa inhibitor [90].

Žula *et al*. [91] synthesized three peptidic compounds (**73-75**) in a six-step protocol starting from L-proline methyl ester or D-leucine, analogs to the natural product spumigin A (**72**), isolated from the cyanobacteria *Nodularia spumigena*. The three peptidic compounds were active as *in vitro* fXa and thrombin inhibitors. It is worth noticing that both the natural scaffold and the derivatives have the guanidine group also present in the direct thrombin inhibitor drug argatroban.

The bis-substituted urea (**77**) was designed and synthesized (using a four-step protocol starting from a protected cyclohexylalanine **76**) by Halland *et al*. [92] as a simplified analog of the natural cyclic peptide anabaenopeptin B (**16**). The simplified derivative was found to be an inhibitor of Activated Thrombin

Activatable Fibrinolysis Inhibitor (TAFIa), being as active as the natural scaffold.

Cephaindole A (**78**), an indole alkaloid found in the Taiwanese orchid *Cephalanceropsis gracilis*, was the inspiration for the synthesis of nitroaromatic derivatives using substituted 3-acetylindoles. Sharma *et al*. [93] reported the synthesis of 15 derivatives, being three (**80-82**) *in vitro* AA-induced platelet aggregation inhibitors. The natural scaffold **78** was also active in this assay, being as active as the derivatives **80-82**.

Hanessian *et al*. [94] obtained, in an 11-step synthesis starting with 4-methylpiperidine (**84**), a dihydropyridine (**85**) analog to the marine sponge metabolite Chlorodysinosin A (**83**). The pyridine was found to be a potent *in vitro* thrombin inhibitor (IC$_{50}$: 3 nM) and more than 90 times less active as a trypsin inhibitor.

De Paula *et al*. [95] synthesized a hemiphtalic ester (**88**) of glycyrrhetinic acid (**87**), designed to be a simplified analog of the natural saponin glycyrrhizin (**86**), a weak indirect thrombin inhibitor. The ester was found to be also an indirect thrombin inhibitor, being more active than the natural saponin.

Two polyphenol esters (**90** and **91**) designed to be simplified analogs of rosmarinic acid (**89**) were obtained by Chapado *et al*. [96], inhibiting thrombin-induced platelet aggregation and thrombin-induced Ca^{2+} mobilization.

Del Turco *et al*. [97] designed and synthesized a pyridopyrimidin-4-one (**92**) as a flavonoid analog. This heterocycle was able to inhibit platelet aggregation induced by collagen and the synthetic Thromboxane A$_2$ analog U46919, but not by thrombin, inhibiting also U46919-induced P-selectin expression.

CONCLUSION

In the past decade, several reports concerning the antithrombotic activity of a diverse range of natural and semi-synthetic products were published. A fair number of these publications (particularly marine and plant-based natural products) reported the biological activities of crude extracts, without any attempts to identify the active compound (or compounds) present in the extract. We ponder that, regarding the importance of the search for new compounds with antithrombotic activity [20 - 22], follow-up studies should be conducted to identify (if possible) the active compound (or compounds) present in these extracts. This information is essential to perform the design and development of a new generation of antithrombotic agents. Furthermore, these studies should also encompass more biological and pharmacological assays with the purpose to assess the potential of these agents in the therapeutics.

Regarding the literature survey presented in this chapter (Tables **1 - 4**), plant-based natural products are the group of natural products with the greatest number of biologically active compounds reported (47), followed by semi-synthetic compounds (18), marine natural products (13) and microorganism-based natural products (11). Marine natural products, in the past few years, have been receiving a great deal of interest regarding the search for new antithrombotic agents. It is expected that, with the approval of marine-based drugs such as trabectedin [98], the interest for marine-based natural products will keep rising.

The compounds reported present a very structurally diverse molecular framework, with terpenes, alkaloids, lignans, anthocyanins, oligo and polysaccharides, linear and cyclic peptides and polyphenols being among the classes presented in this chapter. This is an evidence of the enormous molecular diversity that can arise from the search for new bioactive natural products.

The mechanisms of action of these compounds are also diverse. Most of the compounds act either inhibiting the coagulation cascade or platelet aggregation. Most of the reports discuss the biological effects of these products without defining a key molecular target, pointing, in some cases, if the extrinsical or intrinsical coagulation pathways are being inhibited. Interestingly, some of the compounds highlighted in this chapter are reported presenting new and/or unexplored mechanisms of action, such as the factor XIa inhibitor **7**, factor XII inhibitor **9**, and the TAFIa inhibitors **16-18** and **77**. These new, yet-to-be explored molecular targets can lead to molecules with a new pharmacological profile and, hopefully, less adverse effects when compared with the drugs currently employed.

Most of the compounds presented in this manuscript can be considered weak or moderate agents, exerting their biological activities in concentrations greater than 10 μM. A few compounds, however, exerted potent *in vitro* activities, such as the sulphated oligossacharide **12** (FXase IC_{50}: 597 ng mL^{-1}), the cyclic peptides Anabaenopeptins B, F and C (**16-18**), which inhibited TAFIa (IC_{50}: 1.5, 1.5, and 1.9 nM, respectively), Aeruginosin TR645 (**21**, thrombin IC_{50} = 0.85 μM), Aeruginosin K-139 (**22**, thrombin EC_{50}: 0.66 μM) Kirenol derivatives**68-71** (fXa IC_{50} ranging from 87 nM – 1.7 μM, being the ring-expanded derivative **71** the most potent of the four), the peptide **74** (thrombin Ki: 0.92 μM), the Anabaenopeptin B (**16**) analog **77** (TAFIa IC_{50}: 3 nM), and the Chlorodysinosin A (**83**) analog **85** (thrombin IC_{50}: 3 nM). It is worth noticing that **77** and **85** were designed using the molecular simplification strategy [99], reducing the complexity of the natural scaffolds while keeping the essential features responsible for their biological activities (pharmacophoric groups) and, in both cases, successfully keeping their biological activity profiles and potencies. Also, it is interesting to highlight here compounds **21**, **73-75**, and **85**, all identified as *in* *vitro* thrombin inhibitors, presenting a guanidine, amidine or closely related group in their molecular structures. This is a molecular feature also present in the approved thrombin inhibitor argatroban and it is known that the presence of a guanidine group is crucial to the interaction between thrombin inhibitors and the enzyme [100].

It is also important to notice that the products we consider the most promising (regarding their potencies), the natural marine products **16-18**, and the semi-synthetic derivatives **77** and **85** were tested only in *in vitro* protocols. However, before they could be deemed good enough for further clinical development, more assays (including experimental *in vivo* models) are required to assess their activity profile, oral biodisponibility, toxicity, and safety.

Although, as described in this Chapter's introduction, natural products were, in the past decades, being discarded in favor of fully synthetic compounds, they are still a very significant source of new drugs [10] and, in the past few years, they have been experiencing a resurgence as a source of new hit and lead compounds [13 - 15]. We expect that, as this resurgence trend continues upward, new original natural products with interesting chemical structures and remarkable antithrombotic activities will be reported, leading to new sources of lead compounds and to molecules that can serve as inspiration for the design and development of new antithrombotic agents.

ABBREVIATIONS

AA	arachidonic acid
ADP	adenosine diphosphate
aPTT	activated partial thrombin time
BT	bleeding time
CT	whole blood clotting time
CVD	Cardiovascular diseases
DEP-1	density-enhanced phosphatase 1
ERK	Extracellular signal-regulated kinase
FIB	fibrinogen
fXa	factor Xa
fVII-sTF	factor VII-soluble Tissue Factor
HUVEC	Human umbilical vein endothelial cells
MAPK	mitogen-activated protein kinase
PAC-1	procaspase-activating compound 1
PAF	platelet aggregation factor

PAR-1	Protease-activated Receptor-1
PT	prothrombin time
PLA	platelet-leukocyte aggregate
PTP1B	protein tyrosine phosphatase 1B
TAFIa	thrombin activatable fibrinolysis
TT	thrombin time
WHO	World Health Organization

CONSENT FOR PUBLICATION

Not applicable.

CONFLICT OF INTEREST

The authors declare that there is no conflict of interest.

ACKNOWLEDGEMENT

Declared none.

REFERENCES

[1]   World Health Organization. 2017.https://www.who.int/news-room/fact-sheets/detail/cardiovascul-r-diseases-(cvds)

[2]   Roth GA, Johnson C, Abajobir A, *et al.* Global, regional, and national burden of cardiovascular diseases for 10 causes, 1990 to 2015. J Am Coll Cardiol 2017; 70(1): 1-25.
[http://dx.doi.org/10.1016/j.jacc.2017.04.052] [PMID: 28527533]

[3]   Kaptoge S, Pennells L, De Bacquer D, Cooney MT, Kavousi M, Stevens G, *et al.* WHO CVD Risk Chart Working Group. World Health Organization cardiovascular disease risk charts: revised models to estimate risk in 21 global regions. Lancet Glob Health 2019; 7(10): e1332-45.
[http://dx.doi.org/10.1016/S2214-109X(19)30318-3] [PMID: 31488387]

[4]   GBD 2017 Causes of Death Collaborators.. Global, regional, and national age-sex-specific mortality for 282 causes of death in 195 countries and territories, 1980-2017: a systematic analysis for the Global Burden of Disease Study . Lancet 2018; 392(10159): 88- 1736 .

[5]   Rosengren A, Smyth A, Rangarajan S, *et al.* Socioeconomic status and risk of cardiovascular disease in 20 low-income, middle-income, and high-income countries: the Prospective Urban Rural Epidemiologic (PURE) study. Lancet Glob Health 2019; 7(6): e748-60.
[http://dx.doi.org/10.1016/S2214-109X(19)30045-2] [PMID: 31028013]

[6]   Lee G, Carrington M. Tackling heart disease and poverty. Nurs Health Sci 2007; 9(4): 290-4.
[http://dx.doi.org/10.1111/j.1442-2018.2007.00363.x] [PMID: 17958679]

[7]   Callander EJ, Schofield DJ. The risk of falling into poverty after developing heart disease: a survival analysis. BMC Public Health 2016; 16(1): 570.
[http://dx.doi.org/10.1186/s12889-016-3240-5] [PMID: 27417645]

[8]   Lopez AD, Adair T. Is the long-term decline in cardiovascular-disease mortality in high-income countries over? Evidence from national vital statistics. Int J Epidemiol 2019; 48(6): 1815-23.
[http://dx.doi.org/10.1093/ije/dyz143] [PMID: 31378814]

[9]   Newman DJ, Cragg GM, Snader KM. The influence of natural products upon drug discovery. Nat Prod Rep 2000; 17(3): 215-34.
[http://dx.doi.org/10.1039/a902202c] [PMID: 10888010]

[10]   Newman DJ, Cragg GM. Natural products as sources of new drugs from 1981 to 2014. J Nat Prod 2016; 79(3): 629-61.
[http://dx.doi.org/10.1021/acs.jnatprod.5b01055] [PMID: 26852623]

[11]   Cragg GM, Newman DJ. Natural products: A continuing source of novel drug leads. Biochimica et Biophysica Acta (BBA) -. General Subjects 2013; 1830(6): 3670-95.
[http://dx.doi.org/10.1016/j.bbagen.2013.02.008]

[12]   Calixto JB. The role of natural products in modern drug discovery 2019.
[http://dx.doi.org/10.1590/0001-3765201920190105]

[13]   Shen B. A new golden age of natural products drug discovery. Cell 2015; 163(6): 1297-300.
[http://dx.doi.org/10.1016/j.cell.2015.11.031] [PMID: 26638061]

[14]   Harvey AL, Edrada-Ebel R, Quinn RJ. The re-emergence of natural products for drug discovery in the genomics era. Nat Rev Drug Discov 2015; 14(2): 111-29.
[http://dx.doi.org/10.1038/nrd4510] [PMID: 25614221]

[15]   Li F, Wang Y, Li D, Chen Y, Dou QP. Are we seeing a resurgence in the use of natural products for new drug discovery? Expert Opin Drug Discov 2019; 14(5): 417-20.
[http://dx.doi.org/10.1080/17460441.2019.1582639] [PMID: 30810395]

[16]   Gerwick WH, Moore BS. Lessons from the past and charting the future of marine natural products drug discovery and chemical biology. Chem Biol 2012; 19(1): 85-98.
[http://dx.doi.org/10.1016/j.chembiol.2011.12.014] [PMID: 22284357]

[17]   Li T, Ding T, Li J. Medicinal purposes: bioactive metabolites from marine-derived organisms. Mini Rev Med Chem 2019; 19(2): 138-64.
[http://dx.doi.org/10.2174/1389557517666170927113143] [PMID: 28969543]

[18]   Montaser R, Luesch H. Marine natural products: a new wave of drugs? Future Med Chem 2011; 3(12): 1475-89.
[http://dx.doi.org/10.4155/fmc.11.118] [PMID: 21882941]

[19]   Harter K, Levine M, Henderson SO. Anticoagulation drug therapy: a review. West J Emerg Med 2015; 16(1): 11-7.
[http://dx.doi.org/10.5811/westjem.2014.12.22933] [PMID: 25671002]

[20]   Joppa SA, Salciccioli J, Adamski J, *et al.* A practical review of the emerging direct anticoagulants, laboratory monitoring, and reversal agents. J Clin Med 2018; 7(2): 29.
[http://dx.doi.org/10.3390/jcm7020029] [PMID: 29439477]

[21]   Alquwaizani M, Buckley L, Adams C, Fanikos J. Anticoagulants: A review of the pharmacology, dosing, and complications. Curr Emerg Hosp Med Rep 2013; 1(2): 83-97.
[http://dx.doi.org/10.1007/s40138-013-0014-6] [PMID: 23687625]

[22]   Dangas GD, Tijssen JGP, Wöhrle J, *et al.* GALILEO Investigators. A controlled trial of rivaroxaban after transcatheter aortic-valve replacement. N Engl J Med 2020; 382(2): 120-9.
[http://dx.doi.org/10.1056/NEJMoa1911425] [PMID: 31733180]

[23]   Mousa SA. Antithrombotic effects of naturally derived products on coagulation and platelet function. 2010; 663: pp. 229-40.
[http://dx.doi.org/10.1007/978-1-60761-803-4_9]

[24]   Vilahur G, Badimon L. Antiplatelet properties of natural products. Vascul Pharmacol 2013; 59(3-4): 67-75.
[http://dx.doi.org/10.1016/j.vph.2013.08.002] [PMID: 23994642]

[25]   Chin Y-W, Balunas MJ, Chai HB, Kinghorn AD. Drug discovery from natural sources. AAPS J 2006;

8(2): E239-53.
[http://dx.doi.org/10.1007/BF02854894] [PMID: 16796374]

[26]   Chen C, Yang F-Q, Zhang Q, Wang F-Q, Hu Y-J, Xia Z-N. Natural products for antithrombosis. Evid Based Complement Alternat Med 2015; 2015: 876426.
[http://dx.doi.org/10.1155/2015/876426]

[27]   Karantonis HC, Antonopoulou S, Demopoulos CA. Antithrombotic lipid minor constituents from vegetable oils. Comparison between olive oils and others. J Agric Food Chem 2002; 50(5): 1150-60.
[http://dx.doi.org/10.1021/jf010923t] [PMID: 11853496]

[28]   Barzkar N, Tamadoni Jahromi S, Poorsaheli HB, Vianello F. Metabolites from marine microorganisms, micro, and macroalgae: Immense scope for pharmacology. Mar Drugs 2019; 17(8)E464
[http://dx.doi.org/10.3390/md17080464] [PMID: 31398953]

[29]   Diers JA, Ivey KD, El-Alfy A, *et al.* Identification of antidepressant drug leads through the evaluation of marine natural products with neuropsychiatric pharmacophores. Pharmacol Biochem Behav 2008; 89(1): 46-53.
[http://dx.doi.org/10.1016/j.pbb.2007.10.021] [PMID: 18037479]

[30]   Khotimchenko Y. Pharmacological potential of sea cucumbers. Int J Mol Sci 2018; 19(5): 1342.
[http://dx.doi.org/10.3390/ijms19051342] [PMID: 29724051]

[31]   Ruocco N, Costantini S, Guariniello S, Costantini M. Polysaccharides from the Marine Environment with Pharmacological, Cosmeceutical and Nutraceutical Potential. Molecules 2016; 21(5)E551
[http://dx.doi.org/10.3390/molecules21050551] [PMID: 27128892]

[32]   Molinski TF, Dalisay DS, Lievens SL, Saludes JP. Drug development from marine natural products. Nat Rev Drug Discov 2009; 8(1): 69-85.
[http://dx.doi.org/10.1038/nrd2487] [PMID: 19096380]

[33]   Li G, Guo J, Wang Z, Liu Y, Song H, Wang Q. Marine natural products for drug discovery: first discovery of kealiinines a-c and their derivatives as novel antiviral and antiphytopathogenic fungus agents. J Agric Food Chem 2018; 66(28): 7310-8.
[http://dx.doi.org/10.1021/acs.jafc.8b02238] [PMID: 29975055]

[34]   Thangaraj S, Bragadeeswaran S, Gokula V. Bioactive compounds of sea anemones: a review. Int J Pept Res Ther 2019; 25(4): 1405-16.
[http://dx.doi.org/10.1007/s10989-018-9786-6]

[35]   Mayer AMS, Rodríguez AD, Taglialatela-Scafati O, Fusetani N. Marine pharmacology in 2012-2013: marine compounds with antibacterial, antidiabetic, antifungal, anti-inflammatory, antiprotozoal, antituberculosis, and antiviral activities; affecting the immune and nervous systems, and other miscellaneous mechanisms of action. Mar Drugs 2017; 15(9): 273.
[http://dx.doi.org/10.3390/md15090273] [PMID: 28850074]

[36]   Faioli CN, Domingos TFS, de Oliveira EC, *et al.* Appraisal of antiophidic potential of marine sponges against Bothrops jararaca and Lachesis muta venom. Toxins (Basel) 2013; 5(10): 1799-813.
[http://dx.doi.org/10.3390/toxins5101799] [PMID: 24141284]

[37]   Moura LA, Ortiz-Ramirez F, Cavalcanti DN, *et al.* Evaluation of marine brown algae and sponges from Brazil as anticoagulant and antiplatelet products. Mar Drugs 2011; 9(8): 1346-58.
[http://dx.doi.org/10.3390/md9081346] [PMID: 32143544]

[38]   Mohy El-Din SM, Alagawany NI. Phytochemical constituents and anticoagulation property of marine algae gelidium crinale, sargassum hornschuchii and ulva linza. Thalassas 2019; 35(2): 381-97.
[http://dx.doi.org/10.1007/s41208-019-00142-6]

[39]   Carvalhal F, Cristelo RR, Resende DISP, Pinto MMM, Sousa E, Correia-da-Silva M. Antithrombotics from the sea: polysaccharides and beyond. Mar Drugs 2019; 17(3): 170.
[http://dx.doi.org/10.3390/md17030170] [PMID: 30884850]

[40]   Valcarcel J, Novoa-Carballal R, Pérez-Martín RI, Reis RL, Vázquez JA. Glycosaminoglycans from marine sources as therapeutic agents. Biotechnol Adv 2017; 35(6): 711-25.
[http://dx.doi.org/10.1016/j.biotechadv.2017.07.008] [PMID: 28739506]

[41]   Cheung RCF, Ng TB, Wong JH. Marine peptides: bioactivities and applications. Mar Drugs 2015; 13(7): 4006-43.
[http://dx.doi.org/10.3390/md13074006] [PMID: 26132844]

[42]   de Jesus Raposo MF, de Morais AMB, de Morais RMSC. Marine polysaccharides from algae with potential biomedical applications. Mar Drugs 2015; 13(5): 2967-3028.
[http://dx.doi.org/10.3390/md13052967] [PMID: 25988519]

[43]   Giordano D, Costantini M, Coppola D, et al. Biotechnological applications of bioactive peptides from marine sources. Adv Microb Physiol 2018; 73: 171-220.
[http://dx.doi.org/10.1016/bs.ampbs.2018.05.002] [PMID: 30262109]

[44]   da Silva GA, Domingos TFS, Fonseca RR, Sanchez EF, Teixeira VL, Fuly AL. The red seaweed Plocamium brasiliense shows anti-snake venom toxic effects. J Venom Anim Toxins Incl Trop Dis 2015; 21(1): 2.
[http://dx.doi.org/10.1186/s40409-015-0002-2] [PMID: 25699078]

[45]   de Andrade Moura L, Marqui de Almeida AC, Domingos TFS, et al. Antiplatelet and anticoagulant effects of diterpenes isolated from the marine alga, Dictyota menstrualis. Mar Drugs 2014; 12(5): 2471-84.
[http://dx.doi.org/10.3390/md12052471] [PMID: 24796305]

[46]   Wijesinghe W a. JP, Athukorala Y, Jeon Y-J. Effect of anticoagulative sulfated polysaccharide purified from enzyme-assistant extract of a brown seaweed Ecklonia cava on Wistar rats. Carbohydr Polym 2011; 86(2): 917-21.
[http://dx.doi.org/10.1016/j.carbpol.2011.05.047]

[47]   de Andrade Moura L, Bianco ÉM, Pereira RC, Teixeira VL, Fuly AL. Anticoagulation and antiplatelet effects of a dolastane diterpene isolated from the marine brown alga Canistrocarpus cervicornis. J Thromb Thrombolysis 2011; 31(2): 235-40.
[http://dx.doi.org/10.1007/s11239-010-0545-6] [PMID: 21210185]

[48]   Buchanan MS, Carroll AR, Wessling D, et al. Clavatadine A, a natural product with selective recognition and irreversible inhibition of factor XIa. J Med Chem 2008; 51(12): 3583-7.
[http://dx.doi.org/10.1021/jm800314b] [PMID: 18510371]

[49]   Mohammed BM, Matafonov A, Ivanov I, et al. An update on factor XI structure and function. Thromb Res 2018; 161: 94-105.
[http://dx.doi.org/10.1016/j.thromres.2017.10.008] [PMID: 29223926]

[50]   Roll DM, Ireland CM, Lu HSM, Clardy J. Fascaplysin, an unusual antimicrobial pigment from the marine sponge Fascaplysinopsis sp. J Org Chem 1988; 53(14): 3276-8.
[http://dx.doi.org/10.1021/jo00249a025]

[51]   Ampofo E, Später T, Müller I, Eichler H, Menger MD, Laschke MW. The marine-derived kinase inhibitor fascaplysin exerts anti-thrombotic activity. Mar Drugs 2015; 13(11): 6774-91.
[http://dx.doi.org/10.3390/md13116774] [PMID: 26569265]

[52]   Syed AA, Venkatraman KL, Mehta A. An anticoagulant peptide from Porphyra yezoensis inhibits the activity of factor XIIa: In vitro and in silico analysis. J Mol Graph Model 2019; 89: 225-33.
[http://dx.doi.org/10.1016/j.jmgm.2019.03.019] [PMID: 30921556]

[53]   Yin R, Zhou L, Gao N, z Li, L Zhao , F Shang , et al. Oligosaccharides from depolymerized fucosylated glycosaminoglycan: structures and minimum size for intrinsic factor Xase complex inhibition. J Biol Chem. 2018 Jul 20;jbc.RA118.003809. 2018.

[54]   Restrepo-Espinosa DC, Román Y, Colorado-Ríos J, et al. Structural analysis of a sulfated galactan from the tunic of the ascidian Microcosmus exasperatus and its inhibitory effect of the intrinsic

coagulation pathway. Int J Biol Macromol 2017; 105(Pt 2): 1391-400.
[http://dx.doi.org/10.1016/j.ijbiomac.2017.08.166] [PMID: 28867226]

[55]   Demain AL, Sanchez S. Microbial drug discovery: 80 years of progress. J Antibiot (Tokyo) 2009; 62(1): 5-16.
[http://dx.doi.org/10.1038/ja.2008.16] [PMID: 19132062]

[56]   Yang C, Kwon S, Kim S-J, *et al.* Identification of indothiazinone as a natural antiplatelet agent. Chem Biol Drug Des 2017; 90(5): 873-82.
[http://dx.doi.org/10.1111/cbdd.13008] [PMID: 28432753]

[57]   Jansen R, Mohr KI, Bernecker S, Stadler M, Müller R. Indothiazinone, an indolyl thiazolyl ketone from a novel myxobacterium belonging to the Sorangiineae. J Nat Prod 2014; 77(4): 1054-60.
[http://dx.doi.org/10.1021/np500144t] [PMID: 24697522]

[58]   Wang G, Wu W, Zhu Q, Fu S, Wang X, Hong S, *et al.* Identification and fibrinolytic evaluation of an isoindolone derivative isolated from a rare marine fungus *Stachybotrys longispora* FG216. Chin J Chem 2015; 33(9): 1089-95.
[http://dx.doi.org/10.1002/cjoc.201500176]

[59]   Schreuder H, Liesum A, Lönze P, *et al.* Isolation, co-crystallization and structure-based characterization of anabaenopeptins as highly potent inhibitors of activated thrombin activatable fibrinolysis inhibitor (TAFIa). Sci Rep 2016; 6: 32958.
[http://dx.doi.org/10.1038/srep32958] [PMID: 27604544]

[60]   Zafrir E, Carmeli S. Micropeptins from an Israeli fishpond water bloom of the cyanobacterium Microcystis sp. J Nat Prod 2010; 73(3): 352-8.
[http://dx.doi.org/10.1021/np900546u] [PMID: 20028081]

[61]   Zafrir-Ilan E, Carmeli S. Eight novel serine proteases inhibitors from a water bloom of the cyanobacterium Microcystis sp. Tetrahedron 2010; 66(47): 9194-202.
[http://dx.doi.org/10.1016/j.tet.2010.09.067]

[62]   Hasan-Amer R, Carmeli S. Inhibitors of serine proteases from a microcystis sp. bloom material collected from timurim reservoir, Israel. Mar Drugs 2017; 15(12)E371
[http://dx.doi.org/10.3390/md15120371] [PMID: 29194403]

[63]   Anas ARJ, Mori A, Tone M, *et al.* FVIIa-sTF and thrombin inhibitory activities of compounds isolated from *Microcystis aeruginosa* K-139. Mar Drugs 2017; 15(9): 275.
[http://dx.doi.org/10.3390/md15090275] [PMID: 28867804]

[64]   Gao P, Li S, Liu K, Sun C, Song S, Li L. Antiplatelet aggregation and antithrombotic benefits of terpenes and flavones from hawthorn leaf extract isolated using the activity-guided method. Food Funct 2019; 10(2): 859-66.
[http://dx.doi.org/10.1039/C8FO01862F] [PMID: 30681694]

[65]   Gao P-Y, Li L-Z, Liu K-C, Sun C, Sun X, Wu Y-N, *et al.* Natural terpenoid glycosides with *in vitro/vivo* antithrombotic profiles from the leaves of Crataegus pinnatifida. RSC Advances 2017; 7(76): 48466-74.
[http://dx.doi.org/10.1039/C7RA10768D]

[66]   Zhou C-C, Huang X-X, Gao P-Y, *et al.* Two new compounds from Crataegus pinnatifida and their antithrombotic activities. J Asian Nat Prod Res 2014; 16(2): 169-74.
[http://dx.doi.org/10.1080/10286020.2013.848429] [PMID: 24161196]

[67]   Wang C, Wu Y-B, Wang A-P, Jiang J-D, Kong W-J. Evaluation of anticoagulant and antithrombotic activities of berberine: a focus on the ameliorative effect on blood hypercoagulation. Int J Pharmacol 2018; 14(8): 1087-98.
[http://dx.doi.org/10.3923/ijp.2018.1087.1098]

[68]   Zhang Q, Wang Y-L, Gao D, *et al.* Comparing coagulation activity of *Selaginella tamariscina* before and after stir-frying process and determining the possible active constituents based on compositional

variation. Pharm Biol 2018; 56(1): 67-75.
[http://dx.doi.org/10.1080/13880209.2017.1421673] [PMID: 29295657]

[69]   Lee W, Bae J-S. Antithrombotic and antiplatelet activities of orientin *in vitro* and *in vivo*. J Funct Foods 2015; 17: 388-98.
[http://dx.doi.org/10.1016/j.jff.2015.05.037]

[70]   Lee J-H, Kim M, Chang K-H, *et al.* Antiplatelet effects of *Rhus verniciflua* stokes heartwood and its active constituents--fisetin, butein, and sulfuretin--in rats. J Med Food 2015; 18(1): 21-30.
[http://dx.doi.org/10.1089/jmf.2013.3116] [PMID: 25372471]

[71]   Chen X-Q, Wang X-B, Guan R-F, *et al.* Blood anticoagulation and antiplatelet activity of green tea (-)-epigallocatechin (EGC) in mice. Food Funct 2013; 4(10): 1521-5.
[http://dx.doi.org/10.1039/c3fo60088b] [PMID: 24056410]

[72]   Lee W, Bae J-S. Antithrombotic and antiplatelet activities of vicenin-2. Blood Coagul Fibrinolysis 2015; 26(6): 628-34.
[http://dx.doi.org/10.1097/MBC.0000000000000320] [PMID: 26126169]

[73]   Yoon E-K, Ku S-K, Lee W, *et al.* Antitcoagulant and antiplatelet activities of scolymoside. BMB Rep 2015; 48(10): 577-82.
[http://dx.doi.org/10.5483/BMBRep.2015.48.10.044] [PMID: 25887749]

[74]   Rodrigues CFB, Gaeta HH, Belchor MN, *et al.* Evaluation of Potential Thrombin Inhibitors from the White Mangrove (Laguncularia racemosa (L.) C.F. Gaertn.). Mar Drugs 2015; 13(7): 4505-19.
[http://dx.doi.org/10.3390/md13074505] [PMID: 26197325]

[75]   Ku S-K, Yoon E-K, Lee W, Kwon S, Lee T, Bae J-S. Antithrombotic and antiplatelet activities of pelargonidin *in vivo* and *in vitro*. Arch Pharm Res 2016; 39(3): 398-408.
[http://dx.doi.org/10.1007/s12272-016-0708-x] [PMID: 26762345]

[76]   Lee W, Ku S-K, Kim M-A, Bae J-S. Anti-factor Xa activities of zingerone with anti-platelet aggregation activity. Food Chem Toxicol 2017; 105: 186-93.
[http://dx.doi.org/10.1016/j.fct.2017.04.012] [PMID: 28414123]

[77]   Huang C-H, Chan Y-Y, Kuo P-C, *et al.* The constituents of roots and stems of Illigera luzonensis and their anti-platelet aggregation effects. Int J Mol Sci 2014; 15(8): 13424-36.
[http://dx.doi.org/10.3390/ijms150813424] [PMID: 25089876]

[78]   Choi J-H, Kim S. Mechanisms of attenuation of clot formation and acute thromboembolism by syringic acid in mice. J Funct Foods 2018; 43: 112-22.
[http://dx.doi.org/10.1016/j.jff.2018.02.004]

[79]   Veach D, Hosking H, Thompson K, Santhakumar AB. Anti-platelet and anti-thrombogenic effects of shikimic acid in sedentary population. Food Funct 2016; 7(8): 3609-16.
[http://dx.doi.org/10.1039/C6FO00927A] [PMID: 27480079]

[80]   Zhang HY, Liu H, Yang M, Wei SF. Antithrombotic activities of aqueous extract from *Gardenia jasminoides* and its main constituent. Pharm Biol 2013; 51(2): 221-5.
[http://dx.doi.org/10.3109/13880209.2012.717088] [PMID: 23116215]

[81]   Dahmer T, Berger M, Barlette AG, *et al.* Antithrombotic effect of chikusetsusaponin IVa isolated from *Ilex paraguariensis* (Maté). J Med Food 2012; 15(12): 1073-80.
[http://dx.doi.org/10.1089/jmf.2011.0320] [PMID: 23134458]

[82]   Yang C, An Q, Xiong Z, Song Y, Yu K, Li F. Triterpenes from *Acanthopanax sessiliflorus* fruits and their antiplatelet aggregation activities. Planta Med 2009; 75(6): 656-9.
[http://dx.doi.org/10.1055/s-0029-1185330] [PMID: 19263344]

[83]   Shi Y-M, Wang X-B, Li X-N, *et al.* Lancolides, antiplatelet aggregation nortriterpenoids with tricyclo[6.3.0.0$^{(2,11)}$]undecane-bridged system from *Schisandra lancifolia*. Org Lett 2013; 15(19): 5068-71.
[http://dx.doi.org/10.1021/ol402414z] [PMID: 24059675]

[84]   Ku S-K, Kim JA, Han C-K, Bae J-S. Antithrombotic activities of *epi*-sesamin *in vitro* and *in vivo*. Am J Chin Med 2013; 41(6): 1313-27.
[http://dx.doi.org/10.1142/S0192415X13500882] [PMID: 24228603]

[85]   Shi Y-N, Shi Y-M, Yang L, *et al.* Lignans and aromatic glycosides from Piper wallichii and their antithrombotic activities. J Ethnopharmacol 2015; 162: 87-96.
[http://dx.doi.org/10.1016/j.jep.2014.12.038] [PMID: 25555357]

[86]   Qu W, Xue J, Wu FH, Liang JY. Lignans from Saururus chinensis with Antiplatelet Aggregation and Neuroprotective Activities. Chem Nat Compd 2014; 50(5): 814-8.
[http://dx.doi.org/10.1007/s10600-014-1090-x]

[87]   Shin W, Oh S, Lee S. Synthesis of Substituted Farnesyl Acetone Derivatives and their Inhibitory Activity against Platelet Aggregation. Bull Korean Chem Soc 2019; 40(6): 602-5.
[http://dx.doi.org/10.1002/bkcs.11726]

[88]   Liu J, Sun B, Zhao X, *et al.* Discovery of Potent Orally Active Protease-Activated Receptor 1 (PAR1) Antagonists Based on Andrographolide. J Med Chem 2017; 60(16): 7166-85.
[http://dx.doi.org/10.1021/acs.jmedchem.7b00951] [PMID: 28745507]

[89]   Wang J, Wu M, Gao C, Fu H. Semisynthesis of epoxy-pimarane diterpenoids from kirenol and their FXa inhibition activities. Bioorg Med Chem 2019; 27(7): 1320-6.
[http://dx.doi.org/10.1016/j.bmc.2019.02.032] [PMID: 30792102]

[90]   Wang J, Ma H, Fu H. Semisynthesis of ent-norstrobane diterpenoids as potential inhibitor for factor Xa. Bioorg Med Chem Lett 2018; 28(23-24): 3813-5.
[http://dx.doi.org/10.1016/j.bmcl.2018.05.036] [PMID: 30340898]

[91]   Žula A, Będziak I, Kikelj D, Ilaš J. Synthesis and Evaluation of Spumigin Analogues Library with Thrombin Inhibitory Activity. Mar Drugs 2018; 16(11): 413.
[http://dx.doi.org/10.3390/md16110413] [PMID: 30373260]

[92]   Halland N, Brönstrup M, Czech J, *et al.* Novel Small Molecule Inhibitors of Activated Thrombin Activatable Fibrinolysis Inhibitor (TAFIa) from Natural Product Anabaenopeptin. J Med Chem 2015; 58(11): 4839-44.
[http://dx.doi.org/10.1021/jm501840b] [PMID: 25990761]

[93]   Sharma V, Jaiswal PK, Kumar K, *et al.* An efficient synthesis and biological evaluation of novel analogues of natural product Cephalandole A: A new class of antimicrobial and antiplatelet agents. Fitoterapia 2018; 129: 13-9.
[http://dx.doi.org/10.1016/j.fitote.2018.06.003] [PMID: 29894738]

[94]   Hanessian S, Therrien E, Zhang J, *et al.* From natural products to achiral drug prototypes: potent thrombin inhibitors based on P2/P3 dihydropyrid-2-one core motifs. Bioorg Med Chem Lett 2009; 19(18): 5429-32.
[http://dx.doi.org/10.1016/j.bmcl.2009.07.107] [PMID: 19674897]

[95]   de Paula FT, Frauches PQ, Pedebos C, *et al.* Improving the thrombin inhibitory activity of glycyrrhizin, a triterpenic saponin, through a molecular simplification of the carbohydrate moiety. Chem Biol Drug Des 2013; 82(6): 756-60.
[http://dx.doi.org/10.1111/cbdd.12204] [PMID: 23964664]

[96]   Chapado L, Linares-Palomino PJ, Salido S, Altarejos J, Rosado JA, Salido GM. Synthesis and evaluation of the platelet antiaggregant properties of phenolic antioxidants structurally related to rosmarinic acid. Bioorg Chem 2010; 38(3): 108-14.
[http://dx.doi.org/10.1016/j.bioorg.2009.12.001] [PMID: 20042216]

[97]   Del Turco S, Sartini S, Cigni G, *et al.* Synthetic analogues of flavonoids with improved activity against platelet activation and aggregation as novel prototypes of food supplements. Food Chem 2015; 175: 494-9.
[http://dx.doi.org/10.1016/j.foodchem.2014.12.005] [PMID: 25577111]

[98]   Petek BJ, Loggers ET, Pollack SM, Jones RL. Trabectedin in soft tissue sarcomas. Mar Drugs 2015; 13(2): 974-83.
[http://dx.doi.org/10.3390/md13020974] [PMID: 25686274]

[99]   Wermuth CG, Ed. The practice of medicinal chemistry. Amsterdam: Elsevier, Academic Press 2015.

[100] Karle M, Knecht W, Xue Y. Discovery of benzothiazole guanidines as novel inhibitors of thrombin and trypsin IV. Bioorg Med Chem Lett 2012; 22(14): 4839-43.
[http://dx.doi.org/10.1016/j.bmcl.2012.05.046] [PMID: 22726924]

Transient Receptor Potential Channels: Therapeutic Targets for Cardiometabolic Diseases?

Leidyanne Ferreira Gonçalves, Thereza Cristina Lonzetti Bargut and **Caroline Fernandes-Santos**[*]

Instituto de Saude de Nova Friburgo, Universidade Federal Fluminense, Nova Friburgo, Rio de Janeiro, Brazil

Abstract: Transient receptor potential (TRP) channels are ubiquitously expressed cellular sensors that respond to changes in the cellular environment. They act in nociception, taste perception, thermosensation, mechanosensing, osmolarity sensing, and signal transduction. Mammalian TRP channels comprise 28 members divided into six subfamilies: TRPA (ankyrin), TRPC (canonical), TRPM (melastatin), TRPML (mucolipin), TRPP (polycystin) and TRPV (vanilloid). TRP mutations that result in either gain or loss of function have been linked to several human diseases, among them hypertension, cardiac hypertrophy, obesity, and diabetes. In the myocardium, TRP channels modulate Ca^{+2} handling and are differentially expressed in models of cardiac remodeling and dysfunction. TRP channels are also involved in insulin release from pancreatic beta-cells and glucose tolerance in rodent models of type 2 diabetes. Some of these channels promote thermogenesis and thus prevent diet-induced obesity. How TRP channels are modulated *in vivo* is still unknown since few endogenous ligands were identified so far. However, a wide range of natural products with therapeutic potential activates TRP channels and might serve as models for new drug discovery and development to prevent cardiometabolic morbidity and mortality. Studies with TRP channels show promising results, but the translation to preventive or therapeutic strategies against cardiometabolic diseases is challenging since they are found in multiple tissues and enrolled in several physiological actions, which increases the risk of adverse effects.

Keywords: Adipose tissue, Cardiovascular diseases, Cardiometabolic syndrome, Heart, Obesity, Pancreas, Type 2 diabetes, Transient receptor potential channels, TRPA1, TRPC, TRPM, TRPV.

INTRODUCTION

Cardiometabolic syndrome (CMS), also known as insulin resistance syndrome,

[*] **Corresponding author Caroline Fernandes-Santos:** Instituto de Saude de Nova Friburgo, Universidade Federal Fluminense, Nova Friburgo, Rio de Janeiro, Brazil; Tel: +55 22 2528 7166; E-mail: cf_santos@id.uff.br

Atta-ur-Rahman & M. Iqbal Choudhary (Eds.)

syndrome X, Reaven's syndrome, and Beer belly syndrome, is recognized as a disease [1] and has been defined in several different ways [2]. However, the consensus is that it is a combination of metabolic disorders, such as insulin resistance, impaired glucose tolerance, systemic arterial hypertension, central obesity, and atherogenic dyslipidemia [1, 3]. Around 25% of the adult population worldwide is reportedly suffering from CMS [4].

CMS is commonly associated with the development of cardiovascular diseases, and as obesity increases worldwide, it has become a global pandemic [3]. The western way of life, characterized by a sedentary lifestyle and the increased consumption of high caloric unhealthy foods, has created a positive energy balance environment, increasing the risk for CMS and cardiometabolic diseases [3]. CMS is a significant public health concern owing to the financial impact of higher hospitalization rates due to comorbidities; it also impacts physical well-being and the quality of life and reduces the workforce. Therefore, it is crucial to develop therapeutic strategies focusing on both CMS risk factors and treatment of comorbidities [3].

Transient Receptor Potential (TRP) channels have been identified as potential candidates for the treatment of many diseases, including the cardiometabolic ones, as over the last 15 years supporting evidence has emerged on their role in cardiovascular and metabolic functions. TRP channels are a group of non-selective ion channel sensors that responds to a broad spectrum of physical and chemical stimuli, playing a role in the physiological process of signal transmission [5]. They are primary targets for both endogenous and exogenous substances with therapeutic potential [6]. However, translation to preventive or therapeutic strategies remains challenging as they are present in multiple tissues and thus, are enrolled in several physiological pathways, increasing the risk of adverse effects [6].

Here, we discuss whether TRP channels present an opportunity to combat cardiometabolic diseases, which are a high cost to governments and affect patient's well-being. Evidence shows that TRP channels are relevant as a therapeutic strategy, with additional research necessary to prove their safety and efficacy.

TRP CHANNELS

Cosens and Manning described the first TRP channel in a *Drosophila melanogaster* mutant [7]. From then, until 2017, 28 mammalian TRP channel proteins have been identified. The TRP superfamily of channels is categorized into six families based on amino acid homologies: ankyrin (TRPA), canonical (TRPC), melastatin (TRPM), mucolipin (TRPML), polycystin (TRPP), and vanilloid (TRPV) [5, 8]. The main structure of the TRP channel subunit has six transmembrane domains (TM1 to TM6) that are assembled as homo- or heterotetramers to form selective cation channels with diverse modes of activation and varied permeation properties [9]. They have distinct pharmacological properties, presenting a challenge in drug development [6, 10].

The TRPA family has only one protein identified (TRPA1). The TRPC family contains seven protein members (TRPC1-7), whereas the TRPM family includes eight members (TRPM1-8). The TRPML family contains three members (TRPML1-3), the TRPV family is comprised of six members (TRPV1-6), and the TRPP family has three proteins (TRPP1, TRPP2, and TRPP3) [5]. There is also a family called TRPN (NO-mechano-potential) found in worms, frogs, zebrafish, and *Drosophila,* with no homologous proteins in mammals [5]. TRP channels can be constitutively open or are activated by intracellular cations [5, 10]. While all TRP channels are permeable to cations, two TRP channels are impermeable to Ca^{2+} (TRPM4, TRPM5), and two others are highly Ca^{2+} permeable (TRPV5, TRPV6) [11].

TRP channels are found in the plasma membrane of distinct cell types, and cellular organelles such as lysosomes, endosomes and endoplasmic reticulum (ER), serving as intracellular ion channels [5]. They are activated in response to a variety of stimuli, including temperature, stretch, pressure, chemicals, oxidation/reduction, osmolarity, and pH, and interact with a range of proteins affecting their activity, location, and trafficking [5, 6]. They play a role in the physiological process of signal transmission [5], and are central elements of nociception, converting noxious stimuli into electrical pain signals [8]. Conversely, dysfunction of TRP channels is involved in various pathological conditions such as bladder disorders, cancer, obesity, type 2 diabetes (T2D), heart diseases, respiratory diseases and chronic pain [5]. The main TRP channels expressed in the cardiovascular system, pancreas, and adipose tissue (AT), which are the main focus of this chapter, are shown in Fig. (**1**).

TRPA (ankyrin) Family

The TRPA1 channel is the only member of this family. This chemo-nociceptor is expressed in neurons, C-fibers, and myelinated Aβ-fibers, making it an ideal target for analgesics. It is also found in non-neuronal cells including epithelial cells, melanocytes, mast cells, fibroblasts, and enterochromaffin cells [12].

The TRPA1 channel is activated by various exogenous and endogenous compounds. The exogenous activator ligands are cysteine and lysine reactive electrophilic molecules like the active compound of mustard oil and wasabi (allyl isothiocyanate), cinnamaldehyde extracted from cinnamon, allicin from garlic extract, acrolein from fume exhaust, cannabidiol, menthol, eugenol, and gingerol (ginger) [12, 13]. Examples of some endogenous activator/ligands are bradykinin, hydrogen peroxide (H_2O_2), prostaglandins and nitrated lipids like nitrooleic acid [8, 12].

TRPC (canonical) Family

The canonical family comprises of nonselective Ca^{2+} permeable plasma membrane channels with varying selectivity [12]. They are expressed in excitable and non-excitable cells, as reviewed by Bon *et al.* [14], and most of the TRPCs are spontaneously active [10]. They form two subgroups based on sequence homology, TRPC1/4/5, and TRPC3/6/7 subgroups. TRPC2 is a pseudogene in humans that is expressed in other mammals, and is allocated into the TRPC3/6/7 subgroup [11]. TRPC channels play important roles in different areas, but their importance has mostly been demonstrated in the kidney, cardiovascular system, lung and brain [15, 16].

They are suggested to be store-operated channels (SOCs) activated by the depletion of intracellular Ca^{2+} stores, activated downstream to $G_q/_{11}$-coupled receptors (GPCRs), or receptor tyrosine kinases [11]. Signals from GPCRs to TRPCs are mediated *via* lipid molecules, which can either change channel activity or influence insertion into the plasma membrane [17]. Most TRPCs are inhibited by a Ca^{2+}/calmodulin (CaM)-dependent mechanism [17].

TRPC1 is a prominent member of this family. It remains unclear if TRPC1 forms homomers, but it does form heteromers with TRPC4 and TRPC5. It is also able to interact with other TRP channels like TRPP2 and TRPV6 [11, 18]. It is found in a wide range of tissues, involved in skeletal muscle differentiation, organism growth and development, immune regulation, tumor cell migration and Parkinson's disease [12]. TRPC1 overexpression in endothelial cells can enhance vascular permeability [5], and TRPC1 and TRPC5 are detected in the perivascular adipose tissue (PVAT), negatively contributing as heteromultimers to adiponectin generation in adipocytes [19].

TRPC4 is a homolog of TRPC5, as they share approximately 64% sequence identity. They can form homomultimers as well as heteromultimers with TRPC1, and TRPC3. TRPC4 is widely expressed in the endothelium, smooth muscle cells, brain, and kidney [20]. On the other hand, TRPC5 is not only widely expressed in the brain, where it participates in the formation of transient working memory and is involved in the amygdala function and fear-related behavior [18], but also in the heart, liver, kidney, lung, and uterus [10, 11]. In blood vessels, TRPC5 channels are involved in endothelial cell sprouting, angiogenesis, blood perfusion, and baroreceptor mechanosensation [21, 22]. Thioredoxin, an important redox protein involved in ischemic-reperfusion injury and inflammation, activates TRPC5 and TRPC1 channels in the reduced form [23]. Examples of TRPC5 activators include rosiglitazone (an agonist of peroxisome proliferator-activated receptor-γ [PPARγ]), genistein and daidzein (soy phytoestrogens), and nitric oxide [24]. While ML204 is an exogenous TRPC4 antagonist [6], the TRPC5 ligands with inhibitory action are progesterone and galangin, a flavonoid [8, 11]. A recent study suggested that the TRPC1 channel is a negative regulator of TRPC4/5 since the co-expression of TRPC1 dramatically reduces Ca^{2+} influx through either TRPC4 or TRPC5 homomeric channels [25].

Regarding the TRPC3/6/7 subgroup, TRPC3 is closely related to TRPC6 and TRPC7 (75% of sequence identity), and these channels form both homomultimers and heteromultimers activated by diacylglycerols, with mechanical stretch further activating TRPC6. TRPC3 is expressed in specific regions of the brain, and in the heart [18]. It is also minimally detected in the ovary, colon, small intestine, lung, prostate, placenta, and testis [10]. TRPC6 and TRPC7 are expressed in the retina, and participate in light perception [26]. Furthermore, the kidney and pituitary gland also express TRPC7 [18].

TRPM (melastatin) Family

The TRPM family is implicated in tumorigenesis, proliferation, and differentiation. They are also involved in temperature sensation, magnesium (Mg^{2+}) homeostasis, and taste, and have different modes of activation, cation selectivity, and tissue distribution [12]. They form five subgroups based on sequence homology: TRPM1/3, TRPM2, TRPM4/5, TRPM6/7, and TRPM8 [11].

TRPM1 is expressed in the brain [5], melanocytes, macrophages, and heart, and is a tumor suppressor and a potential prognostic marker for metastatic melanomas [12]. TRPM1 is activated by pregnenolone sulfate, and inhibited by zinc (Zn^{2+}) [11]. On the other hand, TRPM3 channels are expressed in pancreatic beta cells, as well as the brain, pituitary gland, eye, kidney and AT [27, 28]. TRPM3 is activated by sphingolipids, pregnenolone sulfate, and nifedipine [6]. Hypotonic cell swelling and heat (15-25°C) also stimulates this receptor, making it an important mediator of heat sensation in the somatosensory system [12]. TRPM3 channels are blocked by some PPARγ agonists (*e.g.*, rosiglitazone) [29], and naringenin, a flavonoid found in grapefruit and tomato [11].

TRPM2 is a bifunctional protein; it is a cation permeable channel, and also contains functional enzymatic domains on its C-terminal segment. Its endogenous ligands include adenosine diphosphate (ADP) ribose [30], and cyclic ADP ribose (cADP-ribose) [31]. Furthermore, TRPM2 can be chemically activated by reactive oxygen (ROS) and nitrogen species, and physically activated by heat (~35°C)

[11]. TRPM2 is widely expressed, with highest levels detected in the brain, macrophages, and bone marrow [12]. In pancreatic β-cells, TRPM2 is involved in the regulation of insulin secretion [32]. Evidence suggests that this channel is involved in the pathogenesis of bipolar disorders, T2D, cardiovascular, and neurodegenerative diseases [6].

Unlike other TRP channels, TRPM4 and TRPM5 are impermeable to Ca^{2+} and share 40% homology. Since they are permeable to monovalent cations such as sodium (Na^+) and potassium (K^+), these channels are considered Ca^{2+} activated non-specific cation channels. TRPM4 is ubiquitously found throughout the body in tissues such as the heart, brain, skeletal muscle, and AT, and enrolled in cardiac conductance, neurological disturbances, and proinflammatory conditions [11]. TRPM5 is highly expressed in the intestines and taste buds, where it is a transducer of bitter, sweet, and umami taste sensations [12]. Additionally, TRPM5 participates in the regulation of insulin secretion by the pancreatic β-cells [32]. TRPM4 has 3,5-bis(trifluoromethyl)pyrazole derivative BTP2 as an exogenous agonist [33], and 9-phenanthrol as an exogenous antagonist [34], whereas triphenylphosphine oxide is a TRPM5 channel antagonist [35].

TRPM6 and TRPM7 are also bifunctional proteins that form heteromeric channels, and share 50% homology. They are permeable to Mg^{2+}, Zn^{2+}, and Ca^{2+}, playing a role in cellular Mg^{2+} homeostasis. TRPM6 is present in the intestines mediating dietary Mg^{2+} uptake, in the brain, pituitary, and kidney (Mg^{2+} reabsorption), whereas TRPM7 is ubiquitously expressed, especially in the heart, pituitary, bone and AT [12]. TRPM7 is involved in anoxia-induced cell death, transmitter release and embryonic and cardiac morphogenesis [36 - 39]. Mg^{2+} and Ca^{2+} act as TRPM6 and TRPM7 channel blockers [40], while sphingosine [41], carvacrol [42], and waixenicin A are antagonists [43]. Phosphatidylinositol (4,5)-bisphosphate (PIP_2) is a TRPM7 agonist [44].

Finally, TRPM8 is found in the white (WAT) [45] and brown adipose tissue (BAT) [46], and mostly known for thermosensation, but is also involved in pain sensation, bladder function, and cancer [5, 12]. Cold temperatures below 26°C activate TRPM8, and agonists shift temperature sensitivity towards warmer temperatures [47]. It has several ligands, including eucalyptol, icilin, menthol, hydroxycitronellal (exogenous activators), linoleic acid, anandamide (endogenous channel blocker), Δ^9-tetrahydrocannabinol and cannabidiol (exogenous channel blockers), and elismetrep and capsazepine which are synthetic antagonists [6, 8, 11].

TRPML (mucolipin) Family

The mucolipin TRPML family consists of three members, TRPML1, TRPML2, and TRPML3, which can form homomultimers and heteromultimers [12]. TRPMLs are activated by phosphatidyl (3,5) inositol bisphosphate [PI(3,5)P2] and high pH [11]. They are mostly expressed in intracellular vesicles instead of the plasma membrane, and contain targeting motifs for the ER and lysosomes/endosomes [5], and are thus involved in vesicular trafficking events [12].

Mucolipidosis IV is an autosomal recessive lysosomal storage disease, caused by a TRPML1 mutation leading to defective lysosomal function. This channel is ubiquitously expressed, and is involved in membrane trafficking, signal transduction, and late endosome and lysosome ion homeostasis [12]. So far, TRPML2 and TRPML3 have not been implicated in human disease. However, decreased TRPML2 and TRPML3 gene expression has been reported in metabolic syndrome patients [48]. TRPML2 is found in lymphoid and myeloid tissues, with TRPML3 demonstrating higher expression levels in the endocrine system and the kidneys, intestines, and lungs [12].

TRPP (polycystin) Family

This family only contains three members, namely TRPP1, TRPP2, and TRPP3. TRPP1 is a cation channel that forms heteromultimers with the TRPC1 channel. It is widely distributed, with high levels in the kidney, and its mutation attributed to the autosomal dominant polycystic kidney disease 2, affecting 1 in 400-1,000 humans [12]. Furthermore, TRPP2 seems to play a role in kidney and liver function [5]. It is involved in cellular functions, including fertilization, proliferation, mechanosensation, and polarity. Finally, TRPP3 is expressed in neurons, testis, kidney, and non-myocyte cardiac tissue [12]. TRPP channels are activated by ATP [49], and intracellular Ca^{2+} (TRPP1) [50], however TRPP3 ligands need to be investigated.

TRPV (vanilloid) Family

This family name was attributed to the first activation member capsaicin, a vanilloid-like molecule. Members of the TRPV family are divided into TRPV1-4 and TRPV5/6 subgroups. Despite the similarity between them, not all members respond to temperature stimuli. TRPV1-4 have nonselective cation conducting pores, while TRPV5 and TRPV6 are Ca^{2+} selective channels [12].

TRPV1 is the most studied, and well characterized mammalian TRP channel [12]. It forms homomultimers and heteromultimers with TRPV2 and TRPV3. Some examples of tissue expression include the dorsal root neurons, brain, kidney, pancreas, and liver [11]. TRPV1 channels are also expressed in the visceral and subcutaneous WAT [51] and BAT, where they play a role in WAT browning, maintain BAT function, and regulate adipogenesis and inflammation [52 - 54]. They are also expressed in monocytes, macrophages, dendritic cells, lymphocytes, natural killer cells, and neutrophils, playing a pivotal role in inflammation and immunity [55]. TRPV1 is activated by a broad range of endogenous and exogenous agonists like capsaicin, resiniferatoxin, anandamide, allicin, camphor, temperature above 42-43°C, and extracellular protons, making it essential for thermal and chemical nociception [8, 12]. Examples of TRPV1 antagonists include resolvin D2 (endogenous) [56], capsazepine [57], iodo-resiniferatoxin [58] and thapsigargin (exogenous) [59].

TRPV2 is expressed on neuronal and non-neuronal tissues, and is involved in physiological processes and diseases involving nerve growth, and cancer [12]. The endogenous agonists include lysophosphatidylcholine and lysophos-phatidylinositol, while exogenous agonists include cannabidiol, 2-aminoethoxy-diphenyl borate (2-APB), probenecid, and temperature higher than 52°C [6, 60]. Furthermore, tranilast and SKF96365 have been reported as TRPV2 channel blockers [60, 61].

TRPV3 and TRPV4 play a controversial role in thermosensation, however it is well known that TRPV3 is expressed in high levels on skin keratinocytes, and in the oral cavity and gastrointestinal tract. Meanwhile, TRPV4 has different patterns of expression in the body, and responds to both osmotic changes in the cellular environment and mechanical stress, playing a role in osmoregulation and mechanotransduction [12]. TRPV3 is activated by several agonists, for instance, vanillin, cinnamaldehyde, citral, carvacrol, cannabidiol, eugenol, camphor, and menthol, whereas TRPV4 agonists include phorbol 12-myristate 13-acetate, 5,6-epoxyeicosatrienoic acid, and citric acid [6, 8]. Examples of TRPV3 endogenous antagonists include isopentenyl pyrophosphate [62] and resolvin D1 [63], and GRC15300 is an exogenous antagonist [64]. TRPV4 antagonists include resolvin D1 (endogenous) [63], HC-067047 [65], RN-1734 [66] and GSK2193874 (exogenous) [67].

TRPV5 and TRPV6 are distinct from the other TRP channels as they are constitutively active and highly Ca^{2+} selective, contributing to Ca^{2+} homeostasis in the body. They are present in the apical membrane of epithelial cells, and act as active channels when expressed on the plasma membrane. To prevent Ca^{2+} poisoning, these channels are inactivated in the presence of high Ca^{2+} levels [12]. The parathyroid hormone, 17β-estradiol, and 1,25-dihydroxy vitamin D (3) directly activate TRPV5, and also induce its expression [68, 69].

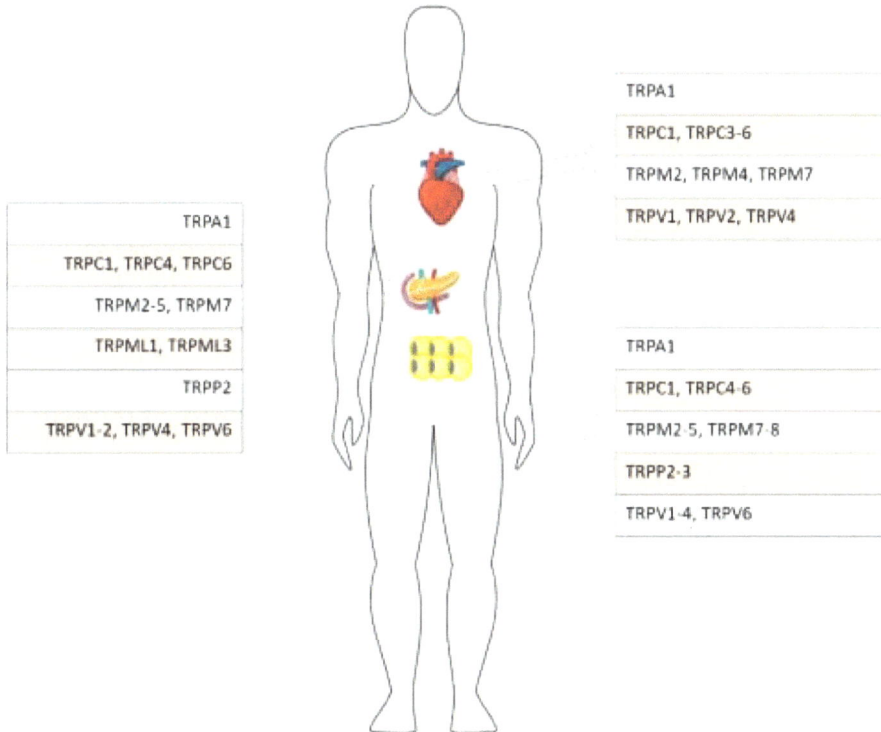

| TRPA1 |
| TRPC1, TRPC3-6 |
| TRPM2, TRPM4, TRPM7 |
| TRPV1, TRPV2, TRPV4 |

| TRPA1 |
| TRPC1, TRPC4, TRPC6 |
| TRPM2-5, TRPM7 |
| TRPML1, TRPML3 |
| TRPP2 |
| TRPV1-2, TRPV4, TRPV6 |

| TRPA1 |
| TRPC1, TRPC4-6 |
| TRPM2-5, TRPM7-8 |
| TRPP2-3 |
| TRPV1-4, TRPV6 |

Fig. (1). TRP channels expression. TRP channels are differentially expressed in the cardiovascular system, adipose tissue and endocrine pancreas. Although their expression in these tissues was already described, the roles of several TRP channels are yet to be fully understood. Abbreviations: TRP, transient receptor potential; TRPA1, transient receptor potential ankyrin 1; TRPC, transient receptor potential canonical; TRPM, transient receptor potential melastatin; TRPML, transient receptor potential mucolipin; TRPP, transient receptor potential polycystin; and TRPV, transient receptor potential vanilloid.

TRP CHANNELS AND CARDIOVASCULAR DISEASES

Cardiac remodeling is commonly associated with chronic hemodynamic alterations. Pathological cardiac hypertrophy can cause sudden death, and is the leading predictor for the development of heart failure (HF) [70]. Mechanical stress over the heart chambers is sensed by the cardiomyocytes and fibroblasts, which adapt through hypertrophy and matrix remodeling, in response to factors such as angiotensin II (Ang II), endothelin 1 (ET-1) and transforming growth factor-β (TGF-β). Abnormal Ca^{2+} handling, characterized by elevated intracellular diastolic Ca^{2+} levels, is noted in cardiac hypertrophy and HF, leading to impairment of the heart contractile function [71]. This response is partly mediated by the Ca^{2+}-activated protein phosphatase calcineurin, which in turn triggers the activation of the transcription factor nuclear factor of activated T cells (NFAT), modulating the expression of hypertrophic genes [72].

TRP Expression

The presence of TRP channels has been demonstrated in cardiac myocytes, fibroblasts, endothelial cells, and vascular smooth muscle cells [73 - 76]. Its expression has been demonstrated in several models of cardiac hypertrophy and fibrosis, hypoxia-induced oxidative stress, hypertrophy and fibrosis, myocardial infarction (MI) and HF. TRP channels modulate the action of some neurohumoral factors such as Ang II, ET-1, and norepinephrine. In vasculature, TRP channels are involved in nitric oxide (NO) release, oxidative stress, endothelial damage, and smooth muscle cell proliferation. Moreover, a role for TRP channels in coagulation and platelets was observed. Most of the evidence has been generated from rodent models of cardiac remodeling and cell culture, with few reports from human cells or tissue biopsies. Here, we focused on studies that investigated the role of TRP channels in cardiac function and adaptive cardiac remodeling. In summary, both the upregulation and downregulation of TRP channels in the heart are associated with pathological, electrical, and signaling of adaptive remodeling. TRPML channels will not be discussed here since despite the expression of TRPML1 and TRPML2 in the heart [77], their role in cardiac function is unknown. Also, there is little evidence of TRPP in heart pathology, and thus its role in cardiac function was not discussed. Table **1** summarizes the main findings regarding TRP expression and modulation in the cardiovascular system.

TRPA1

TRPA1 channels are expressed in the mouse heart, throughout the epicardium, myocardium, and endocardium, at cardiomyocyte costameres, Z-disc and intercalated discs [78]. Its activation has been implicated in animal models of myocardial injury induced by myocardium ischemia-reperfusion (I/R), and pressure overload. Genetic ablation of TRPA1 significantly decreased MI in a mouse model of I/R [79]. Human and mouse hypertrophic hearts also present increased expression of TRPA1 protein [80]. TRPA1 inhibition in mice subjected to transverse aortic constriction (TAC) markedly attenuated interstitial fibrosis, and mRNA expression of hypertrophic markers such as atrial natriuretic peptide (ANP), brain natriuretic peptide (BNP) and β-myosin heavy chain (β-MHC) [80]. The underlying mechanism is the negative regulation of Ca^{2+}/CaM-dependent protein kinase II (CaMKII), and calcineurin signaling pathways by TRPA1 [80]. Previous work from Andrei *et al.* also demonstrated that TRPA1 stimulation in cardiomyocytes activates the CaMKII signaling pathway, increasing intracellular Ca^{+2} availability and handling, thus increasing contractile function [81].

TRPC

Jiang *et al.* investigated the expression of five TRPC channels during the development of the heart in rats (TRPC1, TRPC3, TRPC4, TRPC5, and TRPC6). The time points chosen were embryonic day E18.5, when heart development is almost finished, neonate heart 24 h after birth, and adult eight-week old rat, when the heart phenotype of gene expression becomes relatively constant. All TRPC channels investigated were detected at the three mentioned time points. In fetal/ neonate hearts, TRPC proteins were located in the cytoplasm, and only TRPC3 was detected in the nucleus [73]. In the adult heart, most TRPC channels were found at the T-tubule/Z-line (TRPC1, TRPC3, TRPC5, and TRPC6), and intercalate disk (TRPC1, TRPC3, TRPC4, and TRPC6), whereas the axial component of T-tubule contained TRPC3 and TRPC5 channels. Some regions expressed only one TRPC subtype, such as the two poles of the nucleus (TRPC1), the nucleus (TRPC6) and the M-line (TRPC4).

There are several investigations suggesting that canonical TRP channels are involved in cardiac hypertrophy, and the most prominent evidence has been reported from TRPC1, TRPC3, and TRPC6 studies. TRPC1 protein is increased in the heart of Sprague Dawley rats with TAC-induced left ventricular (LV) hypertrophy [82]. Exposure of H9c2 cells (rat myocardium myoblast) to nicotinamide phosphoribosyltransferase (Nampt), a coenzyme involved in redox reactions, leads to cardiomyocyte hypertrophy and ER stress, and was associated with the increased expression of TRPC1, BNP and markers of ER stress [83]. Knockout of TRPC1 using CRISPR/Cas9 in human pluripotent stem cell lines attenuated cardiomyocyte hypertrophy, whereas TRPC1 overexpression induced cardiomyocyte hypertrophy [84].

In a pressure overload model of TAC, TRPC3 ablation did not affect myocardial cell size, but collagen deposition was markedly reduced in TRPC3 knockout mice [85]. Furthermore, Kitajima *et al.* proved that TRPC3 is involved in pressure overload-induced LV dysfunction in 129 Sv mice, and that TRPC3 is a positive regulator of ROS which stabilizes NADPH oxidase activity [86].

To investigate the role of TRPC channels in pathological cardiac hypertrophy, Wu *et al.* generated transgenic mice by inhibiting TRPC3/6/7 and TRPC1/4/5 subgroups, and subjected these mice to agonist stimulation and pressure overload [87]. After two weeks, transgenic mice expressing the dominant-negative (dn) TRPC3 (dnTRPC3) transgene in the heart and co-infused with phenylephrine (PE) and Ang II showed less cardiac hypertrophy compared to wild type (WT) mice. Also, when dnTRPC3 mice were subjected to TAC for eight weeks, they presented less cardiac hypertrophy than WT mice. Transgenic dnTRPC6 and dnTRPC4 generated mice showed that the expression of these two TRPC channels in the heart is necessary for cardiac hypertrophy, fibrosis, and Ca^{2+} handling. By crossing dnTRPC4 mice with WT TRPC3 transgenic mice, Wu *et al.*

demonstrated that TRPC channels can form complexes in cardiac myocytes across the investigated subgroups, and thus, the expression of any dnTRPC family member renders many potential TRPC tetrameric channel assemblies inactive [87].

Domes *et al*. investigated the involvement of TRPC, in cardiac hypertrophy, in TRPC3 or TRPC6 knockout mice, after the infusion of Ang II by osmotic minipumps for seven days [88]. These mice demonstrated that TRPC3 deletion abolished Ang II-induced cardiac hypertrophy and fibrosis, but the authors were surprised by the discovery that TRPC6 deletion alone did not prevent cardiac hypertrophy, as a previous report had shown the importance of both TRPC3 and TRPC6 in Ang II-induced cardiac hypertrophy [89]. Additionally, Seo *et al*. studied the impact of single and combined suppression of TRPC3 and TRPC6 channels, and found that single channel gene deletion does not provide protection against pressure overload, whereas their combined deletion is protective [90]. A limitation of this study is that the gene knockout was global, and thus the relative contribution of myocytes, fibroblasts, and smooth muscle cells could not be discerned.

Mechanical stretch of the human pluripotent stem cell (PSC)-derived cardiomyocytes increases the expression of connective tissue growth factors (CTGF), TGF-β1 and TGF-β2 mRNAs, but this effect is suppressed by TRPC3 inhibition, indicating a role for this channel in the cardiomyocyte fibrotic response [85]. The expression of CTGF mRNA and α-smooth muscle actin (α-SMA) protein in TGF-β2-stimulated human cardiac fibroblasts was also suppressed by TRPC3 inhibition [85].

Some studies support a role for TRPC3 in cardiac arrhythmia and automacity. Myocardial stretch increases the force of contraction, however the long time-course stretch, over several minutes, reduces it as a result of stress-induced slow increase in Ca^{2+} concentration (SSC). Yamaguchi *et al*. demonstrated that TRPC3 channels are involved in SSC by mediating stretch-induced cation influx (Na^+ and Ca^{2+}) in cardiac myocytes, *via* angiotensin type 1 receptor (AT1R)-induced phospholipase C [91]. Seo *et al*. have also reported the involvement of TRPC6 channels in SSC, and suggested that TRPC3 and TRPC6 can form functional heterotetramers [90], which could provide another source of Ca^{2+} influx, in addition to TRPC3 and TRPC6 monomultimer channels. Doleschal *et al*. demonstrated that the acute activation of TRPC3 channels by either cardiac overexpression or pharmacological activation increases heart contractility and promotes arrhythmias, most likely by a TRPC3/NCX1 interaction [92]. On the other hand, Qi *et al*. demonstrated that TRPC3 positively regulates the diastolic depolarization by increasing LCR and NCX currents in mouse embryonic stem cell-derived cardiomyocytes, suggesting a possible role for this channel as a pacemaker in this cell line [93].

The hypoxia-inducible factor 1 alpha (HIF-1α) regulates the transcription of genes involved in the adaptative response to hypoxia. In a model of mild hypoxia-induced cardiomyocyte hypertrophy (10% O_2) in cell culture, Chu *et al.* showed that HIF-1α promotes cardiac hypertrophy by upregulating TRPC3 and TRPC6 expression, leading to enhanced Ca^{2+}-calcineurin signals [94]. TRPC3 and TRPC6 overexpression, and Ca^{2+}-calcineurin signals are inhibited when HIF-1α is blocked. In this model, hypertrophic changes were determined by β-actin staining, and overexpression of ANP, BNP, and β-MHC.

In humans, recent evidence reported that patients with hypertrophic cardiomyopathy or HF exhibit higher TRPC1 expression compared to the healthy heart [84]. Bush *et al.* showed that failing human hearts, from patients with idiopathic dilated cardiomyopathy, overexpress TRPC5 mRNA and protein compared to nonfailing human hearts [95]. TRPC1, TRPC4, and TRPC6 levels were unchanged between failing and nonfailing human hearts, and the TRPC3 mRNA expression was undetectable [95]. Unlike other TRPC channels, the physiological relevance of TRPC5 expression in the heart remains unclear. Furthermore, adding to the contribution of Bush *et al.*, another research group demonstrated that the functional coupling between inositol-3-phospha-e-responsive TRPC5 channels and endothelial nitric oxide synthase contributes as a negative regulator of hypertrophic signaling induced by ATP in neonatal rat cardiomyocytes [96].

One, two and six weeks after MI, in mice with permanent left main coronary artery (LMCA) occlusion, Makarewich *et al.* reported an increased mRNA expression of TRPC1, TRPC3, TRPC4 and TRPC6 [97]. To investigate the role of TRPC inhibition post-MI, transgenic dnTRPC4 mice, which present reduced activity of both TRPC1/4/5 and TRPC3/6/7 subgroups, were evaluated, revealing that the dnTRPC4 transgene mice do not exhibit TRPC-mediated Ca^{2+} entry after MI, have less pathological hypertrophy, better cardiac performance, less progression to HF, and an increased survival compared to WT mouse [97].

TRPM

TRPM2 has been shown to play an essential role in the susceptibility to oxidative stress and I/R conditions in the heart. TRPM2 are localized in the sarcolemma, and transverse tubules in adult mouse LV myocytes [98]. To investigate the role of TRPM2 channels in the heart, Miller *et al.* generated a global TRPM2 knockout mouse, and performed I/R surgery by LMCA occlusion for 30 minutes. Depletion of TRPM2 channels did not alter the contractile function between WT and knockout sham hearts, however TRPM2 deficiency aggravated the *in vivo* cardiac contractile dysfunction post-I/R injury [98]. Thus, TRPM2 channels protected the heart from I/R injury, a response associated with reduced ROS generation and an increased ROS scavenging capability in adult cardiac myocytes. Further studies from Miller *et al.* reported that the protection of TRPM2 knockout mice from I/R injury is due to attenuation of mitochondrial dysfunction [99]. The underlying mechanism is related to the phosphorylation of proline-rich tyrosine kinase 2 (Pyk2) mediated by Ca^{2+} entry *via* TRPM2, with part of the phosphorylated Pyk2 translocating to the mitochondria to maintain cellular bioenergetics, reducing mitochondrial oxidants and enhancing survival signaling molecules [100].

TRPM4 channels are equally permeable to K^+ and Na^+, and are highly expressed in the Purkinje fibers of the heart [101]. They play an essential role in the human heart conductance system, and TRPM4 is a major gene predisposing to progressive familial heart block type 1B [102]. It is possible that TRPM4 upregulation may be a critical predisposing factor in arrhythmias as its excessive activity can cause arrhythmic changes *in vitro* [103], and influences the action potential of Purkinje cells [101]. A cohort of 178 patients with long QT syndrome reported that TRPM4 variants (p.V441M, p.R499W, p.R499P, and G844D) account for 2.2% of long QT syndrome cases [104]. Additionally, pretreatment of H9c2 cells with 9-phenanthrol (TRPM4 channel inhibitor) prevents cell death in an experimental condition of hypoxia/reoxygenation (H/R) [105].

Sah *et al.* studied the role of TRPM7 in normal ventricular function in cardiac-targeted TRPM7 knockout mice. In summary, they revealed that TRPM7 is extremely important in myocardial proliferation during early cardiogenesis (<E9.0/ mid-gestation), but not in the adult ventricular myocardium under basal conditions (>E12.5) [39]. Early deletion of cardiac TRPM7, before embryonic day E9, results in congestive HF and death by day E11.5 due to myocardium hypoproliferation. TRPM7 deletion at mid-gestation resulted in 50% of mice developing heart block, impaired repolarization, and ventricular arrhythmia. When TRPM7 was deleted in late cardiogenesis, mice were viable and displayed average adult ventricular size and function. Since TRPM7 are permeable by divalent cations, Sah *et al.* investigated the cellular Mg^{2+} and Zn^{2+} content, and detected no differences between WT and knockout mice [39].

TRPM7 is also required for cardiac automaticity. TRPM7 currents are highly substantial in cultured embryonic ventricular myocytes, and isolated sinus atrial node cells compared with quiescent adult ventricular myocytes [106]. Human atrial myocytes express TRPM7 channel proteins, and the expression is increased in the atria of patients with atrial fibrillation [107]. In explanted human hearts,

Parajuli *et al.* reported that patients with nonischemic dilated cardiomyopathy and ventricular tachycardia demonstrate greater TRPM7 expression, cardiac hypertrophy, oxidative stress, and myocardial fibrosis than patients without ventricular tachycardia [108]. Additionally, Macianskiene *et al.* suggested that the density of TRPM7 currents in human atrial cardiomyocytes is based on the underlying pathophysiology, being higher in cells from patients with atrial fibrillation [109].

TRPV

The majority of evidence regarding TRPV role on cardiac function is focused on the TRPV1, TRPV2, and TRPV4 channels. According to Hurt *et al.*, TRPV1 is a low-abundant intracellular protein in cardiomyocytes [110]. It is present throughout the epicardium, myocardium, and endocardium, at cardiomyocyte costameres, Z-discs, and intercalated discs [78]. Ren *et al.* reported that TRPV1 is essential for the bone marrow-derived mesenchymal stem cell (BMSC) differentiation into cardiomyocytes. TRPV1 knockdown, before 5-azacytidin--induced BMSC differentiation, reduced the expression of cardiomyocyte markers like cardiac troponin T (cTnT), cardiac α-actin, and α-MHC [111]. TRPV1 knockdown also downregulates Wnt/β-catenin mRNA and protein expression, a signaling pathway essential to myocardial development [111].

During pressure overload, TRPV1 is increased in mice subjected to TAC-induced cardiac hypertrophy [112, 113]. Capsaicin, a TRPV1 channel agonist, increases cell size in both cultured H9c2 cells and rat neonatal cardiomyocytes, and is related to increase in intracellular Ca^{2+} levels, and CaMKII/MAPK signaling. Additionally, capsazepine, a TRPV1 channel antagonist, prevented TAC-induced cardiac hypertrophy in mice [113]. Overall, this evidence indicates that TRPV1 expression is deleterious to the heart during pressure overload remodeling.

Despite the evidence mentioned above, data in TRPV1 knockout mice are conflicting. Buckley *et al.* first reported that the TRPV1 knockout mice are protected from TAC-induced cardiac hypertrophy, fibrosis, apoptosis, and loss of contractile function [114]. Later, Zhong *et al.* demonstrated that the same animals presented with worsened cardiac hypertrophy when challenged by TAC. Both WT and TRPV1 knockout mice developed cardiac hypertrophy, fibrosis, inflammation and presented increased secretion of tumor necrosis factor α, interleukin-6, and ANP during TAC-induced heart hypertrophy; these changes are worsened in the knockout mice [112].

TRPV2 is another TRP channel with important roles suggested in the heart. Indeed, TRPV2 modulates cardiac inotropy and lusitropy by participating in Ca^{2+} handling. The effects are blunted in knockout mice, indicating an important role of TRPV2 in regulating myocyte contractile function under physiological conditions [115]. In mice models of LV hypertrophy, TAC upregulated TRPV2 expression, but not under β-adrenergic or Ang II stimulation [116]. Additionally, TRPV2 knockout mice displayed reduced LV hypertrophy after TAC, with no response to either β-adrenergic or Ang II stimulation [116]. These channels are also involved in cardiac dystrophic cardiomyopathy [117], and are highly expressed in macrophages infiltrating the peri-infarct zones post-MI in rats [118].

In a mouse model of myocardial I/R injury, both TRPV4 mRNA and protein expression were upregulated. Additionally, inhibition (with the TRPV4 antagonist HC067047) or deletion of TRPV4 channels improved myocardial I/R injury. TRPV4 blockade or absence lead to reduced infarct size, decreased TnT, improved cardiac function, and reduced apoptosis *via* the reperfusion injury salvage kinase (RISK) pathway [119]. Another study from the same group used a H/R model in H9c2 cells and rat neonatal ventricle myocytes to study the mechanisms involved in TRPV4 cardiac injury. H/R increased TRPV4 expression, contributing to Ca^{2+} influx, and cytoplasmic ROS generation [120]. Finally, TRPV4 expression in the heart increases with aging in mice [121].

Table 1. TRP expression and modulation in the cardiovascular system.

Authors	Experimental Model	Intervention	Main findings
TRPA1			
Conklin *et al.*, 2019	Myocardial I/R	TRPA1 knockout	↓ myocardial infarct size after I/R injury
Wang *et al.*, 2018	LV samples from patients with dilated cardiomyopathy	----	↑ TRPA1 protein
	TAC in C57Bl/6J mice	TRPA1 inhibitor (HC030031 and TCS-5861528)	↑ heart TRPA1 protein by TAC, TRPA1 inhibition ↓ CM hypertrophy (CaMKII and calcineurin pathway) and cardiac fibrosis
Andrei *et al.*, 2017	Freshly isolated mouse CMs from C57Bl/6 WT and TRPA1 knockout mice	TRPA1 knockout and TRPA1 activation (allyl isothiocyanate)	TRPA1 stimulation in electrically-stimulated mouse CM increased [Ca^{2+}] and contractile function
Wang *et al.*, 2018	Doxorubicin-induced cardiotoxicity in C57Bl/6J mice	TRPA1 inhibition (HC030031)	Doxorubicin ↑ heart TRPA1 mRNA/protein, and HC030031 attenuated doxorubicin-induced acute cardiotoxicity by ↓ oxidative stress, inflammation, and ER stress
TRPC			

(Table 1) cont.....

Jiang *et al.*, 2014	Heart development in SD rats	----	TRPC1, TRPC3, TRPC4, TRPC5, and TRPC6 were differentially expressed during heart developing in CMs
Mao *et al.*, 2018	TAC in SD rats	----	↑ heart TRPC1 protein
Li *et al.*, 2018	Nampt-induced hypertrophy in H9c2 cells	TRPC1 transient overexpression or inhibition (shRNA)	↑ TRPC1 mRNA/protein in Nampt-induced hypertrophy, and TRPC1 knockdown ↓ CM hypertrophy
Tang *et al.*, 2019	PMA-induced hypertrophy in H9 human ESCs	TRPC1 knockout by CRISPR/Cas9	↓ hypertrophy by TRPC1 knockdown via NF-κB, and ↑ hypertrophy by TRPC1 overexpression
	LV samples from patients with HCM or HF obtained during cardiac surgery	----	↑ TRPC1 mRNA
Numaga-Tomita *et al.*, 2016	TAC in 129Sv mice	TRPC3 knockout	CM hypertrophy by TRPC3 knockdown, but milder fibrosis than WT mice
	Mechanical stretch in human PSC and human cardiac fibroblasts	TRPC3 inhibition (Pyr3)	↓ fibrotic response in human CMs and cardiac fibroblasts
Kitajima *et al.*, 2016	TAC in 129Sv mice	TRPC3 knockout	TRPC3 contributed to pressure overload-induced LV dysfunction, and amplified ROS-dependent maladaptive signaling induced by mechanical stretch
Wu *et al.*, 2010	TAC and Ang II-induced cardiac hypertrophy in transgenic mice	Cardiac-specific dnTRPC3, dnTRPC4, and dnTRPC6	↓ TAC and Ang II-induced cardiac hypertrophy in all transgenic mice
Domes *et al.*, 2014	Ang II-induced cardiac hypertrophy in mice	TRPC3 and TRPC6 knockout	↓ Ang II-induced cardiac hypertrophy in both knockout mice
Onohara *et al.*, 2006	Ang II-induced hypertrophy in rat neonatal CM	TRPC3 and TRPC6 knockdown (siRNA)	TRPC3 and TRPC6 knockdown ↓ CM hypertrophic response
Seo *et al.*, 2014	TAC in C57Bl/6J mice	TRPC3, TRPC6, and TRPC3/6 knockout	Deletion of either TRPC3 or TRPC6 genes did not protect against cardiac hypertrophy, but double deletion was protective, and TRPC6 is involved in SSC
Yamaguchi *et al.*, 2018	Sustained axial stretch in isolated CMs	TRPC3 knockout	TRPC3 is involved in SSC by stretch-induced cation influx (Na^+ and Ca^{2+})

(Table 1) cont.....

Doleschal *et al.*, 2015	Isolated heart and CM from transgenic TRPC3 mice	Cardiac-specific TRPC3 overexpression and TRPC3 agonist (GSK1702934A)	TRPC3 activation ↑ contractility and promotes arrhythmia by TRPC3/NCX1 interaction
Qi *et al.*, 2016	Mouse ESC-CM and HEK293	TRPC3 inhibition (Pyr3), and TRPC3 overexpression or inhibition (dnTRPC3)	TRPC3 contributed to cardiac pacemaker activity by directly evoking membrane depolarization, increasing LCR, and NCX forward mode activation
Chu *et al.*, 2012	Mild hypoxia (10% O_2) in isolated CM from Wistar rats	----	HIF-1α promoted CM hypertrophy by ↑ TRPC3 and TRPC6 mRNA/protein
Bush *et al.*, 2006	Ventricular samples from patients with idiopathic dilated cardiomyopathy	----	↑ TRPC5 mRNA/protein; TRPC1, TRPC4 and TRPC6 levels were unchanged; and TRPC3 was undetectable
Sunggip *et al.*, 2018	Ang II and ET-1-induced CM hypertrophy in rat neonatal CM	TRPC5 knockdown (siRNA)	TRPC5-mediated Ca^{2+} influx negatively regulated ATP-induced CM hypertrophy by modulating NO signaling
Makarewich *et al.*, 2014	MI by permanent LCA occlusion in transgenic mice	Cardiac-specific dnTRPC3, dnTRPC4, and dnTRPC6	↑ TRPC1, TRPC3, TRPC4 and TRPC6 mRNA in the heart of WT mice after MI Mice with dnTRPCs were less responsive to pressure-overloa- -induced hypertrophy
Koitabashi *et al.*, 2010	TAC in C57Bl/6 mice	Sildenafil (PDE5 inhibitor)	Cardiac hypertrophy and ↑ TRPC6 mRNA/protein by TAC which was blocked by sildenafil
Nishida *et al.*, 2010	Ang II and ET-1-induced hypertrophy in rat neonatal CM	Sildenafil (PDE5 inhibitor)	Sildenafil ↓ both agonist-induced and mechanical stretch-induced CM hypertrophy by ↑ TRPC6 protein phosphorylation at Thr[69]
Kiso *et al.*, 2013	ET-1-induced hypertrophy in rat neonatal CM	Sildenafil (PDE5 inhibitor)	Sildenafil ↓ agonist-induced CM hypertrophy by ↓ TRPC1, TRPC3, and TRPC6 mRNA
Kiyonaka *et al.*, 2009	Ang II-induced hypertrophy in rat neonatal CM	TRPC3 inhibition (Pyr3)	Pyr3 ↓ NFAT activation and CM hypertrophy
	TAC in mice	TRPC3 inhibition (Pyr3)	Pyr3 ↓ pressure-overload dilated cardiac hypertrophy and ↓ ANP mRNA

(Table 1) cont.....

Koenig *et al.*, 2013	*Ex vivo* stent implantation into human ascending aorta obtained from routine aortic aneurysmectomy	TRPC3 inhibition (Pyr3)	Pyr3 ↓ stent-induced media hyperplasia
Saliba *et al.*, 2013	L-NAME treated Wistar rats and knockout mice	TRPC3 inhibition (Pyr10) and TRPC3 knockout	TRPC3 inhibition/knockdown ↓ myocardial fibrosis independently of blood pressure
Shimauchi *et al.*, 2017	Doxorubicin-induced cardiotoxicity in 129Sv mice	TRPC3 knockout	TRPC3 participated in doxorubicin-induced myocardial atrophy, oxidative stress, and LV dysfunction
Chen *et al.*, 2017	Doxorubicin-induced cardiotoxicity in SD rats	Salvianolic acid B	Doxorubicin ↑ TRPC3 and TRPC6 protein in isolated adult CM, and Sal B protected against doxorubicin-induced cardiac injury and apoptosis
TRPM			
Miller *et al.*, 2013	Myocardial I/R in C57Bl/6 mice	TRPM2 knockout	TRPM2 is expressed in CM sarcolemma and transverse tubules, and it mediated Ca^{2+} influx in adult mouse CM exposed to H_2O_2 TRPM2 deficiency ↑ cardiac contractile dysfunction post-I/R injury *in vivo*
Miller *et al.*, 2014	Myocardial I/R in C57Bl/6 mice	TRPM2 knockout	TRPM2 protected the heart from I/R injury by ↓ mitochondrial dysfunction and ↓ ROS
Miller *et al.*, 2019	Myocardial I/R in C57Bl/6 mice	TRPM2 knockout	TRPM2-mediated Pyk2 phosphorylation was responsible for the maintenance of mitochondrial function and protection from oxidative injury
Hof *et al.*, 2016	New Zealand rabbits	TRPM4 inhibition (9-phenanthrol)	TRPM4 was expressed in ventricular Purkinje cells and influenced its action potential
Daumy *et al.*, 2016	Peripheral blood lymphocytes from patients with cardiac conduction defects	----	Progressive familial heart block type I was caused by TRPM4 mutation-induced ↑ of expression and function
Hu *et al.*, 2017	Modulation of Ca^{2+} concentration and Ang II in immortalized atrial CM (HL-1) and numerical simulations	TRPM4 knockdown (siRNA)	↑ TRPM4 activity produced arrhythmic changes

(Table 1) cont.....

Hof *et al.*, 2017	Blood samples from patients with long QT syndrome	----	The presence of TRPM4 variants was responsible for 2.2% of long QT syndrome cases
Piao *et al.*, 2015	Myocardial I/R in SD rats	TRPM4 inhibition (9-phenanthrol)	↓ MI size by IV administration of 9-phenanthrol before myocardial I/R
	H/R in H9c2 cells	TRPM4 inhibition (9-phenanthrol)	↓ cell death by 9-phenanthrol treatment before H/R
Sah *et al.*, 2013	129SvEvTac mice	Cardiac-specific TRPM7 knockout	Early deletion of TRPM7 during cardiogenesis produced congestive HF *in utero* In an intermediate time point, it disrupted atrioventricular conduction TRPM7 deletion in late cardiogenesis had no impact on adult ventricular function
Sah *et al.*, 2013	Isolated embryonic, ventricular and sinus atrial node CM, zebrafish, and 129SvEvTac mice	TRPM7 morpholino zebrafish and cardiac-specific TRPM7 knockout	TRPM7 disruption *in vitro* and *in vivo* impairs cardiac automaticity
Parajuli *et al.*, 2015	LV samples from patients with nonischemic dilated cardiomyopathy undergoing heart transplantation	----	↑ TRPM7 mRNA/protein in patients with ventricular tachycardia
Zhang *et al.*, 2012	Right atrial appendage samples from patients undergoing cardiac surgery	----	↑ TRPM7 protein (but not TRPM4 protein) in patients with atrial fibrillation
Macianskiene *et al.*, 2017	Right atrial sample from patients undergoing cardiac surgery	----	TRPM7 current density in human CM was related to the clinical history, being higher in atrial fibrillation
Hoffman *et al.*, 2015	Doxorubicin-induced cardiotoxicity in C57Bl/6 mice	TRPM2 knockout	TRPM2 expression protected mice from doxorubicin-induced death and cardiomyopathy
TRPV			
Ren *et al.*, 2016	BMSCs isolated from the femur and tibia of SD rats	TRPV1 knockdown (siRNA)	TRPV1 is involved in BMSC differentiation into CM
Zhong *et al.*, 2018	TAC in C57Bl/6J mice	TRPV1 knockout	↑ TRPV1 in WT mice and TRPV1 knockdown resulted in more severe ventricular hypertrophy, fibrosis, and dysfunction

(Table 1) cont.....

Chen *et al.*, 2016	H9c2 and rat neonatal CM	TRPV1 agonists (capsaicin and anandamide), antagonist (capsazepine) and knockdown (siRNA)	Capsaicin and anandamide ↓ cell size, capsazepine attenuated this effect, and TRPV1 activation-induced ornithine decarboxylase expression was dependent on CaMKII/MAPK pathway
	TAC in C57Bl/6 mice	TRPV1 inhibition (capsazepine)	↓ TAC-induced cardiac and CM hypertrophy
Buckley *et al.*, 2011	TAC in C57Bl/6J mice	TRPV1 knockout	↓ TAC-induced cardiac hypertrophy, fibrosis, apoptosis, and loss of contractile function
Rubinstein *et al.*, 2014	Mice	TRPV2 knockout and TRPV2 activation (probenecid)	↓ myocardial performance *in vivo* and *ex vivo* by TRPV2 knockdown, and blunted inotropic and lusitropic responses to probenecid
Koch *et al.*, 2017	TAC in mice	TRPV2 knockout	↑ TRPV2 mRNA/protein in WT mice, and ↓ TAC-induced cardiac hypertrophy by TRPV2 knockdown
	Ang II and isoproterenol-induced cardiac hypertrophy in mice	----	Unchanged TRPV2 expression by either Ang II or isoproterenol
Entin-Meer *et al.*, 2014	MI by permanent LCA occlusion in rat	----	↑ TRPV2 in macrophages infiltrating the peri-infarct zone post-MI
Dong *et al.*, 2017	Myocardial I/R in C57Bl/6 mice	TRPV4 inhibition (HC067047) and TRPV4 knockout	↑ TRPV4 mRNA/protein, and TRPV4 inhibition or knockdown improved myocardial I/R injury
Wu *et al.*, 2017	H/R in H9c2 cells and rat neonatal CM	TRPV4 activation (GSK1016790A) and inhibition (HC067047)	↑ TRPV4 mRNA/protein by H/R, contributing to Ca^{2+} overload and cytoplasmic ROS generation
Lang *et al.*, 2015	High-salt diet to WT and knockout C57Bl/6J mice	Capsaicin (TRPV1 agonist) and TRPV1 knockout	Capsaicin ↓ diet-induced cardiac hypertrophy and dysfunction in WT, but not in TRPV1 knockout mice
Hurt *et al.*, 2016	Myocardial I/R in SD rats	Capsaicin (TRPV1 agonist)	Capsaicin ↓ MI size by calcineurin modulation, but ↑ heart rate
Ge *et al.*, 2016	Doxorubicin-induced cardiotoxicity in WT and ALDH2 transgenic mice	TRPV1 agonist (SA13353) and antagonist (capsazepine)	TRPV1 inhibition ↓ doxorubicin-induced cardiac dysfunction and apoptosis

Abbreviations: 9-phe, 9-phenanthrol (TRPM4 inhibitor); ALDH2, aldehyde dehydrogenase; Ang II, angiotensin II; ANP, atrial natriuretic peptide; BMSC, bone marrow-derived mesenchymal stem cell; CaMKII, Ca^{2+}/calmodulin-dependent protein kinase II; CM, cardiomyocyte; dn, dominant negative; ER, endoplasmic reticulum; ESC, embryonic stem cell; ET-1, endothelin 1; HCM, hypertrophic cardiomyopathy; HIF-1α, hypoxia-inducible factor 1α; HF, heart failure; H/R, hypoxia-reoxygenation; I/R, ischemia-reperfusion; IV, intravenous; LCA, left coronary artery; LV, left ventricle; MAPK, mitogen activated protein kinase; MI, myocardial infarction; Nampt, nicotinamide phosphoribosyltransferase; NCX, sodium/calcium exchanger; NFAT, nuclear factor of activated T cells; NO, nitric oxide; PDE5, phosphodiesterase type 5; Pyk2, protein tyrosine kinase 2 β; PMA, phorbol 12-myristate 13-acetate; PNCM, primary neonatal cardiomyocytes; PSC, pluripotent stem cell; Pyr3, pyrazole 3; ROS, reactive oxygen species; Sal B, salvianolic acid B; SD, Sprague-Dawley; SSC, stress-induced slow increase in intracellular Ca^{2+} concentration; TAC, transverse aortic constriction; TRPA1, transient receptor potential ankyrin 1; TRPC, transient receptor potential canonical; TRPM, transient receptor potential melastatin; TRPV, transient receptor potential vanilloid; WT, wild type.

Evidence of TRP Modulation in the Cardiovascular System

TRPC

Sildenafil is a phosphodiesterase type 5 (PDE5) inhibitor used for the treatment of erectile dysfunction, and has indirectly contributed to the treatment of male infertility [122]. PDE5 is also the main cGMP-metabolizing enzyme targeted to clinically treat pulmonary artery hypertension [123].

Mouse heart TRPC6 gene and protein expression are reduced by sildenafil in animals with TAC-induced pressure overload, a response suggested to be dependent on protein kinase G (PKG) activation and NFAT [124]. Nishida *et al.* corroborated this evidence, reporting that PDE5 inhibition suppressed both ET-1/Ang II and mechanical stretch-induced hypertrophy of cultured rat cardiomyocytes, by PKG-dependent phosphorylation of TRPC6 proteins at Thr[69], and inhibition of TRPC6-mediated Ca^{2+} response [125].

Kiso *et al.* showed that other TRPC channels are also modulated by sildenafil. In cultured cardiomyocytes, sildenafil suppresses ET-1-induced hypertrophic responses such as NFAT activation, BNP expression, and cell growth, by decreasing the levels of TRPC1, TRPC3, and TRPC6 mRNA in ET-1-treated cardiomyocytes, whereas TRPC4 and TRPC5 remained unchanged [126]. The authors suggested that sildenafil acts as not only a TRPC6 blocker, but also as an inhibitor of the upregulation of TRPC1, TRPC3 and TRPC6 during the development of cardiac hypertrophy. Based on these reports, sildenafil could be a therapeutic option in cardiac hypertrophy.

Pyrazole is widely used as a template in combinatorial and medicinal chemistry, and various physiological and therapeutic possibilities have so far been explored by incorporating different pharmacophoric groups in this moiety. Drugs based on the pyrazole moiety display fewer side effects, and are being used as antianxiety, anti-inflammatory, antibacterial, antiviral, antipsychotic, anticancer, antiobesity, analgesic and antipyretic [127, 128]. The pyrazole-derived compounds ethyl 1-[--(trichloroprop-2-enamide)phenyl]-5-(trifluoromethyl)-1H-pyrazole-4-carboxylate (Pyr3) and N-[4-[3,5-bis(trifluoromethyl)pyrazol-1-yl]phenyl]-4-methylbenzenesulfonamide (Pyr10) are selective blockers of the TRPC3 channel [129, 130], and there is some evidence supporting their beneficial cardiac effects.

In vitro, Pyr3 suppressed Ang II-induced NFAT translocation, mechanical stretch-induced NFAT activation, actin reorganization, BNP expression, and protein synthesis in rat neonatal cardiomyocytes [129]. Additionally, concentric and dilated cardiac hypertrophy was attenuated by Pyr3 in mice subjected to TAC, followed by the reduced expression of ANP mRNA, a marker of cardiac hypertrophy [129]. In-stent restenosis is the result of a healing process which comprises vascular smooth muscle phenotype switching from contractile to a synthetic form, and Koening *et al.* demonstrated that Pyr3 inhibits smooth muscle cell proliferation and suppresses proliferative markers when implanted in a stent prototype into the human aorta [131].

To date, there is one single and recent report on the effects of Pyr10 on cardiac hypertrophy and fibrosis. When administered to L-NAME-treated mice, Pyr10 does not affect blood pressure, but completely abrogates myocardial fibrosis, impairs coronary vessel thickening, and reduces necrotic regions as replacement collagen was absent [76]. According to Seo *et al.*, agents that target only one TRP channel subtype will similarly affect the other subtypes in heterotetramers [90]. This hypothesis may explain the efficacy of Pyr3 and Pyr10, despite its sole action on the TRPC3 channel, considering that other TRPC channels have been implicated in cardiac hypertrophy, as mentioned previously.

TRPV

Capsaicin inhibits the development of cardiac hypertrophy when administered for six months to WT mice fed a high-salt diet, a protective effect that was blunted in TRPV1 knockout mice. This amelioration of cardiac dysfunction was associated with an increase in endurance capacity, energy expenditure, and physical performance [132]. In another study, using a rodent model of I/R, capsaicin reduced myocardial infarct size through a calcineurin-dependent mechanism, by altering mitochondrial membrane potential, although observed in only a narrow therapeutic window. Despite this beneficial effect, capsaicin increases the heart rate in a dose-dependent manner [110]. To overcome this issue, the authors developed a peptide (V1-cal) that mimics the calcineurin site on TRPV1, and revealed that it did not influence body temperature and heart rate [110].

Modulating TRPV1 channels is a promising therapeutic strategy, and current antihyperalgesics with TRPV1 antagonist action could serve as new therapeutic strategies against cardiac hypertrophy. However, previously attempts highlighted important issues, such as sudden myocardial infarction due to coronary vasospasm following excessive capsaicin consumption [133, 134], and hyperthermia in humans mediated *via* TRPV1 antagonism [135]. Also, activation of TRPV1 channels leads to a painful sensation [136]. Capsaicin is a promising therapeutic agent in cardiac hypertrophy and metabolic dysfunction (as discussed later), however the cardiovascular physiological safety needs further investigation.

Doxorubicin-induced Cardiotoxicity

Doxorubicin is an anthracycline drug routinely used in the treatment of several cancers, and known for its dose-dependent cardiotoxicity, with multifactorial mechanisms involved. The available literature asserts that doxorubicin metabolites interfere with iron and Ca^{2+} homeostasis, generates ROS or nitrogen intermediate species, and disrupts mitochondrial respiration [137]. Patients undergoing doxorubicin treatment may present LV wall stress, reduced ejection fraction, arrhythmias, and congestive HF. In late treatment phases, the agent causes the heart to shrink due to myocardial apoptosis and fibrosis during dilated cardiomyopathy [138].

Since some TRP channels are involved in maladaptive cardiac remodeling, drugs targeting these channels could provide protection from doxorubicin-induced cardiotoxicity. Mice treated with doxorubicin have presented a decrease in body weight (BW) and heart weight (HW), accompanied by a substantial increase in myocardial TRPA1 mRNA and protein [139]. Although the use of a TRPA1-specific inhibitor five days before and after doxorubicin failed to protect from BW- and HW-induced changes, it lowered serum enzymes associated with cardiotoxicity, including creatine kinase-myocardial band (CK-MB) and lactate dehydrase. Moreover, TRPA1 inhibition prevents doxorubicin-induced cardiomyocyte apoptosis by inhibiting oxidative stress, inflammation, and ER stress [139].

Shimauch *et al.* reported that mice treated with doxorubicin demonstrated a severe reduction in HW and cardiomyocyte size, with an increase in the levels of TRPC3. However, doxorubicin is unable to induce these responses in TRPC3 knockout mice. Moreover, the LV systolic and diastolic dysfunction, observed in WT mice treated with doxorubicin, are abolished in TRPC3 knockout animals [140]. Overall, the authors suggest that there is a functional coupling of TRPC3 and NADPH oxidase, which is essential for doxorubicin-induced cell atrophy and ROS production in cardiomyocytes [140].

Salvianolic acid B (Sal B) is the most abundant bioactive compound extracted from the root of *Salvia miltiorrhiza Bunge* (Lamiaceae). It is widely distributed in China and Japan, and has been used for the treatment of various diseases. There is strong evidence suggesting that Sal B has a cardiovascular protective effect; this has been demonstrated in doxorubicin-induced cardiac dysfunction, and has been associated with the inhibition of ER stress mediated cardiomyocyte apoptosis [141]. In male Sprague Dawley rats, Sal B was found to reduce doxorubicin-induced ER stress by inhibiting TRPC3 and TRPC6 mediated Ca^{+2} overload in rat cardiomyocytes. Sal B also prevented doxorubicin-induced cardiac injury and apoptosis in the rat heart, and cardiac myocyte contractile dysfunction [142].

Studies on TRPM2 indicate that the TRPM2 knockout mice present lower survival when treated with doxorubicin. The TRPM2 knockout mouse heart exhibits lower maximal first time derivative of LV pressure rise, even lower under doxorubicin treatment [143]. Finally, the TRPV1 agonist SA13353 reversed doxorubicin-induced cardiac functional defects and apoptosis [144]. Overall, rodent studies have suggested that modulation of TRP channels may protect from doxorubicin-induced cardiotoxicity.

OBESITY AND DIABETES

Obesity is defined as an excessive BW, due to AT accumulation, which is usually associated with the development of T2D and cardiovascular diseases. Although obesity has a multifactorial etiology, it is usually accepted that it develops from an imbalance between energy intake and expenditure. In obesity, the AT expands, increasing the release of proinflammatory mediators, and reducing the production and secretion of anti-inflammatory molecules, thus generating a state of low-grade inflammation. This condition is closely related to the development of insulin resistance in peripheral tissues, culminating in T2D in long term [145].

There are two types of AT: WAT and BAT. While WAT is responsible for energy storage, BAT dissipates energy as heat (*e.g.*, nonshivering thermogenesis) [146, 147]. Importantly, both tissues are now recognized for their endocrine functions, releasing a range of bioactive compounds, usually known as adipokines and batokines, respectively [148]. In the recent years, beige (or brite) adipocytes were described, and are characterized as white adipocytes that under stimuli acquire a brown-like phenotype, in a process called WAT browning [149, 150]. Aside from the type of AT, its location is also crucial for body metabolism. Importantly, WAT can be found both at the subcutaneous and visceral regions, with the first being linked to benefits in body metabolism including browning of AT, and the second associated with inflammation and development of comorbidities such as insulin resistance [146].

Based on the contribution of AT to obesity development, and the impact of obesity on insulin resistance and the further development of T2D, this section will focus on the role of TRP channels on WAT, BAT, and the endocrine pancreas. A summary of the studies on AT and endocrine pancreas reported in the next sections are presented in Table **2** and Table **3**, respectively. Although the expression of TRP channels in other metabolically active tissues such as liver, small intestine, skeletal muscle, and their sensory innervation is undoubtedly important to obesity and its comorbidities, they will not be discussed here as we consider AT and endocrine pancreas as the central players in the development of these diseases (for a review of their implication in obesity and comorbidities, please see references [151, 152]).

TRP Expression

The first evidence of TRP channels in AT was reported in 2007 by Zhang *et al.* who revealed TRPV1 mRNA and protein expression in mice and humans visceral AT, and 3T3-L1 preadipocytes [51]. Thereafter, several other TRP channels have been described [153, 154]. In the AT, TRP channels control intracellular Ca^{+2} levels, involved in the regulation of differentiation and physiological functions in adipocytes. Consequently, these channels have an essential role in mediating adipocyte function, adiposity, and obesity [151].

Regarding the endocrine pancreas, several TRP channels have already been identified in a range of pancreatic cell lines [152, 155 - 157]. As the secretion of insulin by its endocrine cells involves oscillations in Ca^{+2} levels within the pancreatic β-cells, TRP channels may be implicated in the regulation of insulin secretion [157].

Although reportedly expressed in AT and pancreas, many of the TRP functions have not yet been fully demonstrated and thus, remain to be investigated. Moreover, in the pancreas and β-cells, the majority of studies used cell (*in vitro*) experiments, while *in vivo* models are scarce, thus creating a gap in knowledge necessitating appropriate research.

TRPA1

TRPA1 mRNA expression is present in 3T3-L1 adipocytes, visceral, and subcutaneous WAT and BAT of mice [153, 154]. In the AT, incubation of a TRPA1 activator with 3T3-L1 cells inhibited lipid accumulation, and reduced PPARγ expression in these cells. Importantly, TRPA1 blockade during differentiation of the 3T3-L1 adipocytes reduced the inhibition of lipid storage [158]. TRPA1 expression was confirmed in RINm5F cells (a rat pancreatic β-cell line), and freshly isolated rat pancreatic β-cells [155, 156]. Endogenous and exogenous agonists of TRPA1 stimulated insulin secretion in rat pancreatic β-cells, a phenomenon that was inhibited by TRPA1 antagonists [155]. Similar results are observed when RINm5F cells are used [156]. Thus, TRPA1 channels appear to have beneficial roles in AT and endocrine pancreas, and could counteract obesity and T2D.

TRPC

Gene expression of TRPC1, TRPC4, and TRPC6 is detected on 3T3-L1 adipocytes, and in mouse visceral WAT and BAT. Interestingly, TRPC4 and TRPC6 are present at higher levels in preadipocytes compared to adipocytes, suggesting that these channels might have a role in adipogenesis [153]. TRPC1 and TRPC5 are also identified in 3T3-L1 adipocytes and human PVAT. In adipocytes, the knockdown of these receptors increases adiponectin production [19], indicating a detrimental role in the development of obesity and insulin resistance. Additionally, TRPC6 expression is increased in BAT in comparison to WAT, demonstrating its possible role in this tissue [153]. Also, TRPC1 knockout mice fed high-fat diets display decreased BW, and fat mass when compared to WT animals. The introduction of exercise in both groups improve insulin resistance. The study suggests that TRPC1 may regulate adiposity, by regulating autophagy and apoptosis in the AT [159].

In the endocrine pancreas, TRPC1, TRPC4, and TRPC6 are identified in different cell lines, and TRPC1 is observed in human β-cells [152, 157, 160]. Nevertheless, little is known of their effects on pancreatic β-cells. A single report revealed that TRPC4 knockout mice did not present alterations in glucose homeostasis after glucose tolerance tests, nor following an intraperitoneal glucose challenge [161].

TRPM

TRPM2 and TRPM8 expression are detected in 3T3-L1 adipocytes, and in mouse visceral and subcutaneous WAT and BAT [153, 154], while TRPM3, TRPM4, and TRPM5 are present in subcutaneous WAT and BAT from mice [154]. TRPM7 is also identified in 3T3-L1 adipocytes, and human preadipocytes [162, 163]. In the AT, studies investigated mainly TRPM2 and TRPM5, although there are reports on TRPM4, TRPM7, and TRPM8. TRPM2 knockout mice exhibit improved glucose metabolism in peripheral tissues, leading to enhanced insulin sensitivity. When submitted to a high-fat diet, these mice are resistant to obesity, through increased energy expenditure, and a further improvement in AT inflammation [164]. Moreover, diet-induced obesity and *db/db* mice present reduced gene expression of TRPM2 in the subcutaneous WAT [154]. Although TRPM5 knockout mice are protected against a cafeteria diet (*i.e.*, obesogenic diet), characterized by reduced BW and adiposity, and an improvement in insulin resistance, these effects are suggested to be a consequence of the reduced calorie intake due to altered TRPM5-mediated taste signaling and palatability [165]. These events are also demonstrated in mice fed a sucrose diet [166].

Inhibition of TRPM4 in the human adipose-derived stem cells promotes a reduction of lipid droplet accumulation, and triggers the expression of adipogenic genes, including CCAAT-enhancer-binding proteins alpha (C/EBPα), C/EBPβ and PPARγ, thus, indicating a potential role for TRPM4 in adipogenesis [167]. Additionally, TRPM7 is implicated in adipogenesis, as its silencing decreases adipogenic differentiation [162]. Furthermore, TRPM7 promotes cell proliferation in 3T3-L1 preadipocytes, while its knockdown inhibits adipogenesis [163]. Also, TRPM8 knockout mice housed at cold temperatures become obese, and have dysfunctional glucose metabolism associated with daytime hyperphagia and diminished fat oxidation [168]. Moreover, TRPM8 expression is higher in preadipocytes than adipocytes, indicating a possible role for this receptor in adipogenesis [153]. Interestingly, in obese Thai subjects, a whole exome sequencing of protein-coding regions in the total genome also identified TRPM8 as a gene involved in obesity development, by regulating feeding behavior and energy expenditure [169]. Moreover, Tabur *et al.* found that TRPM8 and TRPM5 gene polymorphisms in a Turkish population could contribute to individual susceptibility to CMS [48].

TRPM2, TRPM3, TRPM4, and TRPM5 expressions are present in a range of pancreatic cell lines, while TRPM2, TRPM3, TRPM4 and TRPM7 are also described in human β-cells [157, 160]. Several studies in the endocrine pancreas have investigated TRPM2, TRPM4, and TRPM5 channels. In pancreatic rat islands, a glucagon-like peptide-1 (GLP-1) agonist is able to induce insulin secretion in a TRPM2-dependent manner, whereas knockdown markedly reduced insulin secretion [170]. Consequently, TRPM2 knockout mice present impaired glucose-stimulated insulin secretion, resulting in elevated basal glucose levels and glucose intolerance [171]. Moreover, TRPM2 was suggested to be involved in β-cell apoptosis. Activation of TRPM2 mediates β-cell death [172] and, on conversely, its suppression protects these cells from death [173].

Regarding the role of TRPM4 in the endocrine pancreas, studies are controversial. In mice lacking TRPM4, there were no differences in glucose-induced insulin secretion and no signs of impaired glucose tolerance [174]. Nevertheless, GLP--stimulated insulin secretion has proven to be at least partially dependent on TRPM4 activation [175], as TRPM4 inhibition decreases its levels in pancreatic β-cells [176]. TRPM5 knockout mice present elevated blood glucose after glucose tolerance tests, though displaying normal insulin sensitivity. In addition, insulin secretion is reduced in isolated pancreatic β-cells [177]. In accordance, *ob/ob* and *db/db* mice present diminished TRPM5 gene expression in pancreatic islets, and murine β-cell line insulin downregulated TRPM5 expression, indicating that the increased leptin levels may be linked to impaired TRPM5 expression [178]. Another study demonstrated the downregulation of TRPM5 in *ob/ob* mice and proved that TRPM5 rescue through dietary taurine is accompanied by an improvement in glucose homeostasis [179].

Aside from TRPM2, TRPM4, and TRPM5 that were reported in both AT and pancreas, TRPM3 is also studied in pancreatic cells. When activated by a synthetic agonist (CIM0216), TRPM3 triggers insulin secretion in pancreatic β-cells [180]. With regard to TRPM8, its knockdown in mice results in an increased insulin sensitivity without effects on glucose tolerance, due to a compensatory mechanism of enhanced insulin clearance in the liver [181]. However, Fonfria *et al*. failed to observe TRPM8 expression in the endocrine pancreas [182].

TRPML and TRPP

TRPP2 gene expression is present in 3T3-L1 adipocytes, and mouse visceral WAT and BAT [153]. Meanwhile, TRPP3 expression is found in human adipocytes [183]. Also, TRPP2, TRPML1, and TRPML3 expressions are described in human pancreatic β-cells [160]. Little is known of TRPP and TRPML role on obesity and T2D, and there is limited literature on their significance in AT and endocrine pancreas. In one study, adipocyte knockdown of TRPP3 repressed the expression of genes that characterize a brown fat signature, like uncoupling protein 1 (UCP1) and PPARγ coactivator 1 alpha (PGC1α), though other general adipogenic genes remained unaltered, suggesting a possible role for TRPP3 in mitochondrial function [183]. On the other hand, the role of TRPP2 in AT and endocrine pancreas, and of TRPML1 and TRPML3 in pancreatic β-cells remains to be elucidated.

TRPV

TRPV1, TRPV2, TRPV3, and TRPV4 are expressed in 3T3-L1 adipocytes, visceral and subcutaneous WAT from mice and also in BAT from mice. TRPV6 has been identified in adipocytes and mouse visceral WAT and BAT [153, 154]. TRPV2 and TRPV4 are also expressed in human preadipocytes [162]. There are several reports on the role of TRPV1-4 channels in the AT. TRPV1 expression is reduced in visceral AT in obese *ob/ob* and *db/db* mice and obese men, compared to their lean counterparts [51]. The same decrease in TRPV1 expression and activity was confirmed in the visceral and subcutaneous WAT and BAT of mice with diet-induced obesity [52, 53]. Knockdown of TRPV1 channel has also been investigated, though with discrepant results. Motter *et al*. reports that TRPV1 null mice fed an obesogenic diet had less BW gain and adiposity when compared to WT animals. This difference was reportedly not related to energy intake or absorption, but rather to an increase in thermogenic capacity probably through modulation of AT neurons [184].

Another study with high-fat diet-induced obesity demonstrated that TRPV1 knockdown provides no protection against BW gain, but improves glucose tolerance and the profile of proinflammatory cytokines (*e.g.*, leptin) when compared to WT mice, indicating a possible role of TRPV1 in the development of T2D [185]. Nevertheless, in the same model, TRPV1 knockouts promote obesity through the stimulation of positive energy balance and leptin resistance, and also induce insulin resistance in both WAT and BAT [186]. Lastly, TRPV1 is an essential modulator of BAT clock gene oscillations, thus, suggesting a role for this channel in BAT thermogenesis [187].

Following the same trend, TRPV3 was proven to have similar effects as TRPV1. In diet-induced obese, *ob/ob,* and *db/db* mice, TRPV3 expression is reduced in visceral WAT [188]. TRPV1 and TRPV3 expressions are higher in preadipocytes, suggesting their participation in adipogenesis [153]. Interestingly, diet-induced obese and *db/db* mice present modulation of not only TRPV1, but also TRPV3 gene expression, in both WAT and BAT. On the contrary, TRPV2 and TRPV4 mRNA expression increases in both tissues and animal models (*i.e.*, high-fat and *db/db* mice) [154].

In this sense, cultured brown adipocytes and the BAT from TRPV2 knockout mice show diminished expression of thermogenic genes. Mice also present larger adipocytes in BAT, cold intolerance, reduced elevation of BAT temperature under adrenergic stimuli, and higher amounts of WAT. When challenged with a high-fat diet, these animals present elevated BW and adiposity [189]. The same research group also demonstrated that TRPV2 expression increases during brown adipocytes differentiation. Additionally, while TRPV2 agonists inhibit adipocyte differentiation, its antagonists restore this process. Importantly, TRPV2 agonism in brown cells from knockout mice have a minor effect in inhibiting adipocyte differentiation [190].

In a mouse model of fetal programming in which females were fed a high-fat diet, male pups show increased TRPV4 mRNA expression in both visceral WAT and BAT, together with increased BW and fat. All these changes are tackled when females are switched to a standard-chow diet during pregnancy [191]. TRPV4 knockout mice fed a high-fat diet are shown to be protected from obesity, with smaller adipocytes in visceral WAT and BAT, and no changes in food intake [192]. Accordingly, TRPV4 knockdown in adipocytes upregulates the expression of PGC1α mRNA and protein, and other thermogenic and mitochondrial genes like UCP1 as well, thus, suggesting the browning of these cells may happen in the absence of TRPV4. Moreover, TRPV4 knockdown further reduces the expression of proinflammatory genes involved in the development of insulin resistance. When TRPV4 knockout mice were investigated, the authors observed an increase in UCP1 gene and protein expression associated with other genes involved in subcutaneous WAT browning. When these mice were challenged with a high-fat diet, they were protected from obesity, AT inflammation and insulin resistance

[193]. Nevertheless, despite this evidence, another study demonstrated that high-fat diet fed TRPV4 knockout mice showed increased BW and adiposity [194]. Bishnoi *et al.* suggested that TRPV4 and TRPV6 might represent important roles in WAT, since their expression is prevalent in this tissue compared to BAT [153]. Both TRPV2 and TRPV4 are involved in adipogenesis, since gene silencing decreased adipogenic differentiation [162]. Lastly, genotypes at the TRPV4 locus are shown to independently affect the obesity status in Taiwanese subjects [195].

Regarding the endocrine pancreas, TRPV1, TRPV2, TRPV4, and TRPV6 were found in different pancreatic cell lines [152, 157]. In this sense, while TRPV1 expression is controversial, TRPV2 and TRPV4 have also been studied [157]. Treatment of *ob/ob* mice with a TRPV1 antagonist (*N*-(4-*tert*-butylphenyl)-4-(3-chloropyridin-2-yl)tetrahydropyrazine-1(2*H*)-carboxamidte monohydro- chloride) enhances insulin secretion and reduces insulin resistance [196]. Although one study did report the TRPV1 expression in pancreatic β-cells [197], the majority of the reports indicate that its expression is restricted to TRPV1-positive neurons innervating the pancreas [157, 198]. Regarding TRPV2, its inhibition reduces insulin autocrine actions in pancreatic β-cells [199]. Lastly, activation of TRPV4 in pancreatic β-cells enhances glucose-stimulated insulin release [200] and, on the other hand, the reduced TRPV4 expression protects pancreatic β-cells against apoptosis [201].

In summary, modulating TRPV1, TRPV2, and TRPV3 expression in the AT may be beneficial for combating obesity and its comorbidities, though some results remain controversial for TRPV1. Meanwhile, TRPV4 may stimulate adiposity and weight gain. In the endocrine pancreas, TRPV1 and TRPV4 appear to have beneficial effects through the increased insulin secretion and reduced apoptosis, respectively; TRPV2 may reduce the action of insulin.

Table 2. TRP expression and modulation in the adipose tissue.

Authors	Experimental Model	Intervention	Main Findings
TRPA1			
Lieder *et al.*, 2017	3T3-L1 adipocytes	*trans*-pellitorine	TRPA1-dependent ↓ lipid accumulation and PPARγ mRNA/protein expression
Tamura *et al.*, 2012	DIO in C57Bl/6 mice	TRPA1 agonist (cinnamaldehyde)	↓ visceral AT and ↑ UCP1 protein in BAT

(Table 2) cont.....

Khare *et al.*, 2016	DIO in swiss albino mice	TRPA1 agonist (cinnamaldehyde)	↓ BM gain, ↑ lipolytic gene expression, and ↓ inflammatory gene expression in visceral WAT
	3T3-L1 preadipocytes		↓ lipid accumulation and favored gene expression toward a lipolytic phenotype
TRPC			
Sukumar *et al.*, 2012	3T3-L1 adipocytes and transgenic mice	Channel blockade by antibodies, TRPC1-TRPC5 knockdown *in vitro*, or conditional disruption of Ca^{2+} permeability in TRPC5 incorporating channels *in vivo*	↑ adiponectin production
	HEK 293 cells and 3T3-L1 adipocytes	α-linolenic acid and ω-3 fatty acids	Inhibition of TRPC1 and TRPC5 channels, and linolenic acid ↑ adiponectin production
Krout *et al.*, 2017	DIO and exercise (voluntary wheel running)	TRPC1 knockout mice	↓ fat mass, adipocyte number, and fasting glucose, associated with ↓ autophagy markers and ↑ apoptosis markers in sWAT
TRPM			
Zhang *et al.*, 2012	DIO in mice	TRPM2 knockout mice	Resistance to obesity, with ↑ EE, ↑ expression of genes involved in lipid metabolism and mitochondrial function in WAT, ↑ insulin sensitivity and ↓ AT inflammation
Larsson *et al.*, 2015	DIO in mice	TRPM5 knockout mice	↓ body and fat mass gain and ↑ glucose tolerance, which was associated with changes in the taste signaling system
Glendinning *et al.*, 2012	DIO in mice	TRPM5 knockout mice	↓ BM gain
Tran *et al.*, 2014	Human adipose-derived stem cells	TRPM4 knockdown (shRNA)	↓ lipid droplet accumulation and adipogenesis gene expression
Che *et al.*, 2014	Human white preadipocytes	TRPM7 knockdown (shRNA)	↓ adipogenic differentiation
Chen *et al.*, 2014	3T3-L1 preadipocytes	TRPM7 knockdown (siRNA)	↓ proliferation and adipogenesis
Reimúndez *et al.*, 2018	Mice raised at mild cold temperature	TRPM8 knockout mice	Obesity and dysfunctional glucose metabolism associated with daytime hyperphagia and ↓ fat oxidation

(Table 2) cont.....

Ma et al., 2012	Mouse brown adipocytes	TRPM8 agonist (menthol)	↑ UCP1 protein expression
	DIO in C57Bl/6 mice		↑ core temperature and prevented obesity and glucose intolerance
Goralczyk et al., 2017	Human progenitors-derived white adipocytes	TRPM8 agonist (menthol)	↑ UCP1 protein expression and uncoupled respiration, indicative of browning
Rossato et al., 2014	Human white adipocytes	TRPM8 agonist (menthol and icilin)	↑ UCP1 mRNA/protein expression, glucose uptake and heat production, indicative of browning
Jiang et al., 2017	Mouse white adipocytes	TRPM8 agonist (menthol)	↑ thermogenic genes expression
	DIO in C57Bl/6 mice		↓ BM gain and adiposity, and ↑ glucose metabolism ↑ thermogenic genes expression in sWAT, indicative of browning
Khare et al., 2019	Swiss albino mice	TRPM8 agonist (menthol)	Induction of a brown fat-like phenotype in sWAT
TRPV			
Baskaran et al., 2016	DIO in TRPV1 knockout mice	TRPV1 agonist (capsaicin)	Browning of sWAT, counteracting obesity, and it was abolished in TRPV1 knockout mice
Baskaran et al., 2017	DIO in TRPV1 knockout mice	TRPV1 agonist (capsaicin)	↑ thermogenic genes (*e.g.*, UCP1) in BAT, associated with BM loss, and these effects were absent in TRPV1 knockout mice
Motter and Ahern, 2008	DIO in mice	TRPV1 knockout mice	↑ BM gain and adiposity with ↑ thermogenic capacity
Marshall et al., 2013	DIO in mice	TRPV1 knockout mice	↑ glucose tolerance and cytokine profile without BM change
Lee et al., 2015	DIO in mice	TRPV1 knockout mice	↑ BM gain and insulin resistance, with altered energy balance and leptin resistance
Moraes et al., 2017	Mice kept in constant darkness or a light-dark cycle	TRPV1 knockout mice	Modulation of BAT clock gene oscillations
Sun et al., 2016	Mice	TRPV2 knockout mice	↑ adipocyte size in BAT, ↑ WAT mass, and cold intolerance
Sun et al., 2016	Mouse brown adipocytes	TRPV2 agonists (2-APB and LPC)	Inhibited brown adipocytes differentiation
		TRPV2 antagonist (SKF96365)	Restored brown adipocytes differentiation

(Table 2) cont.....

Kusudo *et al.*, 2012	DIO in mice	TRPV4 knockout mice	Protection from obesity with ↓ adipocyte size in visceral WAT and BAT
Ye *et al.*, 2012	3T3-F442A adipocytes and mouse white adipocytes	TRPV4 knockdown (shRNA)	↑ thermogenic and mitochondrial genes (*e.g.*, UCP1), suggestive of browning
	DIO in mice	TRPV4 knockout mice	↑ thermogenesis in AT and protect against obesity, AT inflammation and insulin resistance
O'Conor *et al.*, 2013	DIO in mice	TRPV4 knockout mice	↑ BM gain and adiposity
Che *et al.*, 2014	Human white preadipocytes	TRPV2 and TRPV4 knockdown (shRNA)	↓ adipogenic differentiation
Rigamonti *et al.*, 2018	Young obese subjects	TRPV1 agonist (capsaicin)	↑ EE
Yoneshiro *et al.*, 2012	Healthy men	TRPV1 agonist (capsinoids)	↑ EE through BAT activation
Inoue *et al.*, 2007	Men and postmenopausal women with a BMI > 23 kg/m^2	TRPV1 agonist (capsinoids)	↑ EE and fat oxidation
Iwasaki *et al.*, 2011	DIO in C57Bl/6 mice	TRPV1 agonist (monoacylglycerols)	↑ UCP1 protein expression in BAT and ↓ visceral WAT mass
Cheung *et al.*, 2015	3T3-L1 preadipocytes	TRPV3 agonist (-)- epicatechin	↓ lipid accumulation and adipogenesis
	DIO in C57Bl/6 mice		↓ adipogenesis and BM gain

Abbreviations: 2-APB, 2-aminoethoxydiphenyl borate; AT, adipose tissue; BAT, brown adipose tissue; BM, body mass; BMI, body mass index; DIO, diet-induced obesity; EE, energy expenditure; LPC, lysophosphatidylcholine; PPARγ, peroxisome proliferator-activated receptor gamma; sWAT, subcutaneous white adipose tissue; TRPA1, transient receptor potential ankyrin 1; TRPC, transient receptor potential canonical; TRPM, transient receptor potential melastatin; TRPV, transient receptor potential vanilloid; UCP1, uncoupling protein 1; WAT, white adipose tissue.

Table 3. TRP expression and modulation in the endocrine pancreas.

Authors	Experimental Model	Intervention	Main Findings
TRPA1			
Cao *et al.*, 2012	Rat pancreatic β-cells and RINm5F cells (rat β-cell line)	TRPA1 agonists (allyl isothiocyanate, 4-hydroxynonenal, cyclopentenone prostaglandins, and methylglyoxal)	↑ insulin release
		TRPA1 antagonists (HC030031 and AP-18) and TRPA1 knockdown (siRNA)	↓ insulin release

(Table 3) cont.....

Numazawa *et al.*, 2012	RINm5F cells	TRPA1 agonists (allyl isothiocyanate and 15-deoxy-Δ12,14-prostaglandin J2)	↑ Ca^{2+} influx, suggestive of insulin secretion stimulation
		TRPA1 antagonist (HC030031)	↓ Ca^{2+} influx, suggestive of insulin secretion inhibition
TRPC			
Novelli *et al.*, 2016	INS-1E cells (rat β-cell line)	Hyperforin (TRPC6 agonist)	↓ inflammatory and apoptotic genes expression
TRPM			
Togashi *et al.*, 2006	RINm5F cells and rat pancreatic islets	TRPM2 knockdown (siRNA)	↓ insulin release
Uchida *et al.*, 2011	Mice (*in vivo*) and mouse pancreatic islets (*in vitro*)	TRPM2 knockout mice	↑ basal blood glucose and after GTT and ↓ insulin secretion
Vennekens *et al.*, 2007	Mice	TRPM4 knockout mice	Unchanged glucose-stimulated insulin secretion and no signs of impaired glucose tolerance
Shigeto *et al.*, 2015	Mouse pancreatic islets	TRPM4 and TRPM5 knockout mice	↓ GLP-1-stimulated insulin secretion
Marigo *et al.*, 2009	INS-1E cells	TRPM4 inhibition (dnTRPM4)	↓ insulin secretion
Brixel *et al.*, 2010	Mice (*in vivo*) and mouse pancreatic islets (*in vitro*)	TRPM5 knockout mice	↑ blood glucose after a GTT and ↓ insulin secretion
Held *et al.*, 2015	Mouse pancreatic islets	TRPM3 agonist (CIM0216)	↑ insulin release
McCoy *et al.*, 2013	Mice	TRPM8 knockout mice	A normal response to glucose challenge, but prolonged hypoglycemia in response to insulin with ↑ rates of insulin clearance
Philippaert *et al.*, 2017	Mouse pancreatic islets	Steviol glycosides	TRPM5-dependent ↑ glucose-stimulated insulin secretion
	DIO in C57Bl/6 mice		TRPM5-dependent protection against hyperglycemia
TRPV			
Tanaka *et al.*, 2011	*ob/ob* mice	TRPV1 antagonist (BCTC)	↓ fasting glucose and insulin, and ↑ plasma insulin secretion after OGTT

(Table 3) cont.....

Hisanaga *et al.*, **2011**	MIN6 cells (mouse β-cell line)	TRPV2 knockdown (shRNA)	↓ insulin secretion
Skrzypski *et al.*, **2013**	INS-1E cells	TRPV4 agonist (4α-PDD)	↑ glucose-stimulated insulin secretion
Casas *et al.*, **2008**	MIN6 cells	TRPV4 knockdown (siRNA)	↓ cell death
Akiba *et al.* **2004**	RINm5F cells	TRPV1 agonist (capsaicin)	↑ insulin secretion
	SD rats		↑ plasma insulin
Wang *et al.*, **2012**	*db/db* mice	TRPV1 agonist (capsaicin)	↑ glucose homeostasis, and ↑ plasmatic GLP-1
	TRPV1 knockout mice		Capsaicin ↑ GLP-1 and insulin secretion and ↑ glucose tolerance in WT mice, which was absent in knockout mice
Mori *et al.*, **2018**	Mouse pancreatic islets	TRPA1 agonist (allyl isothiocyanate)	↑ insulin secretion
	TRPV1 knockout mice		↑ blood insulin in WT mice, but not in knockout mice

<u>Abbreviations</u>: 4α-PDD, 4α-phorbol 12,13-didecanoate; BCTC, *N*-(4-*tert*-butylphenyl)-4-(3-chloropyri-in-2-yl)tetrahydropyrazine-1(2*H*)-carboxamidte monohydrochloride; DIO, diet-induced obesity; dnTRPM4, dominant-negative construct ΔN TRPM4; GLP-1, glucagon-like peptide-1; GTT, glucose tolerance test; OGTT, oral glucose tolerance test; SD, Sprague-Dawley; TRPA1, transient receptor potential ankyrin 1; TRPC, transient receptor potential canonical; TRPM, transient receptor potential melastatin; TRPV, transient receptor potential vanilloid; WT, wild type.

Modulation of TRP Expression in the Adipose Tissue and Endocrine Pancreas

TRP channels are modulated by a wide range of endogenous and exogenous ligands [6]. Here we will focus on exogenous chemicals and natural compounds that have an impact on AT and endocrine pancreas function, and thus may have a role in the development of drugs and food strategies to tackle obesity and T2D.

TRPA1

Several exogenous ligands of TRPA1 have been identified, including cinnamaldehyde. Cinnamaldehyde is a pungent compound found in cinnamon or dried barks of cassia, known as a TRPA1 agonist. In mice pair-fed with an obesogenic diet (*i.e.*, high-fat high-sucrose diet), cinnamaldehyde supplementation reduces visceral AT and increases UCP1 protein expression in BAT [202]. Similarly, cinnamaldehyde prevents high-fat induced weight gain, decreases leptin levels, increases lipolytic gene expression, and decreases inflammatory gene expression in visceral WAT. Nevertheless, these effects are concomitant with a decrease in fasting-induced hyperphagia. In 3T3-L1 preadipocytes, cinnamaldehyde also prevents lipid accumulation favoring a lipolytic phenotype [203].

TRPC

Studies using the exogenous ligands of TRPC5 and TRPC6 are scarce, but may have a potential impact on the AT and endocrine pancreas. N-3 polyunsaturated fatty acids (*i.e.*, α-linolenic acid) are found to stimulate adiponectin production in a mechanism dependent on TRPC5 modulation [19]. Although hyperforin — a constituent of St. John's wort — is known to be an exogenous activator of TRPC6 that modulates pancreatic β-cells inflammation and apoptosis [204, 205], its role in insulin resistance, T2D and obesity remains elusive.

TRPM

Two TRPM channels have agonists that display effects on AT and endocrine pancreas: TRPM5 and TRPM8. Steviol glycosides are natural non-caloric sweet-tasting molecules, present in extracts of the scrub plant *Stevia rebaudiana,* shown to potentiate the activity of TRPM5 and enhance glucose-induced insulin secretion in a TRPM5-dependent manner. In high-fat diet fed mice, steviol glycosides ameliorate glucose metabolism, and this effect is abolished in knockout mice [206].

Among TRPM8 exogenous agonists, menthol, a cooling agent from the mint plant, is well investigated. Brown adipocytes challenged with menthol increase UCP1 expression. Also, chronic treatment with dietary menthol provided to diet-induced obese mice increases core temperature and locomotor activity, and is associated with improved BW and glucose homeostasis. Importantly, these effects are absent in TRPM8 null mice [46]. In white adipocytes, menthol increases UCP-1 expression and uncouples respiration, thus indicating a role for inducing browning. Nevertheless, in this study, the same phenomenon was not observed in brown adipocytes [183].

Additionally, in human white adipocytes, treatment with menthol and icillin (a synthetic TRPM8 agonist) induces a brown-like phenotype, increasing UCP1 expression, glucose uptake, and heat production, and supporting its role in the counteraction of obesity and T2D [45]. In accordance, activation of TRPM8 by menthol enhances the expression of thermogenic genes in cultured white adipocytes, and dietary menthol administered to diet-induced obese mice enhances WAT browning and improves glucose metabolism [207]. Recently, a single oral and topical menthol administration was proved sufficient to induce a brown-like phenotype in subcutaneous WAT [208].

TRPV

Capsaicin is found in chili peppers, and is the most studied nutritional compound that activates TRP channels, that may have beneficial effects on obesity and its comorbidities [151]. Capsaicin was shown to prevent adipogenesis in 3T3-L1 preadipocytes, and TRPV1 knockdown abolished this effect. Similarly, capsaicin administration for 120 days prevents diet-induced obesity in WT mice, but not in TRPV1 knockout animals [51]. More recently, capsaicin triggered WAT browning in mice *via* TRPV1, by increasing the expression of important brown fat and thermogenic markers, such as UCP1, PGC1α, and PR domain containing 16 (PRDM16) [53]. Along with subcutaneous WAT browning, capsaicin modulates BAT since it prevents, through TRPV1 activation, the reduction of critical thermogenic mediators (*e.g.*, PGC1α and PRDM16) in mice fed with a high-fat diet [52]. These beneficial effects are accompanied by a reduction in weight gain, and enhancement in metabolic activity, and are abolished in TRPV1 knockout mice [52, 53].

In the endocrine pancreas, capsaicin has been known to increase insulin secretion in pancreatic β-cells in a TRPV1-dependent manner, proved by the abolishment of this effect following the administration of the TRPV1 inhibitor, capsazepine. Capsaicin can also increase plasma insulin levels in rats [197]. Similarly, mice treated with capsaicin demonstrate an increased postprandial insulin secretion. However as stated before, this effect was not associated with a direct secretagogue action, and is attributed to GLP-1-increased incretin secretion. Importantly, the insulin increase is abolished in TRPV1 knockout mice [209].

In humans, capsaicin increases energy expenditure without affecting energy intake in young obese subjects [210]. Similarly, capsinoids, which are nonpungent analogs of capsaicin, increase energy expenditure through the activation of BAT in healthy men [211]. Similarly, they increase energy expenditure and fat oxidation, and these effects are enhanced in subjects with high body mass index scores [212]. Lastly, a recent meta-analysis confirms that capsaicin or capsinoids are relevant in promoting weight loss in subjects with elevated body mass index, through a negative energy balance and increase in fat oxidation [213].

Aside from capsaicin, other TRPV agonists have already been studied. Dietary monoacylglycerols are novel TRPV1 agonists which were shown to increase the UCP1 content in BAT, and reduce visceral WAT mass in mice fed a high-fat high-sucrose diet [214]. Allyl isothiocyanate is a natural compound found in plants belonging to the family Cruciferae, which is the pungent ingredient found in mustard, horseradish, and wasabi. It enhances insulin secretion in pancreatic islands, an effect abolished in cells from TRPV1 knockout mice [215].

Both (-)-epicatechin, a green tea polyphenol, and diphenylborinic anhydride, an established TRPV3 agonist, impair the expression of adipogenic genes, including PPARγ and C/EBPα, thus inhibiting adipogenesis. These results have been confirmed in diet-induced obese mice, where weight gain and adipogenesis were prevented [188].

FUTURE PERSPECTIVES

CMS combines several metabolic dysfunctions, presenting a treatment challenge. Currently, many drugs that dealing with individual conditions, such as high blood pressure, blood glucose, and lipids, are available. However, a single therapy to solve all these issues is yet to be developed. Patients are often subjected to many pills, leading to poor treatment adherence and high treatment costs. In this direction, the approval for a polypill — a fixed-dose combination treatment — for cardiovascular diseases has been made available in several countries, but its implementation in the clinical practice has proven challenging. The literature shows that polypills have benefits on cardiovascular diseases [216], but little is known about their role in obesity, as an antiobesity agent is not present in the formula. Since TRPs channels have been correlated with some aspects of CMS, as detailed in this chapter and in Fig. (2), they appear to present a potential new target for CMS treatment. However, further studies need to thoroughly investigate the relationship between these channels in tissue function and disease development, in order to design new drugs for treatment or prevention of CMS, and thus improve patient well-being and health status. Capsaicin is a promising strategy to combat CMS as a monotherapy, as it possesses a broad range of beneficial effects on the cardiovascular system and metabolism. However, further studies are necessary since capsaicin has dose-dependent side effects concerning cardiovascular physiology. On the other hand, other substances such as cinnamaldehyde, pyrazole, and menthol could be used in combination to well-established therapies, to treat CMS manifestations, however further studies need to evaluate pharmacological interactions and safety. Finally, both the molecular structure of these compounds and the known biological effects, known to be possessed as shown in several studies, will serve as a direction toward the discovery of new TRP channel modulators to treat CMS.

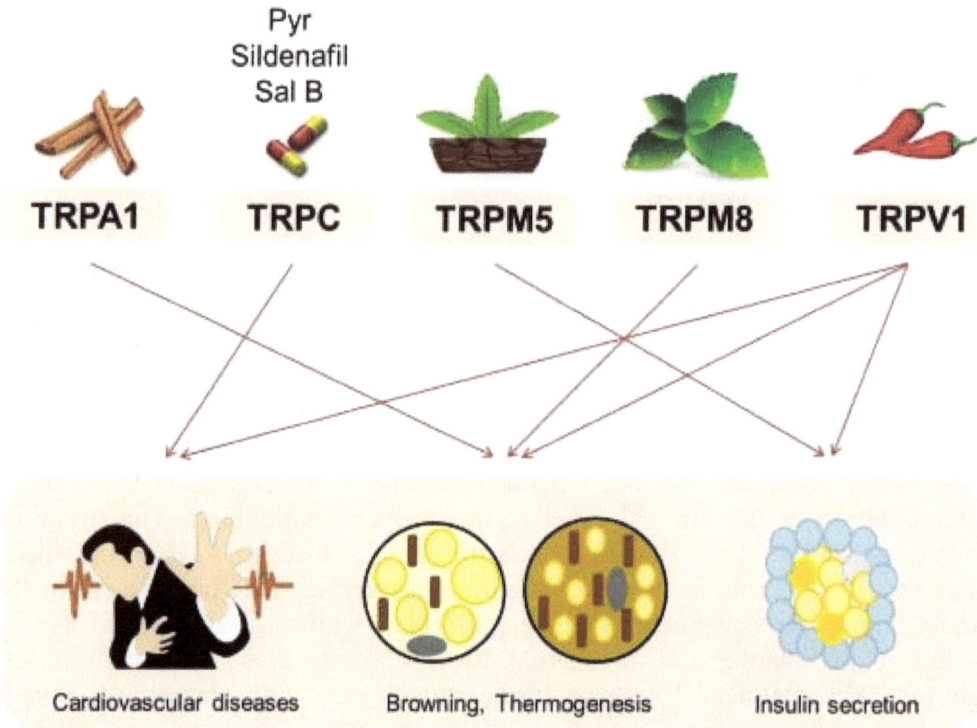

Fig. (2). TRP channels activation and their effect on tissues that are involved in cardiometabolic syndrome. TRPA1 can be activated by cinnamaldehyde, which is the pungent compound in cinnamon, with effects on the adipose tissue that encompasses reduced fat accumulation and BAT thermogenesis. In relation to TRPC, some drugs already known by their pharmacological action, such as sildenafil (phosphodiesterase type 5 inhibitor), pyrazole, and the medicinal root *Salvia miltiorrhiza Bunge* are selective blockers of TRPC channels such as TRPC3 and TRPC6, protecting against cardiac injury. TRPM5 can be activated by the use of steviol glycosides, natural non-caloric sweet-tasting molecules that ameliorate insulin secretion, while menthol (a cooling agent from the mint plant) is the most well investigated TRPM8 agonist, inducing a brown-like phenotype in WAT. Lastly, TRPV1 is classically known to be activated by capsaicin, found in chili peppers, promoting WAT browning and increased thermogenesis in BAT, stimulating insulin secretion in pancreas, and protecting from cardiac injury. The modulation of these TRP channels on the cardiovascular system, adipose tissue and endocrine pancreas may contribute to the beneficial effects on cardiovascular diseases, obesity and diabetes, thus culminating in improvements in the cardiometabolic syndrome. Abbreviations: BAT, brown adipose tissue; Pyr, pyrazole; TRP, transient receptor potential; TRPA1, transient receptor potential ankyrin 1; TRPC, transient receptor potential canonical; TRPM, transient receptor potential melastatin; TRPV, transient receptor potential vanilloid; and WAT, white adipose tissue.

CONCLUSION

Studies investigating TRP channels demonstrate promising results, but translation in to preventive or therapeutic strategies against cardiometabolic diseases is challenging due to their presence in multiple tissues and role in several physiological actions, which increases the risk of adverse effects.

CONSENT FOR PUBLICATION

Not applicable.

CONFLICT OF INTEREST

The authors confirm that they have no conflict of interest to declare for this publication.

ACKNOWLEDGEMENTS

Declare none.

REFERENCES

[1]   Srivastava AK. Challenges in the treatment of cardiometabolic syndrome. Indian J Pharmacol 2012; 44(2): 155-6.
[http://dx.doi.org/10.4103/0253-7613.93579] [PMID: 22529466]

[2]   Ash-Bernal R, Peterson LR. The cardiometabolic syndrome and cardiovascular disease. J Cardiometab Syndr 2006; 1(1): 25-8.
[http://dx.doi.org/10.1111/j.0197-3118.2006.05452.x] [PMID: 17675903]

[3]   Kelli HM, Kassas I, Lattouf OM. Cardio Metabolic Syndrome: A Global Epidemic. J Diabetes Metab 2015; 6(3)
[http://dx.doi.org/10.4172/2155-6156.1000513] [PMID: 29480368]

[4]   Saljoughian M. Cardiometabolic Syndrome: A Global Health Issue. US Pharm 2016; 41(2): HS19-21.

[5]   Ma J, Yang L, Ma Y, Wang X, Ren J, Yang J. Targeting transient receptor potential channels in cardiometabolic diseases and myocardial ischemia reperfusion injury. Curr Drug Targets 2017; 18(15): 1733-45.
[http://dx.doi.org/10.2174/1389450116666151019102052] [PMID: 26477459]

[6]   Kaneko Y, Szallasi A. Transient receptor potential (TRP) channels: A clinical perspective. Br J Pharmacol 2014; 171(10): 2474-507.
[http://dx.doi.org/10.1111/bph.12414] [PMID: 24102319]

[7]   Cosens DJ, Manning A. Abnormal electroretinogram from a Drosophila mutant. Nature 1969; 224(5216): 285-7.
[http://dx.doi.org/10.1038/224285a0] [PMID: 5344615]

[8]   Basso L, Altier C. Transient Receptor Potential Channels in neuropathic pain. Curr Opin Pharmacol 2017; 32: 9-15.
[http://dx.doi.org/10.1016/j.coph.2016.10.002] [PMID: 27835802]

[9]   Owsianik G, Talavera K, Voets T, Nilius B. Permeation and selectivity of TRP channels. Annu Rev Physiol 2006; 68: 685-717.
[http://dx.doi.org/10.1146/annurev.physiol.68.040204.101406] [PMID: 16460288]

[10] Feng S. TRPC Channel Structure and Properties. Adv Exp Med Biol 2017; 976: 9-23.
[http://dx.doi.org/10.1007/978-94-024-1088-4_2] [PMID: 28508309]

[11] Blair NT, Carvacho I, Chaudhuri D, Clapham DE, DeCaen P, Delling M, *et al.* Transient Receptor Potential channels IUPHAR/BPS Guide to PHARMACOLOGY 2019.

[12] Samanta A, Hughes TET, Moiseenkova-Bell VY. Transient Receptor Potential (TRP) Channels. Subcell Biochem 2018; 87: 141-65.
[http://dx.doi.org/10.1007/978-981-10-7757-9_6] [PMID: 29464560]

[13]   Vriens J, Nilius B, Vennekens R. Herbal compounds and toxins modulating TRP channels. Curr Neuropharmacol 2008; 6(1): 79-96.
[http://dx.doi.org/10.2174/157015908783769644] [PMID: 19305789]

[14]   Bon RS, Beech DJ. In pursuit of small molecule chemistry for calcium-permeable non-selective TRPC channels -- mirage or pot of gold? Br J Pharmacol 2013; 170(3): 459-74.
[http://dx.doi.org/10.1111/bph.12274] [PMID: 23763262]

[15]   Tai Y, Yang S, Liu Y, Shao W. TRPC Channels in Health and Disease. Adv Exp Med Biol 2017; 976: 35-45.
[http://dx.doi.org/10.1007/978-94-024-1088-4_4] [PMID: 28508311]

[16]   Sharma S, Hopkins CR. Review of Transient Receptor Potential Canonical (TRPC5) Channel Modulators and Diseases. J Med Chem 2019; 62(17): 7589-602.
[http://dx.doi.org/10.1021/acs.jmedchem.8b01954] [PMID: 30943030]

[17]   Nilius B, Szallasi A. Transient receptor potential channels as drug targets: From the science of basic research to the art of medicine. Pharmacol Rev 2014; 66(3): 676-814.
[http://dx.doi.org/10.1124/pr.113.008268] [PMID: 24951385]

[18]   Li H. TRP Channel Classification. Adv Exp Med Biol 2017; 976: 1-8.
[http://dx.doi.org/10.1007/978-94-024-1088-4_1] [PMID: 28508308]

[19]   Sukumar P, Sedo A, Li J, *et al.* Constitutively active TRPC channels of adipocytes confer a mechanism for sensing dietary fatty acids and regulating adiponectin. Circ Res 2012; 111(2): 191-200.
[http://dx.doi.org/10.1161/CIRCRESAHA.112.270751] [PMID: 22668831]

[20]   Pedersen SF, Owsianik G, Nilius B. TRP channels: An overview. Cell Calcium 2005; 38(3-4): 233-52.
[http://dx.doi.org/10.1016/j.ceca.2005.06.028] [PMID: 16098585]

[21]   Lau OC, Shen B, Wong CO, *et al.* TRPC5 channels participate in pressure-sensing in aortic baroreceptors. Nat Commun 2016; 7: 11947.
[http://dx.doi.org/10.1038/ncomms11947] [PMID: 27411851]

[22]   Zhu Y, Gao M, Zhou T, *et al.* The TRPC5 channel regulates angiogenesis and promotes recovery from ischemic injury in mice. J Biol Chem 2019; 294(1): 28-37.
[http://dx.doi.org/10.1074/jbc.RA118.005392] [PMID: 30413532]

[23]   Xu SZ, Sukumar P, Zeng F, *et al.* TRPC channel activation by extracellular thioredoxin. Nature 2008; 451(7174): 69-72.
[http://dx.doi.org/10.1038/nature06414] [PMID: 18172497]

[24]   Mizoguchi Y, Monji A. TRPC Channels and Brain Inflammation. Adv Exp Med Biol 2017; 976: 111-21.
[http://dx.doi.org/10.1007/978-94-024-1088-4_10] [PMID: 28508317]

[25]   Kim J, Ko J, Myeong J, Kwak M, Hong C, So I. TRPC1 as a negative regulator for TRPC4 and TRPC5 channels. Pflugers Arch 2019; 471(8): 1045-53.
[http://dx.doi.org/10.1007/s00424-019-02289-w] [PMID: 31222490]

[26]   Poletini MO, Moraes MN, Ramos BC, Jerônimo R, Castrucci AM. TRP channels: A missing bond in the entrainment mechanism of peripheral clocks throughout evolution. Temperature (Austin) 2015; 2(4): 522-34.
[http://dx.doi.org/10.1080/23328940.2015.1115803] [PMID: 27227072]

[27]   Oberwinkler J, Philipp SE. TRPM3. Handb Exp Pharmacol 2014; 222: 427-59.
[http://dx.doi.org/10.1007/978-3-642-54215-2_17] [PMID: 24756716]

[28]   Thiel G, Müller I, Rössler OG. Signal transduction *via* TRPM3 channels in pancreatic β-cells. J Mol Endocrinol 2013; 50(3): R75-83.
[http://dx.doi.org/10.1530/JME-12-0237] [PMID: 23511953]

[29]   Majeed Y, Bahnasi Y, Seymour VA, *et al.* Rapid and contrasting effects of rosiglitazone on transient

receptor potential TRPM3 and TRPC5 channels. Mol Pharmacol 2011; 79(6): 1023-30.
[http://dx.doi.org/10.1124/mol.110.069922] [PMID: 21406603]

[30]   Perraud AL, Takanishi CL, Shen B, *et al.* Accumulation of free ADP-ribose from mitochondria
        mediates oxidative stress-induced gating of TRPM2 cation channels. J Biol Chem 2005; 280(7): 6138-
        48.
        [http://dx.doi.org/10.1074/jbc.M411446200] [PMID: 15561722]

[31]   Kolisek M, Beck A, Fleig A, Penner R. Cyclic ADP-ribose and hydrogen peroxide synergize with
        ADP-ribose in the activation of TRPM2 channels. Mol Cell 2005; 18(1): 61-9.
        [http://dx.doi.org/10.1016/j.molcel.2005.02.033] [PMID: 15808509]

[32]   Zhu Z, Luo Z, Ma S, Liu D. TRP channels and their implications in metabolic diseases. Pflugers Arch
        2011; 461(2): 211-23.
        [http://dx.doi.org/10.1007/s00424-010-0902-5] [PMID: 21110037]

[33]   Grand T, Demion M, Norez C, *et al.* 9-phenanthrol inhibits human TRPM4 but not TRPM5 cationic
        channels. Br J Pharmacol 2008; 153(8): 1697-705.
        [http://dx.doi.org/10.1038/bjp.2008.38] [PMID: 18297105]

[34]   Takezawa R, Cheng H, Beck A, *et al.* A pyrazole derivative potently inhibits lymphocyte Ca^{2+} influx
        and cytokine production by facilitating transient receptor potential melastatin 4 channel activity. Mol
        Pharmacol 2006; 69(4): 1413-20.
        [http://dx.doi.org/10.1124/mol.105.021154] [PMID: 16407466]

[35]   Palmer RK, Atwal K, Bakaj I, *et al.* Triphenylphosphine oxide is a potent and selective inhibitor of the
        transient receptor potential melastatin-5 ion channel. Assay Drug Dev Technol 2010; 8(6): 703-13.
        [http://dx.doi.org/10.1089/adt.2010.0334] [PMID: 21158685]

[36]   Aarts M, Iihara K, Wei WL, *et al.* A key role for TRPM7 channels in anoxic neuronal death. Cell
        2003; 115(7): 863-77.
        [http://dx.doi.org/10.1016/S0092-8674(03)01017-1] [PMID: 14697204]

[37]   Krapivinsky G, Mochida S, Krapivinsky L, Cibulsky SM, Clapham DE. The TRPM7 ion channel
        functions in cholinergic synaptic vesicles and affects transmitter release. Neuron 2006; 52(3): 485-96.
        [http://dx.doi.org/10.1016/j.neuron.2006.09.033] [PMID: 17088214]

[38]   Jin J, Desai BN, Navarro B, Donovan A, Andrews NC, Clapham DE. Deletion of Trpm7 disrupts
        embryonic development and thymopoiesis without altering Mg^{2+} homeostasis. Science 2008;
        322(5902): 756-60.
        [http://dx.doi.org/10.1126/science.1163493] [PMID: 18974357]

[39]   Sah R, Mesirca P, Mason X, *et al.* Timing of myocardial trpm7 deletion during cardiogenesis variably
        disrupts adult ventricular function, conduction, and repolarization. Circulation 2013; 128(2): 101-14.
        [http://dx.doi.org/10.1161/CIRCULATIONAHA.112.000768] [PMID: 23734001]

[40]   Kraft R, Harteneck C. The mammalian melastatin-related transient receptor potential cation channels:
        An overview. Pflugers Arch 2005; 451(1): 204-11.
        [http://dx.doi.org/10.1007/s00424-005-1428-0] [PMID: 15895246]

[41]   Qin X, Yue Z, Sun B, *et al.* Sphingosine and FTY720 are potent inhibitors of the transient receptor
        potential melastatin 7 (TRPM7) channels. Br J Pharmacol 2013; 168(6): 1294-312.
        [http://dx.doi.org/10.1111/bph.12012] [PMID: 23145923]

[42]   Parnas M, Peters M, Dadon D, *et al.* Carvacrol is a novel inhibitor of Drosophila TRPL and
        mammalian TRPM7 channels. Cell Calcium 2009; 45(3): 300-9.
        [http://dx.doi.org/10.1016/j.ceca.2008.11.009] [PMID: 19135721]

[43]   Zierler S, Yao G, Zhang Z, *et al.* Waixenicin A inhibits cell proliferation through magnesium-
        dependent block of transient receptor potential melastatin 7 (TRPM7) channels. J Biol Chem 2011;
        286(45): 39328-35.
        [http://dx.doi.org/10.1074/jbc.M111.264341] [PMID: 21926172]

[44]   Runnels LW, Yue L, Clapham DE. TRP-PLIK, a bifunctional protein with kinase and ion channel activities. Science 2001; 291(5506): 1043-7.
[http://dx.doi.org/10.1126/science.1058519] [PMID: 11161216]

[45]   Rossato M, Granzotto M, Macchi V, *et al.* Human white adipocytes express the cold receptor TRPM8 which activation induces UCP1 expression, mitochondrial activation and heat production. Mol Cell Endocrinol 2014; 383(1-2): 137-46.
[http://dx.doi.org/10.1016/j.mce.2013.12.005] [PMID: 24342393]

[46]   Ma S, Yu H, Zhao Z, *et al.* Activation of the cold-sensing TRPM8 channel triggers UCP1-dependent thermogenesis and prevents obesity. J Mol Cell Biol 2012; 4(2): 88-96.
[http://dx.doi.org/10.1093/jmcb/mjs001] [PMID: 22241835]

[47]   McKemy DD, Neuhausser WM, Julius D. Identification of a cold receptor reveals a general role for TRP channels in thermosensation. Nature 2002; 416(6876): 52-8.
[http://dx.doi.org/10.1038/nature719] [PMID: 11882888]

[48]   Tabur S, Oztuzcu S, Duzen IV, *et al.* Role of the transient receptor potential (TRP) channel gene expressions and TRP melastatin (TRPM) channel gene polymorphisms in obesity-related metabolic syndrome. Eur Rev Med Pharmacol Sci 2015; 19(8): 1388-97.
[PMID: 25967713]

[49]   Traynor D, Kay RR. A polycystin-type transient receptor potential (Trp) channel that is activated by ATP. Biol Open 2017; 6(2): 200-9.
[http://dx.doi.org/10.1242/bio.020685] [PMID: 28011630]

[50]   Koulen P, Cai Y, Geng L, *et al.* Polycystin-2 is an intracellular calcium release channel. Nat Cell Biol 2002; 4(3): 191-7.
[http://dx.doi.org/10.1038/ncb754] [PMID: 11854751]

[51]   Zhang LL, Yan Liu D, Ma LQ, *et al.* Activation of transient receptor potential vanilloid type-1 channel prevents adipogenesis and obesity. Circ Res 2007; 100(7): 1063-70.
[http://dx.doi.org/10.1161/01.RES.0000262653.84850.8b] [PMID: 17347480]

[52]   Baskaran P, Krishnan V, Fettel K, *et al.* TRPV1 activation counters diet-induced obesity through sirtuin-1 activation and PRDM-16 deacetylation in brown adipose tissue. Int J Obes 2017; 41(5): 739-49.
[http://dx.doi.org/10.1038/ijo.2017.16] [PMID: 28104916]

[53]   Baskaran P, Krishnan V, Ren J, Thyagarajan B. Capsaicin induces browning of white adipose tissue and counters obesity by activating TRPV1 channel-dependent mechanisms. Br J Pharmacol 2016; 173(15): 2369-89.
[http://dx.doi.org/10.1111/bph.13514] [PMID: 27174467]

[54]   Baskaran P, Markert L, Bennis J, Zimmerman L, Fox J, Thyagarajan B. Assessment of Pharmacology, Safety, and Metabolic activity of Capsaicin Feeding in Mice. Sci Rep 2019; 9(1): 8588.
[http://dx.doi.org/10.1038/s41598-019-45050-0] [PMID: 31197191]

[55]   Omari SA, Adams MJ, Geraghty DP. TRPV1 Channels in Immune Cells and Hematological Malignancies. Adv Pharmacol 2017; 79: 173-98.
[http://dx.doi.org/10.1016/bs.apha.2017.01.002] [PMID: 28528668]

[56]   Park CK, Xu ZZ, Liu T, Lü N, Serhan CN, Ji RR. Resolvin D2 is a potent endogenous inhibitor for transient receptor potential subtype V1/A1, inflammatory pain, and spinal cord synaptic plasticity in mice: distinct roles of resolvin D1, D2, and E1. J Neurosci 2011; 31(50): 18433-8.
[http://dx.doi.org/10.1523/JNEUROSCI.4192-11.2011] [PMID: 22171045]

[57]   Dickenson AH, Dray A. Selective antagonism of capsaicin by capsazepine: evidence for a spinal receptor site in capsaicin-induced antinociception. Br J Pharmacol 1991; 104(4): 1045-9.
[http://dx.doi.org/10.1111/j.1476-5381.1991.tb12547.x] [PMID: 1810591]

[58]   Seabrook GR, Sutton KG, Jarolimek W, *et al.* Functional properties of the high-affinity TRPV1 (VR1)

vanilloid receptor antagonist (4-hydroxy-5-iodo-3-methoxyphenylacetate ester) iodo-resiniferatoxin. J Pharmacol Exp Ther 2002; 303(3): 1052-60.
[http://dx.doi.org/10.1124/jpet.102.040394] [PMID: 12438527]

[59]   Tóth A, Kedei N, Szabó T, Wang Y, Blumberg PM. Thapsigargin binds to and inhibits the cloned vanilloid receptor-1. Biochem Biophys Res Commun 2002; 293(2): 777-82.
[http://dx.doi.org/10.1016/S0006-291X(02)00293-0] [PMID: 12054538]

[60]   Juvin V, Penna A, Chemin J, Lin YL, Rassendren FA. Pharmacological characterization and molecular determinants of the activation of transient receptor potential V2 channel orthologs by 2-aminoethoxydiphenyl borate. Mol Pharmacol 2007; 72(5): 1258-68.
[http://dx.doi.org/10.1124/mol.107.037044] [PMID: 17673572]

[61]   Nie L, Oishi Y, Doi I, Shibata H, Kojima I. Inhibition of proliferation of MCF-7 breast cancer cells by a blocker of Ca($^{2+}$)-permeable channel. Cell Calcium 1997; 22(2): 75-82.
[http://dx.doi.org/10.1016/S0143-4160(97)90107-X] [PMID: 9292225]

[62]   Bang S, Yoo S, Yang TJ, Cho H, Hwang SW. Isopentenyl pyrophosphate is a novel antinociceptive substance that inhibits TRPV3 and TRPA1 ion channels. Pain 2011; 152(5): 1156-64.
[http://dx.doi.org/10.1016/j.pain.2011.01.044] [PMID: 21353389]

[63]   Bang S, Yoo S, Yang TJ, Cho H, Kim YG, Hwang SW. Resolvin D1 attenuates activation of sensory transient receptor potential channels leading to multiple anti-nociception. Br J Pharmacol 2010; 161(3): 707-20.
[http://dx.doi.org/10.1111/j.1476-5381.2010.00909.x] [PMID: 20880407]

[64]   Khairatkar NJ, Maharaj N, Thomas A. The TRPV3 Receptor as a Pain Target: A Therapeutic Promise or Just Some More New Biology? Open Drug Discov J 2010; 2: 89-97.
[http://dx.doi.org/10.2174/1877381801002030089]

[65]   Everaerts W, Zhen X, Ghosh D, *et al.* Inhibition of the cation channel TRPV4 improves bladder function in mice and rats with cyclophosphamide-induced cystitis. Proc Natl Acad Sci USA 2010; 107(44): 19084-9.
[http://dx.doi.org/10.1073/pnas.1005333107] [PMID: 20956320]

[66]   Vincent F, Acevedo A, Nguyen MT, *et al.* Identification and characterization of novel TRPV4 modulators. Biochem Biophys Res Commun 2009; 389(3): 490-4.
[http://dx.doi.org/10.1016/j.bbrc.2009.09.007] [PMID: 19737537]

[67]   Huh D, Leslie DC, Matthews BD, *et al.* A human disease model of drug toxicity-induced pulmonary edema in a lung-on-a-chip microdevice. Sci Transl Med 2012; 4(159)159ra147
[http://dx.doi.org/10.1126/scitranslmed.3004249] [PMID: 23136042]

[68]   de Groot T, Lee K, Langeslag M, *et al.* Parathyroid hormone activates TRPV5 via PKA-dependent phosphorylation. J Am Soc Nephrol 2009; 20(8): 1693-704.
[http://dx.doi.org/10.1681/ASN.2008080873] [PMID: 19423690]

[69]   Irnaten M, Blanchard-Gutton N, Praetorius J, Harvey BJ. Rapid effects of 17beta-estradiol on TRPV5 epithelial Ca^{2+} channels in rat renal cells. Steroids 2009; 74(8): 642-9.
[http://dx.doi.org/10.1016/j.steroids.2009.02.002] [PMID: 19463684]

[70]   Levy D, Garrison RJ, Savage DD, Kannel WB, Castelli WP. Prognostic implications of echocardiographically determined left ventricular mass in the Framingham Heart Study. N Engl J Med 1990; 322(22): 1561-6.
[http://dx.doi.org/10.1056/NEJM199005313222203] [PMID: 2139921]

[71]   Frey N, McKinsey TA, Olson EN. Decoding calcium signals involved in cardiac growth and function. Nat Med 2000; 6(11): 1221-7.
[http://dx.doi.org/10.1038/81321] [PMID: 11062532]

[72]   Houser SR, Molkentin JD. Does contractile Ca^{2+} control calcineurin-NFAT signaling and pathological hypertrophy in cardiac myocytes? Sci Signal 2008; 1(25): pe31.

[http://dx.doi.org/10.1126/scisignal.125pe31] [PMID: 18577756]

[73]   Jiang Y, Huang H, Liu P, *et al.* Expression and localization of TRPC proteins in rat ventricular myocytes at various developmental stages. Cell Tissue Res 2014; 355(1): 201-12.
[http://dx.doi.org/10.1007/s00441-013-1733-4] [PMID: 24146259]

[74]   Beech DJ. Characteristics of transient receptor potential canonical calcium-permeable channels and their relevance to vascular physiology and disease. Circ J 2013; 77(3): 570-9.
[http://dx.doi.org/10.1253/circj.CJ-13-0154] [PMID: 23412755]

[75]   Cioffi DL, Wu S, Alexeyev M, Goodman SR, Zhu MX, Stevens T. Activation of the endothelial store-operated ISOC Ca^{2+} channel requires interaction of protein 4.1 with TRPC4. Circ Res 2005; 97(11): 1164-72.
[http://dx.doi.org/10.1161/01.RES.0000193597.65217.00] [PMID: 16254212]

[76]   Saliba Y, Jebara V, Hajal J, *et al.* Transient Receptor Potential Canonical 3 and Nuclear Factor of Activated T Cells C3 Signaling Pathway Critically Regulates Myocardial Fibrosis. Antioxid Redox Signal 2019; 30(16): 1851-79.
[http://dx.doi.org/10.1089/ars.2018.7545] [PMID: 30318928]

[77]   Samie MA, Grimm C, Evans JA, *et al.* The tissue-specific expression of TRPML2 (MCOLN-2) gene is influenced by the presence of TRPML1. Pflugers Arch 2009; 459(1): 79-91.
[http://dx.doi.org/10.1007/s00424-009-0716-5] [PMID: 19763610]

[78]   Andrei SR, Sinharoy P, Bratz IN, Damron DS. TRPA1 is functionally co-expressed with TRPV1 in cardiac muscle: Co-localization at z-discs, costameres and intercalated discs. Channels (Austin) 2016; 10(5): 395-409.
[http://dx.doi.org/10.1080/19336950.2016.1185579] [PMID: 27144598]

[79]   Conklin DJ, Guo Y, Nystoriak MA, *et al.* TRPA1 channel contributes to myocardial ischemia-reperfusion injury. Am J Physiol Heart Circ Physiol 2019; 316(4): H889-99.
[http://dx.doi.org/10.1152/ajpheart.00106.2018] [PMID: 30735434]

[80]   Wang Z, Xu Y, Wang M, *et al.* TRPA1 inhibition ameliorates pressure overload-induced cardiac hypertrophy and fibrosis in mice. EBioMedicine 2018; 36: 54-62.
[http://dx.doi.org/10.1016/j.ebiom.2018.08.022] [PMID: 30297144]

[81]   Andrei SR, Ghosh M, Sinharoy P, Dey S, Bratz IN, Damron DS. TRPA1 ion channel stimulation enhances cardiomyocyte contractile function via a CaMKII-dependent pathway. Channels (Austin) 2017; 11(6): 587-603.
[http://dx.doi.org/10.1080/19336950.2017.1365206] [PMID: 28792844]

[82]   Mao ZJ, Zhang QL, Shang J, Gao T, Yuan WJ, Qin LP. Shenfu Injection attenuates rat myocardial hypertrophy by up-regulating miR-19a-3p expression. Sci Rep 2018; 8(1): 4660.
[http://dx.doi.org/10.1038/s41598-018-23137-4] [PMID: 29549288]

[83]   Li J, Wu W, Zhao M, Liu X. Involvement of TRPC1 in Nampt-induced cardiomyocyte hypertrophy through the activation of ER stress. Cell Mol Biol 2017; 63(4): 33-7.
[http://dx.doi.org/10.14715/cmb/2017.63.4.6] [PMID: 28478801]

[84]   Tang L, Yao F, Wang H, *et al.* Inhibition of TRPC1 prevents cardiac hypertrophy via NF-κB signaling pathway in human pluripotent stem cell-derived cardiomyocytes. J Mol Cell Cardiol 2019; 126: 143-54.
[http://dx.doi.org/10.1016/j.yjmcc.2018.10.020] [PMID: 30423318]

[85]   Numaga-Tomita T, Kitajima N, Kuroda T, *et al.* TRPC3-GEF-H1 axis mediates pressure overload-induced cardiac fibrosis. Sci Rep 2016; 6: 39383.
[http://dx.doi.org/10.1038/srep39383] [PMID: 27991560]

[86]   Kitajima N, Numaga-Tomita T, Watanabe M, *et al.* TRPC3 positively regulates reactive oxygen species driving maladaptive cardiac remodeling. Sci Rep 2016; 6: 37001.
[http://dx.doi.org/10.1038/srep37001] [PMID: 27833156]

[87]   Wu X, Eder P, Chang B, Molkentin JD. TRPC channels are necessary mediators of pathologic cardiac hypertrophy. Proc Natl Acad Sci USA 2010; 107(15): 7000-5.
[http://dx.doi.org/10.1073/pnas.1001825107] [PMID: 20351294]

[88]   Domes K, Patrucco E, Loga F, *et al.* Murine cardiac growth, TRPC channels, and cGMP kinase I. Pflugers Arch 2015; 467(10): 2229-34.
[http://dx.doi.org/10.1007/s00424-014-1682-0] [PMID: 25547873]

[89]   Onohara N, Nishida M, Inoue R, *et al.* TRPC3 and TRPC6 are essential for angiotensin II-induced cardiac hypertrophy. EMBO J 2006; 25(22): 5305-16.
[http://dx.doi.org/10.1038/sj.emboj.7601417] [PMID: 17082763]

[90]   Seo K, Rainer PP, Shalkey Hahn V, *et al.* Combined TRPC3 and TRPC6 blockade by selective small-molecule or genetic deletion inhibits pathological cardiac hypertrophy. Proc Natl Acad Sci USA 2014; 111(4): 1551-6.
[http://dx.doi.org/10.1073/pnas.1308963111] [PMID: 24453217]

[91]   Yamaguchi Y, Iribe G, Kaneko T, *et al.* TRPC3 participates in angiotensin II type 1 receptor-dependent stress-induced slow increase in intracellular Ca^{2+} concentration in mouse cardiomyocytes. J Physiol Sci 2018; 68(2): 153-64.
[http://dx.doi.org/10.1007/s12576-016-0519-3] [PMID: 28105583]

[92]   Doleschal B, Primessnig U, Wölkart G, *et al.* TRPC3 contributes to regulation of cardiac contractility and arrhythmogenesis by dynamic interaction with NCX1. Cardiovasc Res 2015; 106(1): 163-73.
[http://dx.doi.org/10.1093/cvr/cvv022] [PMID: 25631581]

[93]   Qi Z, Wong CK, Suen CH, *et al.* TRPC3 regulates the automaticity of embryonic stem cell-derived cardiomyocytes. Int J Cardiol 2016; 203: 169-81.
[http://dx.doi.org/10.1016/j.ijcard.2015.10.018] [PMID: 26512833]

[94]   Chu W, Wan L, Zhao D, *et al.* Mild hypoxia-induced cardiomyocyte hypertrophy via up-regulation of HIF-1α-mediated TRPC signalling. J Cell Mol Med 2012; 16(9): 2022-34.
[http://dx.doi.org/10.1111/j.1582-4934.2011.01497.x] [PMID: 22129453]

[95]   Bush EW, Hood DB, Papst PJ, *et al.* Canonical transient receptor potential channels promote cardiomyocyte hypertrophy through activation of calcineurin signaling. J Biol Chem 2006; 281(44): 33487-96.
[http://dx.doi.org/10.1074/jbc.M605536200] [PMID: 16950785]

[96]   Sunggip C, Shimoda K, Oda S, *et al.* TRPC5-eNOS Axis Negatively Regulates ATP-Induced Cardiomyocyte Hypertrophy. Front Pharmacol 2018; 9: 523.
[http://dx.doi.org/10.3389/fphar.2018.00523] [PMID: 29872396]

[97]   Makarewich CA, Zhang H, Davis J, *et al.* Transient receptor potential channels contribute to pathological structural and functional remodeling after myocardial infarction. Circ Res 2014; 115(6): 567-80.
[http://dx.doi.org/10.1161/CIRCRESAHA.115.303831] [PMID: 25047165]

[98]   Miller BA, Wang J, Hirschler-Laszkiewicz I, *et al.* The second member of transient receptor potential-melastatin channel family protects hearts from ischemia-reperfusion injury. Am J Physiol Heart Circ Physiol 2013; 304(7): H1010-22.
[http://dx.doi.org/10.1152/ajpheart.00906.2012] [PMID: 23376831]

[99]   Miller BA, Hoffman NE, Merali S, *et al.* TRPM2 channels protect against cardiac ischemia-reperfusion injury: Role of mitochondria. J Biol Chem 2014; 289(11): 7615-29.
[http://dx.doi.org/10.1074/jbc.M113.533851] [PMID: 24492610]

[100]   Miller BA, Wang J, Song J, *et al.* Trpm2 enhances physiological bioenergetics and protects against pathological oxidative cardiac injury: Role of Pyk2 phosphorylation. J Cell Physiol 2019.
[http://dx.doi.org/10.1002/jcp.28146] [PMID: 30637731]

[101]   Hof T, Sallé L, Coulbault L, *et al.* TRPM4 non-selective cation channels influence action potentials in

rabbit Purkinje fibres. J Physiol 2016; 594(2): 295-306.
[http://dx.doi.org/10.1113/JP271347] [PMID: 26548780]

[102] Daumy X, Amarouch MY, Lindenbaum P, *et al.* Targeted resequencing identifies TRPM4 as a major gene predisposing to progressive familial heart block type I. Int J Cardiol 2016; 207: 349-58.
[http://dx.doi.org/10.1016/j.ijcard.2016.01.052] [PMID: 26820365]

[103] Hu Y, Duan Y, Takeuchi A, *et al.* Uncovering the arrhythmogenic potential of TRPM4 activation in atrial-derived HL-1 cells using novel recording and numerical approaches. Cardiovasc Res 2017; 113(10): 1243-55.
[http://dx.doi.org/10.1093/cvr/cvx117] [PMID: 28898995]

[104] Hof T, Liu H, Sallé L, *et al.* TRPM4 non-selective cation channel variants in long QT syndrome. BMC Med Genet 2017; 18(1): 31.
[http://dx.doi.org/10.1186/s12881-017-0397-4] [PMID: 28315637]

[105] Piao H, Takahashi K, Yamaguchi Y, Wang C, Liu K, Naruse K. Transient receptor potential melastatin-4 is involved in hypoxia-reoxygenation injury in the cardiomyocytes. PLoS One 2015; 10(4)e0121703
[http://dx.doi.org/10.1371/journal.pone.0121703] [PMID: 25836769]

[106] Sah R, Mesirca P, Van den Boogert M, *et al.* Ion channel-kinase TRPM7 is required for maintaining cardiac automaticity. Proc Natl Acad Sci USA 2013; 110(32): E3037-46.
[http://dx.doi.org/10.1073/pnas.1311865110] [PMID: 23878236]

[107] Zhang YH, Sun HY, Chen KH, *et al.* Evidence for functional expression of TRPM7 channels in human atrial myocytes. Basic Res Cardiol 2012; 107(5): 282.
[http://dx.doi.org/10.1007/s00395-012-0282-4] [PMID: 22802050]

[108] Parajuli N, Valtuille L, Basu R, *et al.* Determinants of ventricular arrhythmias in human explanted hearts with dilated cardiomyopathy. Eur J Clin Invest 2015; 45(12): 1286-96.
[http://dx.doi.org/10.1111/eci.12549] [PMID: 26444674]

[109] Mačianskienė R, Almanaitytė M, Jekabsone A, Mubagwa K. Modulation of Human Cardiac TRPM7 Current by Extracellular Acidic pH Depends upon Extracellular Concentrations of Divalent Cations. PLoS One 2017; 12(1)e0170923
[http://dx.doi.org/10.1371/journal.pone.0170923] [PMID: 28129376]

[110] Hurt CM, Lu Y, Stary CM, *et al.* Transient Receptor Potential Vanilloid 1 Regulates Mitochondrial Membrane Potential and Myocardial Reperfusion Injury. J Am Heart Assoc 2016; 5(9)e003774
[http://dx.doi.org/10.1161/JAHA.116.003774] [PMID: 27671317]

[111] Ren M, Wang T, Huang L, *et al.* Role of VR1 in the differentiation of bone marrow-derived mesenchymal stem cells into cardiomyocytes associated with Wnt/β-catenin signaling. Cardiovasc Ther 2016; 34(6): 482-8.
[http://dx.doi.org/10.1111/1755-5922.12228] [PMID: 27662603]

[112] Zhong B, Rubinstein J, Ma S, Wang DH. Genetic ablation of TRPV1 exacerbates pressure overload-induced cardiac hypertrophy. Biomed Pharmacother 2018; 99: 261-70.
[http://dx.doi.org/10.1016/j.biopha.2018.01.065] [PMID: 29334670]

[113] Chen M, Xin J, Liu B, *et al.* Mitogen-Activated Protein Kinase and Intracellular Polyamine Signaling Is Involved in TRPV1 Activation-Induced Cardiac Hypertrophy. J Am Heart Assoc 2016; 5(8)e003718
[http://dx.doi.org/10.1161/JAHA.116.003718] [PMID: 27473037]

[114] Buckley CL, Stokes AJ. Mice lacking functional TRPV1 are protected from pressure overload cardiac hypertrophy. Channels (Austin) 2011; 5(4): 367-74.
[http://dx.doi.org/10.4161/chan.5.4.17083] [PMID: 21814047]

[115] Rubinstein J, Lasko VM, Koch SE, *et al.* Novel role of transient receptor potential vanilloid 2 in the regulation of cardiac performance. Am J Physiol Heart Circ Physiol 2014; 306(4): H574-84.

[http://dx.doi.org/10.1152/ajpheart.00854.2013] [PMID: 24322617]

[116]   Koch SE, Mann A, Jones S, *et al.* Transient receptor potential vanilloid 2 function regulates cardiac hypertrophy via stretch-induced activation. J Hypertens 2017; 35(3): 602-11.
[http://dx.doi.org/10.1097/HJH.0000000000001213] [PMID: 28009703]

[117]   Lorin C, Vögeli I, Niggli E. Dystrophic cardiomyopathy: Role of TRPV2 channels in stretch-induced cell damage. Cardiovasc Res 2015; 106(1): 153-62.
[http://dx.doi.org/10.1093/cvr/cvv021] [PMID: 25616416]

[118]   Entin-Meer M, Levy R, Goryainov P, *et al.* The transient receptor potential vanilloid 2 cation channel is abundant in macrophages accumulating at the peri-infarct zone and may enhance their migration capacity towards injured cardiomyocytes following myocardial infarction. PLoS One 2014; 9(8)e105055
[http://dx.doi.org/10.1371/journal.pone.0105055] [PMID: 25136832]

[119]   Dong Q, Li J, Wu QF, *et al.* Blockage of transient receptor potential vanilloid 4 alleviates myocardial ischemia/reperfusion injury in mice. Sci Rep 2017; 7: 42678.
[http://dx.doi.org/10.1038/srep42678] [PMID: 28205608]

[120]   Wu QF, Qian C, Zhao N, *et al.* Activation of transient receptor potential vanilloid 4 involves in hypoxia/reoxygenation injury in cardiomyocytes. Cell Death Dis 2017; 8(5)e2828
[http://dx.doi.org/10.1038/cddis.2017.227] [PMID: 28542130]

[121]   Jones JL, Peana D, Veteto AB, *et al.* TRPV4 increases cardiomyocyte calcium cycling and contractility yet contributes to damage in the aged heart following hypoosmotic stress. Cardiovasc Res 2019; 115(1): 46-56.
[http://dx.doi.org/10.1093/cvr/cvy156] [PMID: 29931225]

[122]   Scherzer ND, Le TV, Hellstrom WJG. Sildenafil's impact on male infertility: What has changed in 20 years? Int J Impot Res 2019; 31(2): 71-3.
[http://dx.doi.org/10.1038/s41443-018-0067-x] [PMID: 30837720]

[123]   Igarashi A, Inoue S, Ishii T, Tsutani K, Watanabe H. Comparative Effectiveness of Oral Medications for Pulmonary Arterial Hypertension. Int Heart J 2016; 57(4): 466-72.
[http://dx.doi.org/10.1536/ihj.15-459] [PMID: 27385603]

[124]   Koitabashi N, Aiba T, Hesketh GG, *et al.* Cyclic GMP/PKG-dependent inhibition of TRPC6 channel activity and expression negatively regulates cardiomyocyte NFAT activation Novel mechanism of cardiac stress modulation by PDE5 inhibition. J Mol Cell Cardiol 2010; 48(4): 713-24.
[http://dx.doi.org/10.1016/j.yjmcc.2009.11.015] [PMID: 19961855]

[125]   Nishida M, Watanabe K, Sato Y, *et al.* Phosphorylation of TRPC6 channels at Thr69 is required for anti-hypertrophic effects of phosphodiesterase 5 inhibition. J Biol Chem 2010; 285(17): 13244-53.
[http://dx.doi.org/10.1074/jbc.M109.074104] [PMID: 20177073]

[126]   Kiso H, Ohba T, Iino K, *et al.* Sildenafil prevents the up-regulation of transient receptor potential canonical channels in the development of cardiomyocyte hypertrophy. Biochem Biophys Res Commun 2013; 436(3): 514-8.
[http://dx.doi.org/10.1016/j.bbrc.2013.06.002] [PMID: 23764398]

[127]   Dwivedi J, Sharma S, Jain S, Singh A. The Synthetic and Biological Attributes of Pyrazole Derivatives: A Review. Mini Rev Med Chem 2018; 18(11): 918-47.
[http://dx.doi.org/10.2174/1389557517666170927160919] [PMID: 28971774]

[128]   Ganguly S, Jacob SK. Therapeutic Outlook of Pyrazole Analogs: A Mini Review. Mini Rev Med Chem 2017; 17(11): 959-83.
[http://dx.doi.org/10.2174/1389557516666151120115302] [PMID: 26586126]

[129]   Kiyonaka S, Kato K, Nishida M, *et al.* Selective and direct inhibition of TRPC3 channels underlies biological activities of a pyrazole compound. Proc Natl Acad Sci USA 2009; 106(13): 5400-5.
[http://dx.doi.org/10.1073/pnas.0808793106] [PMID: 19289841]

[130] Schleifer H, Doleschal B, Lichtenegger M, *et al.* Novel pyrazole compounds for pharmacological discrimination between receptor-operated and store-operated Ca(2+) entry pathways. Br J Pharmacol 2012; 167(8): 1712-22.
[http://dx.doi.org/10.1111/j.1476-5381.2012.02126.x] [PMID: 22862290]

[131] Koenig S, Schernthaner M, Maechler H, *et al.* A TRPC3 blocker, ethyl-1-(4-(2,-,3-trichloroacrylamide)phenyl)-5-(trifluoromethyl)-1H-pyrazole-4-carboxylate (Pyr3), prevents stent-induced arterial remodeling. J Pharmacol Exp Ther 2013; 344(1): 33-40.
[http://dx.doi.org/10.1124/jpet.112.196832] [PMID: 23010361]

[132] Lang H, Li Q, Yu H, *et al.* Activation of TRPV1 attenuates high salt-induced cardiac hypertrophy through improvement of mitochondrial function. Br J Pharmacol 2015; 172(23): 5548-58.
[http://dx.doi.org/10.1111/bph.12987] [PMID: 25339153]

[133] Sogut O, Kaya H, Gokdemir MT, Sezen Y. Acute myocardial infarction and coronary vasospasm associated with the ingestion of cayenne pepper pills in a 25-year-old male. Int J Emerg Med 2012; 5: 5.
[http://dx.doi.org/10.1186/1865-1380-5-5] [PMID: 22264348]

[134] Sayin MR, Karabag T, Dogan SM, Akpinar I, Aydin M. A case of acute myocardial infarction due to the use of cayenne pepper pills. Wien Klin Wochenschr 2012; 124(7-8): 285-7.
[http://dx.doi.org/10.1007/s00508-012-0163-8] [PMID: 22527825]

[135] Gavva NR, Treanor JJ, Garami A, *et al.* Pharmacological blockade of the vanilloid receptor TRPV1 elicits marked hyperthermia in humans. Pain 2008; 136(1-2): 202-10.
[http://dx.doi.org/10.1016/j.pain.2008.01.024] [PMID: 18337008]

[136] Stucky CL, Dubin AE, Jeske NA, Malin SA, McKemy DD, Story GM. Roles of transient receptor potential channels in pain. Brain Res Brain Res Rev 2009; 60(1): 2-23.
[http://dx.doi.org/10.1016/j.brainresrev.2008.12.018] [PMID: 19203589]

[137] Thorn CF, Oshiro C, Marsh S, *et al.* Doxorubicin pathways: Pharmacodynamics and adverse effects. Pharmacogenet Genomics 2011; 21(7): 440-6.
[http://dx.doi.org/10.1097/FPC.0b013e32833ffb56] [PMID: 21048526]

[138] Cove-Smith L, Woodhouse N, Hargreaves A, *et al.* An integrated characterization of serological, pathological, and functional events in doxorubicin-induced cardiotoxicity. Toxicol Sci 2014; 140(1): 3-15.
[http://dx.doi.org/10.1093/toxsci/kfu057] [PMID: 24675088]

[139] Wang Z, Wang M, Liu J, *et al.* Inhibition of TRPA1 Attenuates Doxorubicin-Induced Acute Cardiotoxicity by Suppressing Oxidative Stress, the Inflammatory Response, and Endoplasmic Reticulum Stress. Oxid Med Cell Longev 2018; 20185179468
[http://dx.doi.org/10.1155/2018/5179468] [PMID: 29682158]

[140] Shimauchi T, Numaga-Tomita T, Ito T, *et al.* TRPC3-Nox2 complex mediates doxorubicin-induced myocardial atrophy. JCI Insight 2017; 2(15): 93358.
[http://dx.doi.org/10.1172/jci.insight.93358] [PMID: 28768915]

[141] Chen R, Sun G, Yang L, Wang J, Sun X. Salvianolic acid B protects against doxorubicin induced cardiac dysfunction *via* inhibition of ER stress mediated cardiomyocyte apoptosis. Toxicol Res (Camb) 2016; 5(5): 1335-45.
[http://dx.doi.org/10.1039/C6TX00111D] [PMID: 30090438]

[142] Chen RC, Sun GB, Ye JX, Wang J, Zhang MD, Sun XB. Salvianolic acid B attenuates doxorubicin-induced ER stress by inhibiting TRPC3 and TRPC6 mediated Ca^{2+} overload in rat cardiomyocytes. Toxicol Lett 2017; 276: 21-30.
[http://dx.doi.org/10.1016/j.toxlet.2017.04.010] [PMID: 28495616]

[143] Hoffman NE, Miller BA, Wang J, *et al.* Ca^{2+} entry via Trpm2 is essential for cardiac myocyte bioenergetics maintenance. Am J Physiol Heart Circ Physiol 2015; 308(6): H637-50.

[http://dx.doi.org/10.1152/ajpheart.00720.2014] [PMID: 25576627]

[144] Ge W, Yuan M, Ceylan AF, Wang X, Ren J. Mitochondrial aldehyde dehydrogenase protects against doxorubicin cardiotoxicity through a transient receptor potential channel vanilloid 1-mediated mechanism. Biochim Biophys Acta 2016; 1862(4): 622-34.
[http://dx.doi.org/10.1016/j.bbadis.2015.12.014] [PMID: 26692169]

[145] González-Muniesa P, Mártinez-González MA, Hu FB, *et al.* Obesity. Nat Rev Dis Primers 2017; 3: 17034.
[http://dx.doi.org/10.1038/nrdp.2017.34] [PMID: 28617414]

[146] Cinti S. The adipose organ. Prostaglandins Leukot Essent Fatty Acids 2005; 73(1): 9-15.
[http://dx.doi.org/10.1016/j.plefa.2005.04.010] [PMID: 15936182]

[147] Baboota RK, Sarma SM, Boparai RK, Kondepudi KK, Mantri S, Bishnoi M. Microarray based gene expression analysis of murine brown and subcutaneous adipose tissue: Significance with human. PLoS One 2015; 10(5)e0127701
[http://dx.doi.org/10.1371/journal.pone.0127701] [PMID: 26010905]

[148] Scheideler M, Herzig S, Georgiadi A. Endocrine and autocrine/paracrine modulators of brown adipose tissue mass and activity as novel therapeutic strategies against obesity and type 2 diabetes. Horm Mol Biol Clin Investig 2017; 31(2): /j/hmbci.2017.31.issue-2/hmbci-2017-0043/hmbci-2017-0043.xml.
[http://dx.doi.org/10.1515/hmbci-2017-0043] [PMID: 28850545]

[149] Wu J, Boström P, Sparks LM, *et al.* Beige adipocytes are a distinct type of thermogenic fat cell in mouse and human. Cell 2012; 150(2): 366-76.
[http://dx.doi.org/10.1016/j.cell.2012.05.016] [PMID: 22796012]

[150] Lee P, Werner CD, Kebebew E, Celi FS. Functional thermogenic beige adipogenesis is inducible in human neck fat. Int J Obes 2014; 38(2): 170-6.
[http://dx.doi.org/10.1038/ijo.2013.82] [PMID: 23736373]

[151] Gao P, Yan Z, Zhu Z. The role of adipose TRP channels in the pathogenesis of obesity. J Cell Physiol 2019; 234(8): 12483-97.
[http://dx.doi.org/10.1002/jcp.28106] [PMID: 30618095]

[152] Bishnoi M, Khare P, Brown L, Panchal SK. Transient receptor potential (TRP) channels: a metabolic TR(i)P to obesity prevention and therapy. Obes Rev 2018; 19(9): 1269-92.
[http://dx.doi.org/10.1111/obr.12703] [PMID: 29797770]

[153] Bishnoi M, Kondepudi KK, Gupta A, Karmase A, Boparai RK. Expression of multiple Transient Receptor Potential channel genes in murine 3T3-L1 cell lines and adipose tissue. Pharmacol Rep 2013; 65(3): 751-5.
[http://dx.doi.org/10.1016/S1734-1140(13)71055-7] [PMID: 23950600]

[154] Sun W, Li C, Zhang Y, *et al.* Gene expression changes of thermo-sensitive transient receptor potential channels in obese mice. Cell Biol Int 2017; 41(8): 908-13.
[http://dx.doi.org/10.1002/cbin.10783] [PMID: 28464448]

[155] Cao DS, Zhong L, Hsieh TH, *et al.* Expression of transient receptor potential ankyrin 1 (TRPA1) and its role in insulin release from rat pancreatic beta cells. PLoS One 2012; 7(5)e38005
[http://dx.doi.org/10.1371/journal.pone.0038005] [PMID: 22701540]

[156] Numazawa S, Takase M, Ahiko T, Ishii M, Shimizu S, Yoshida T. Possible involvement of transient receptor potential channels in electrophile-induced insulin secretion from RINm5F cells. Biol Pharm Bull 2012; 35(3): 346-54.
[http://dx.doi.org/10.1248/bpb.35.346] [PMID: 22382320]

[157] Philippaert K, Vennekens R. The Role of TRP Channels in the Pancreatic Beta-Cell. 2017.
[http://dx.doi.org/10.4324/9781315152837-12] [PMID: 29356488]]

[158] Lieder B, Zaunschirm M, Holik AK, *et al.* The Alkamide *trans*-Pellitorine Targets PPARγ via TRPV1 and TRPA1 to Reduce Lipid Accumulation in Developing 3T3-L1 Adipocytes. Front Pharmacol 2017;

8: 316.
[http://dx.doi.org/10.3389/fphar.2017.00316] [PMID: 28620299]

[159]   Krout D, Schaar A, Sun Y, *et al.* The TRPC1 Ca^{2+}-permeable channel inhibits exercise-induced protection against high-fat diet-induced obesity and type II diabetes. J Biol Chem 2017; 292(50): 20799-807.
[http://dx.doi.org/10.1074/jbc.M117.809954] [PMID: 29074621]

[160]   Marabita F, Islam MS. Expression of Transient Receptor Potential Channels in the Purified Human Pancreatic β-Cells. Pancreas 2017; 46(1): 97-101.
[http://dx.doi.org/10.1097/MPA.0000000000000685] [PMID: 27464700]

[161]   Freichel M, Philipp S, Cavalie A, Flockerzi V. TRPC4 and TRPC4-deficient mice. Novartis Found Symp 2004; 258: 189-99. discussion 99-203, 63-6.
[http://dx.doi.org/10.1002/0470862580.ch14] [PMID: 15104183]]

[162]   Che H, Yue J, Tse HF, Li GR. Functional TRPV and TRPM channels in human preadipocytes. Pflugers Arch 2014; 466(5): 947-59.
[http://dx.doi.org/10.1007/s00424-013-1355-4] [PMID: 24057349]

[163]   Chen KH, Xu XH, Liu Y, Hu Y, Jin MW, Li GR. TRPM7 channels regulate proliferation and adipogenesis in 3T3-L1 preadipocytes. J Cell Physiol 2014; 229(1): 60-7.
[http://dx.doi.org/10.1002/jcp.24417] [PMID: 23765921]

[164]   Zhang Z, Zhang W, Jung DY, *et al.* TRPM2 Ca^{2+} channel regulates energy balance and glucose metabolism. Am J Physiol Endocrinol Metab 2012; 302(7): E807-16.
[http://dx.doi.org/10.1152/ajpendo.00239.2011] [PMID: 22275755]

[165]   Larsson MH, Håkansson P, Jansen FP, Magnell K, Brodin P. Ablation of TRPM5 in Mice Results in Reduced Body Weight Gain and Improved Glucose Tolerance and Protects from Excessive Consumption of Sweet Palatable Food when Fed High Caloric Diets. PLoS One 2015; 10(9)e0138373
[http://dx.doi.org/10.1371/journal.pone.0138373] [PMID: 26397098]

[166]   Glendinning JI, Gillman J, Zamer H, Margolskee RF, Sclafani A. The role of T1r3 and Trpm5 in carbohydrate-induced obesity in mice. Physiol Behav 2012; 107(1): 50-8.
[http://dx.doi.org/10.1016/j.physbeh.2012.05.023] [PMID: 22683548]

[167]   Tran TD, Zolochevska O, Figueiredo ML, *et al.* Histamine-induced Ca^{2+} signalling is mediated by TRPM4 channels in human adipose-derived stem cells. Biochem J 2014; 463(1): 123-34.
[http://dx.doi.org/10.1042/BJ20140065] [PMID: 25001294]

[168]   Reimúndez A, Fernández-Peña C, García G, *et al.* Deletion of the Cold Thermoreceptor TRPM8 Increases Heat Loss and Food Intake Leading to Reduced Body Temperature and Obesity in Mice. J Neurosci 2018; 38(15): 3643-56.
[http://dx.doi.org/10.1523/JNEUROSCI.3002-17.2018] [PMID: 29530988]

[169]   Kaewsutthi S, Santiprabhob J, Phonrat B, Tungtrongchitr A, Lertrit P, Tungtrongchitr R. Exome sequencing in Thai patients with familial obesity. Genet Mol Res 2016; 15(2)
[http://dx.doi.org/10.4238/gmr.15028311] [PMID: 27421018]

[170]   Togashi K, Hara Y, Tominaga T, *et al.* TRPM2 activation by cyclic ADP-ribose at body temperature is involved in insulin secretion. EMBO J 2006; 25(9): 1804-15.
[http://dx.doi.org/10.1038/sj.emboj.7601083] [PMID: 16601673]

[171]   Uchida K, Dezaki K, Damdindorj B, *et al.* Lack of TRPM2 impaired insulin secretion and glucose metabolisms in mice. Diabetes 2011; 60(1): 119-26.
[http://dx.doi.org/10.2337/db10-0276] [PMID: 20921208]

[172]   Ishii M, Shimizu S, Hara Y, *et al.* Intracellular-produced hydroxyl radical mediates H2O2-induced Ca^{2+} influx and cell death in rat beta-cell line RIN-5F. Cell Calcium 2006; 39(6): 487-94.
[http://dx.doi.org/10.1016/j.ceca.2006.01.013] [PMID: 16546253]

[173]   Lange I, Yamamoto S, Partida-Sanchez S, Mori Y, Fleig A, Penner R. TRPM2 functions as a

lysosomal Ca2+-release channel in beta cells. Sci Signal 2009; 2(71): ra23.
[http://dx.doi.org/10.1126/scisignal.2000278] [PMID: 19454650]

[174] Vennekens R, Olausson J, Meissner M, *et al.* Increased IgE-dependent mast cell activation and anaphylactic responses in mice lacking the calcium-activated nonselective cation channel TRPM4. Nat Immunol 2007; 8(3): 312-20.
[http://dx.doi.org/10.1038/ni1441] [PMID: 17293867]

[175] Shigeto M, Ramracheya R, Tarasov AI, *et al.* GLP-1 stimulates insulin secretion by PKC-dependent TRPM4 and TRPM5 activation. J Clin Invest 2015; 125(12): 4714-28.
[http://dx.doi.org/10.1172/JCI81975] [PMID: 26571400]

[176] Marigo V, Courville K, Hsu WH, Feng JM, Cheng H. TRPM4 impacts on Ca^{2+} signals during agonist-induced insulin secretion in pancreatic beta-cells. Mol Cell Endocrinol 2009; 299(2): 194-203.
[http://dx.doi.org/10.1016/j.mce.2008.11.011] [PMID: 19063936]

[177] Brixel LR, Monteilh-Zoller MK, Ingenbrandt CS, *et al.* TRPM5 regulates glucose-stimulated insulin secretion. Pflugers Arch 2010; 460(1): 69-76.
[http://dx.doi.org/10.1007/s00424-010-0835-z] [PMID: 20393858]

[178] Colsoul B, Jacobs G, Philippaert K, *et al.* Insulin downregulates the expression of the Ca^{2+}-activated nonselective cation channel TRPM5 in pancreatic islets from leptin-deficient mouse models. Pflugers Arch 2014; 466(3): 611-21.
[http://dx.doi.org/10.1007/s00424-013-1389-7] [PMID: 24221356]

[179] Santos-Silva JC, Ribeiro RA, Vettorazzi JF, *et al.* Taurine supplementation ameliorates glucose homeostasis, prevents insulin and glucagon hypersecretion, and controls β, α, and δ-cell masses in genetic obese mice. Amino Acids 2015; 47(8): 1533-48.
[http://dx.doi.org/10.1007/s00726-015-1988-z] [PMID: 25940922]

[180] Held K, Kichko T, De Clercq K, *et al.* Activation of TRPM3 by a potent synthetic ligand reveals a role in peptide release. Proc Natl Acad Sci USA 2015; 112(11): E1363-72.
[http://dx.doi.org/10.1073/pnas.1419845112] [PMID: 25733887]

[181] McCoy DD, Zhou L, Nguyen AK, Watts AG, Donovan CM, McKemy DD. Enhanced insulin clearance in mice lacking TRPM8 channels. Am J Physiol Endocrinol Metab 2013; 305(1): E78-88.
[http://dx.doi.org/10.1152/ajpendo.00542.2012] [PMID: 23651844]

[182] Fonfria E, Murdock PR, Cusdin FS, Benham CD, Kelsell RE, McNulty S. Tissue distribution profiles of the human TRPM cation channel family. J Recept Signal Transduct Res 2006; 26(3): 159-78.
[http://dx.doi.org/10.1080/10799890600637506] [PMID: 16777713]

[183] Goralczyk A, van Vijven M, Koch M, *et al.* TRP channels in brown and white adipogenesis from human progenitors: New therapeutic targets and the caveats associated with the common antibiotic, streptomycin. FASEB J 2017; 31(8): 3251-66.
[http://dx.doi.org/10.1096/fj.201601081RR] [PMID: 28416581]

[184] Motter AL, Ahern GP. TRPV1-null mice are protected from diet-induced obesity. FEBS Lett 2008; 582(15): 2257-62.
[http://dx.doi.org/10.1016/j.febslet.2008.05.021] [PMID: 18503767]

[185] Marshall NJ, Liang L, Bodkin J, *et al.* A role for TRPV1 in influencing the onset of cardiovascular disease in obesity. Hypertension 2013; 61(1): 246-52.
[http://dx.doi.org/10.1161/HYPERTENSIONAHA.112.201434] [PMID: 23150506]

[186] Lee E, Jung DY, Kim JH, *et al.* Transient receptor potential vanilloid type-1 channel regulates diet-induced obesity, insulin resistance, and leptin resistance. FASEB J 2015; 29(8): 3182-92.
[http://dx.doi.org/10.1096/fj.14-268300] [PMID: 25888600]

[187] Moraes MN, Mezzalira N, de Assis LV, Menaker M, Guler A, Castrucci AM. TRPV1 participates in the activation of clock molecular machinery in the brown adipose tissue in response to light-dark cycle. Biochim Biophys Acta Mol Cell Res 2017; 1864(2): 324-35.

[http://dx.doi.org/10.1016/j.bbamcr.2016.11.010] [PMID: 27864077]

[188]   Cheung SY, Huang Y, Kwan HY, Chung HY, Yao X. Activation of transient receptor potential vanilloid 3 channel suppresses adipogenesis. Endocrinology 2015; 156(6): 2074-86.
[http://dx.doi.org/10.1210/en.2014-1831] [PMID: 25774551]

[189]   Sun W, Uchida K, Suzuki Y, *et al.* Lack of TRPV2 impairs thermogenesis in mouse brown adipose tissue. EMBO Rep 2016; 17(3): 383-99.
[http://dx.doi.org/10.15252/embr.201540819] [PMID: 26882545]

[190]   Sun W, Uchida K, Takahashi N, *et al.* Activation of TRPV2 negatively regulates the differentiation of mouse brown adipocytes. Pflugers Arch 2016; 468(9): 1527-40.
[http://dx.doi.org/10.1007/s00424-016-1846-1] [PMID: 27318696]

[191]   Janoschek R, Bae-Gartz I, Vohlen C, Alcazar MA, Dinger K, Appel S, *et al.* Dietary intervention in obese dams protects male offspring from WAT induction of TRPV4, adiposity, and hyperinsulinemia. Obesity Silver Spring, Md 2016; 24(6)1266
[http://dx.doi.org/10.1002/oby.21486] [PMID: 27106804]

[192]   Kusudo T, Wang Z, Mizuno A, Suzuki M, Yamashita H. TRPV4 deficiency increases skeletal muscle metabolic capacity and resistance against diet-induced obesity. J Appl Physiol (1985) 2012; 112(7): 1223-32.
[http://dx.doi.org/10.1152/japplphysiol.01070.2011] [PMID: 22207724]

[193]   Ye L, Kleiner S, Wu J, *et al.* TRPV4 is a regulator of adipose oxidative metabolism, inflammation, and energy homeostasis. Cell 2012; 151(1): 96-110.
[http://dx.doi.org/10.1016/j.cell.2012.08.034] [PMID: 23021218]

[194]   O'Conor CJ, Griffin TM, Liedtke W, Guilak F. Increased susceptibility of Trpv4-deficient mice to obesity and obesity-induced osteoarthritis with very high-fat diet. Ann Rheum Dis 2013; 72(2): 300-4.
[http://dx.doi.org/10.1136/annrheumdis-2012-202272] [PMID: 23178209]

[195]   Duan DM, Wu S, Hsu LA, *et al.* Associations between TRPV4 genotypes and body mass index in Taiwanese subjects. Mol Genet Genomics 2015; 290(4): 1357-65.
[http://dx.doi.org/10.1007/s00438-015-0996-8] [PMID: 25647731]

[196]   Tanaka H, Shimaya A, Kiso T, Kuramochi T, Shimokawa T, Shibasaki M. Enhanced insulin secretion and sensitization in diabetic mice on chronic treatment with a transient receptor potential vanilloid 1 antagonist. Life Sci 2011; 88(11-12): 559-63.
[http://dx.doi.org/10.1016/j.lfs.2011.01.016] [PMID: 21277869]

[197]   Akiba Y, Kato S, Katsube K, *et al.* Transient receptor potential vanilloid subfamily 1 expressed in pancreatic islet beta cells modulates insulin secretion in rats. Biochem Biophys Res Commun 2004; 321(1): 219-25.
[http://dx.doi.org/10.1016/j.bbrc.2004.06.149] [PMID: 15358238]

[198]   Gram DX, Ahrén B, Nagy I, *et al.* Capsaicin-sensitive sensory fibers in the islets of Langerhans contribute to defective insulin secretion in Zucker diabetic rat, an animal model for some aspects of human type 2 diabetes. Eur J Neurosci 2007; 25(1): 213-23.
[http://dx.doi.org/10.1111/j.1460-9568.2006.05261.x] [PMID: 17241282]

[199]   Hisanaga E, Nagasawa M, Ueki K, Kulkarni RN, Mori M, Kojima I. Regulation of calcium-permeable TRPV2 channel by insulin in pancreatic beta-cells. Diabetes 2009; 58(1): 174-84.
[http://dx.doi.org/10.2337/db08-0862] [PMID: 18984736]

[200]   Skrzypski M, Kakkassery M, Mergler S, *et al.* Activation of TRPV4 channel in pancreatic INS-1E beta cells enhances glucose-stimulated insulin secretion via calcium-dependent mechanisms. FEBS Lett 2013; 587(19): 3281-7.
[http://dx.doi.org/10.1016/j.febslet.2013.08.025] [PMID: 23999312]

[201]   Casas S, Novials A, Reimann F, Gomis R, Gribble FM. Calcium elevation in mouse pancreatic beta cells evoked by extracellular human islet amyloid polypeptide involves activation of the

mechanosensitive ion channel TRPV4. Diabetologia 2008; 51(12): 2252-62.
[http://dx.doi.org/10.1007/s00125-008-1111-z] [PMID: 18751967]

[202] Tamura Y, Iwasaki Y, Narukawa M, Watanabe T. Ingestion of cinnamaldehyde, a TRPA1 agonist, reduces visceral fats in mice fed a high-fat and high-sucrose diet. J Nutr Sci Vitaminol (Tokyo) 2012; 58(1): 9-13.
[http://dx.doi.org/10.3177/jnsv.58.9] [PMID: 23007061]

[203] Khare P, Jagtap S, Jain Y, *et al.* Cinnamaldehyde supplementation prevents fasting-induced hyperphagia, lipid accumulation, and inflammation in high-fat diet-fed mice. Biofactors 2016; 42(2): 201-11.
[http://dx.doi.org/10.1002/biof.1265] [PMID: 26893251]

[204] Leuner K, Kazanski V, Müller M, *et al.* Hyperforin--a key constituent of St. John's wort specifically activates TRPC6 channels. FASEB J 2007; 21(14): 4101-11.
[http://dx.doi.org/10.1096/fj.07-8110com] [PMID: 17666455]

[205] Novelli M, Menegazzi M, Beffy P, Porozov S, Gregorelli A, Giacopelli D, *et al.* St. John's wort extract and hyperforin inhibit multiple phosphorylation steps of cytokine signaling and prevent inflammatory and apoptotic gene induction in pancreatic beta cells. Int J Biochem Cell Biol 2016; 81(Pt A): 92-104.
[http://dx.doi.org/10.1016/j.biocel.2016.10.017] [PMID: 27780755]

[206] Philippaert K, Pironet A, Mesuere M, *et al.* Steviol glycosides enhance pancreatic beta-cell function and taste sensation by potentiation of TRPM5 channel activity. Nat Commun 2017; 8: 14733.
[http://dx.doi.org/10.1038/ncomms14733] [PMID: 28361903]

[207] Jiang C, Zhai M, Yan D, *et al.* Dietary menthol-induced TRPM8 activation enhances WAT "browning" and ameliorates diet-induced obesity. Oncotarget 2017; 8(43): 75114-26.
[http://dx.doi.org/10.18632/oncotarget.20540] [PMID: 29088850]

[208] Khare P, Chauhan A, Kumar V, *et al.* Bioavailable Menthol (Transient Receptor Potential Melastatin-8 Agonist) Induces Energy Expending Phenotype in Differentiating Adipocytes. Cells 2019; 8(5)E383
[http://dx.doi.org/10.3390/cells8050383] [PMID: 31027377]

[209] Wang P, Yan Z, Zhong J, *et al.* Transient receptor potential vanilloid 1 activation enhances gut glucagon-like peptide-1 secretion and improves glucose homeostasis. Diabetes 2012; 61(8): 2155-65.
[http://dx.doi.org/10.2337/db11-1503] [PMID: 22664955]

[210] Rigamonti AE, Casnici C, Marelli O, *et al.* Acute administration of capsaicin increases resting energy expenditure in young obese subjects without affecting energy intake, appetite, and circulating levels of orexigenic/anorexigenic peptides. Nutr Res 2018; 52: 71-9.
[http://dx.doi.org/10.1016/j.nutres.2018.02.002] [PMID: 29530622]

[211] Yoneshiro T, Aita S, Kawai Y, Iwanaga T, Saito M. Nonpungent capsaicin analogs (capsinoids) increase energy expenditure through the activation of brown adipose tissue in humans. Am J Clin Nutr 2012; 95(4): 845-50.
[http://dx.doi.org/10.3945/ajcn.111.018606] [PMID: 22378725]

[212] Inoue N, Matsunaga Y, Satoh H, Takahashi M. Enhanced energy expenditure and fat oxidation in humans with high BMI scores by the ingestion of novel and non-pungent capsaicin analogues (capsinoids). Biosci Biotechnol Biochem 2007; 71(2): 380-9.
[http://dx.doi.org/10.1271/bbb.60341] [PMID: 17284861]

[213] Zsiborás C, Mátics R, Hegyi P, *et al.* Capsaicin and capsiate could be appropriate agents for treatment of obesity: A meta-analysis of human studies. Crit Rev Food Sci Nutr 2018; 58(9): 1419-27.
[http://dx.doi.org/10.1080/10408398.2016.1262324] [PMID: 28001433]

[214] Iwasaki Y, Tamura Y, Inayoshi K, *et al.* TRPV1 agonist monoacylglycerol increases UCP1 content in brown adipose tissue and suppresses accumulation of visceral fat in mice fed a high-fat and high-sucrose diet. Biosci Biotechnol Biochem 2011; 75(5): 904-9.
[http://dx.doi.org/10.1271/bbb.100850] [PMID: 21597186]

[215] Mori N, Kurata M, Yamazaki H, *et al.* Allyl isothiocyanate increases carbohydrate oxidation through enhancing insulin secretion by TRPV1. Biosci Biotechnol Biochem 2018; 82(4): 698-708.
[http://dx.doi.org/10.1080/09168451.2017.1407234] [PMID: 29207921]

[216] Huffman MD, Xavier D, Perel P. Uses of polypills for cardiovascular disease and evidence to date. Lancet 2017; 389(10073): 1055-65.
[http://dx.doi.org/10.1016/S0140-6736(17)30553-6] [PMID: 28290995]

CHAPTER 5

Treatment of Raynaud's Phenomenon

Sevdalina Nikolova Lambova[*]

Medical University - Plovdiv, Faculty of Medicine, Department of Propaedeutics of Internal Diseases, Bulgaria

Abstract: Raynaud's phenomenon (RP) represents a clinical expression of recurrent vasospasm of the small arteries and arterioles of the acral parts (most commonly fingers and toes) provoked by cold exposure and emotional stress. Here, the therapeutic strategies in primary and secondary RP in systemic sclerosis (SSc) are discussed that are based on the evolving knowledge about different pathogenic pathways of the peripheral vascular syndrome. The vasospasm in primary RP is reversible while the secondary SSc-related RP is associated with endothelial injury and subsequent structural abnormalities that lead to tissue damage. The disbalance between vasodilators (nitric oxide - NO, prostacycline) and vasoconstrictors (endothelin-1, angiotensin) is the major consequence of the endothelial injury in secondary SSc-related RP. Therapeutic options in primary RP patients include administration of oral, well-tolerated drugs such as herbal extracts from Ginkgo biloba, pentoxifyllin, or calcium channel blockers. European League Against Rheumatism recommends standardised therapeutic approach for management of SSc-related RP that includes administration of dihydropyridine-type calcium channel blockers, fluoxetine, phosphodiesterase type 5 inhibitors and intravenous iloprost. Other approaches have been also studied such as inhibition of renin-angiotensin system, statins, botulinum toxin but currently there is not enough evidence for their use. Scientific knowledge about mechanisms of action of different drugs corresponding to the underlying pathogenesis are discussed as well as available experience in RP regarding efficacy and safety profile. Individualization of therapy with using complex approach and drug combinations in resistant cases of severe RP and digital ulcers are presented.

Keywords: Angiotensin, Antiplatelet drugs, Aspirin, Bosentan, Endothelin, Digital ulcers, Fluoxetine, Iloprost, Nitric oxide, Nifedipine, Pathogenesis, Pentoxifyllin, Phosphodiesterase inhibitors, Prostacyclin, Raynaud's phenomenon, Serotonin, Sildenafil, Systemic sclerosis, Treatment.

Raynaud's phenomenon (RP) represents a clinical expression of recurrent vasospasm of the small arteries, arterioles and arteriovenous shunts of the acral

[*] **Corresponding author Sevdalina Nikolova Lambova:** Medical University - Plovdiv, Faculty of Medicine, Department of Propaedeutics of Internal Diseases, Bulgaria

Atta-ur-Rahman & M. Iqbal Choudhary (Eds.)

parts (most commonly fingers and toes) provoked by cold exposure and emotional stress [1]. It manifests usually in three phases with phasic skin colour changes *i.e.,* white discoloration in the phase of ischaemia, blue – in the subsequent phase of asphyxia and finally red discoloration - in the phase of reactive hyperemia. Skin colour changes are reversible and differ with distinct demarcation between the affected and unaffected area.

RP is classified into two subtypes - primary and secondary RP [1 - 4] that differ in pathogenic, clinical and prognostic aspects and require different therapeutic approaches. Primary RP is not associated with an underlying disease, differs with female predominance, family history, younger age at onset (below 30 years, mainly at puberty), but this phenomenon should be interpreted with caution as primary RP with late onset (above the age of 40) is also possible [5]. Prevalence of primary RP varying from 1.6 to 7.2% (calculated pooled prevalence 4.85%) was reported in a recent systematic literature review [6]. Clinically, primary RP is characterized with benign course, absence of digital ulcers, lack of symptoms and signs of underlying systemic autoimmune disease. Its diagnosis is generally based on the following criteria *i.e.,* **1)** vasospastic attacks precipitated by cold or emotional stress; **2)** symmetry of attacks; **3)** absence of digital ulcerations or gangrenes; **4)** normal erythrocyte sedimentation rate; **5)** negative test for antinuclear autoantibodies; **6)** normal capillaroscopic findings [7].

Contrary, secondary RP is a syndrome in the context of underlying disease. Secondary RP is a common clinical symptom in systemic autoimmune rheumatic disease and differs with highest prevalence of approximately 95% in systemic sclerosis (SSc)/scleroderma [2, 4, 8]. Secondary RP in rheumatic diseases is characterized by later age of onset above 30 years, presence of signs of connective tissue disease, more severe course with development of digital ulcers in a part of the cases, thumb involvement [2, 4, 9] (Fig. **1**). Differential diagnosis of RP in rheumatic disease is broad and includes a spectrum of diseases that are characterized with varying prevalence of RP *i.e.*, SSc, mixed connective tissue disease, undifferentiated connective tissue disease, systemic lupus erythematosus, Sjögren syndrome, dermatomyositis, polymyositis, rheumatoid arthritis, systemic vasculitides (Buerger disease, Takayasu arteritis, polyarteritis nodosa, granulomatosis with polyangiitis, *etc.*), fibromyalgia, cryoglobulinaemia. RP could also be a sign of a spectrum of non-rheumatic pathology that also should be recognized and properly differentiated by the rheumatologists in routine clinical practice and includes cases of drug-induced RP by beta blockers, cytotoxic drugs – vinblastine, bleomycin, interferon, *etc.*; paraneoplastic RP – associated with solid tumours and haematological malignancies; vibration-induced white finger; hypothyroidism; carpal tunnel syndrome, *etc.* [2, 4, 8 - 15].

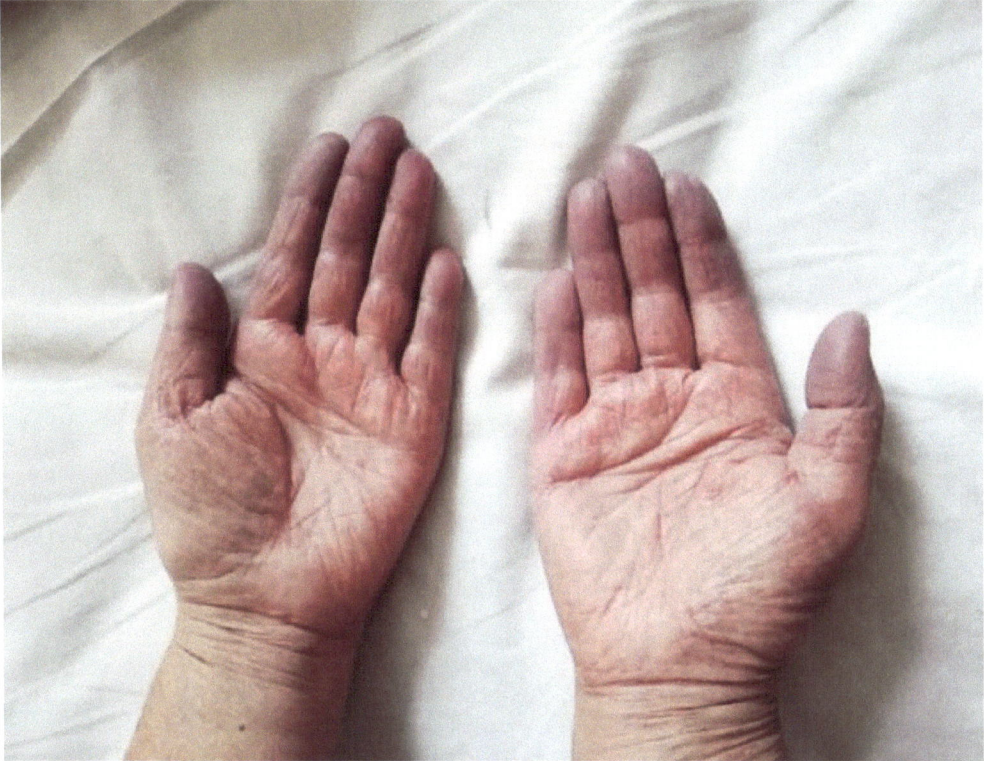

Fig. (1). Vasospastic attack in secondary SSc-related RP, phase of asphyxia with blue discoloration of the fingers; involvement of the thumbs is evident.

Different pathogenesis of primary and secondary RP results in different clinical course, severity, prognosis and respectively requires different therapeutic regimens. Here, the therapeutic strategies in primary and secondary RP in SSc are discussed. The vasospasm in primary RP is reversible while the secondary SSc-related RP is associated with endothelial injury and subsequent structural abnormalities that lead to tissue damage.

PRIMARY RAYNAUD'S PHENOMENON

Non-pharmacological measures represent an integral part of the complex care for RP patients. Patients should be instructed to avoid cold exposure, to wear warm clothes and gloves, and to stop smoking. Moreover, in milder forms of primary RP, these measures may be enough to control the symptoms. In cases of specific exposures that are known to induce peripheral vasospasm, the contact should be restricted such as reduction of caffeine consumption, avoidance of known causative agents *i.e.,* beta blockers, interferons, use of protective devices by patients working with vibration [10].

In primary RP patients, symptoms are mild without development of trophic changes *i.e.*, digital ulcers and necrotic lesions. Drug therapy should be initiated when non-pharmacological measures are ineffective and the attacks of RP are more pronounced and affect quality of life. The variable clinical course, high rate of a placebo effect, and the lack of standard outcome measures are the limiting factors for establishing precise recommendations for treatment of primary RP patients [4]. Therapeutic options in primary RP patients include administration of oral, well-tolerated drugs such as herbal extract from Ginkgo biloba, pentoxifyllin, calcium channel blockers (CCBs).

Ginkgo Biloba

Pharmacology

It has been suggested that Ginkgo biloba acts not only as a vasodilator but also possesses antiplatelet and radical scavenging effects that may be additional mechanisms that influence symptoms in RP patients.

Clinical Trials

Therapeutic effect of Ginkgo biloba has been evaluated in 22 primary RP patients in a double-blind, placebo-controlled trial. Ginkgo biloba was administered at a high dosage of 120 mg three times daily (total 360mg per day). The number of attacks per week has decreased significantly in patients treated with Ginkgo biloba *vs* placebo group after a 10-week therapeutic course. Administration of Ginkgo biloba was not associated with significant side effects or with withdrawal from the study due to side effects [16]. However, in 41 patients with primary RP, 10-week treatment with Ginkgo biloba (120 twice daily) did not lead to statistically significant reduction in frequency, duration, and severity of vasospastic attacks *vs* placebo [17]. Thus, in mild forms of primary RP, administration of Ginkgo biloba is a possible, well-tolerated therapeutic option. However, the evidence for its efficacy is limited and should be assessed in future placebo-controlled clinical trials.

The mechanism of action and considerations for clinical use of pentoxifyllin and CCBs in primary RP are given below in the sections presenting these drugs for use in secondary RP in SSc.

SECONDARY RAYNAUD'S PHENOMENON IN SYSTEMIC SCLEROSIS

Therapeutic influence on different levels of vascular function have been studied in SSc based on the current knowledge about the underlying pathogenic mechanisms of vascular pathology *i.e.,* interventions that influence calcium channels, endothelial function, neurogenic vascular control, blood rheology, platelet function, *etc.* The endothelium is active tissue that is involved in control of blood vessel tone. It produces both vasodilative (nitric oxide/NO, prostacycline/PgI_2) and vasoconstrictive substances (endothelin-1/ET-1, angiotensin) [18]. In SSc, profound endothelial damage occurs as a result of the action of various factors *i.e.,* free oxygen radicals produced as a result of recurrent ischaemia and reperfusion, anti-endothelial antibodies, *etc.* Clinically, the endothelial injury in SSc is manifested by severe RP that is frequently accompanied by digital ulcers. Among the major consequences of the endothelial damage in secondary SSc-related RP is the disbalance between vasodilators and vasoconstrictors [11, 19]. Increased levels of asymmetric dimethylarginine, that is an endogeneous NO synthesis inhibitor produced by endothelial cells, have been observed in secondary RP in SSc. While, ET-1, a potent vasoconstrictor, has been found to be elevated in the plasma of SSc patients *vs* primary RP [20]. In addition, increased expression of ET-1 in the skin of scleroderma patients has been also detected [21]. ET-1 has been suggested to play a role also in the pathogenesis of primary RP but the evidence is weaker in comparison with SSc [11, 22]. The major pathogenically-oriented therapeutic approaches in SSc-related secondary RP are presented below (Fig. **2**).

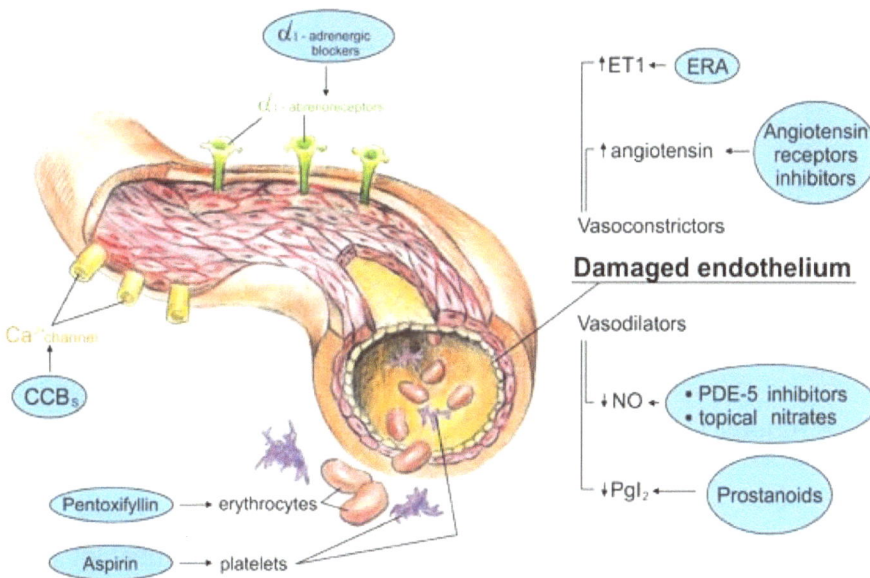

Fig. (2). Pathogenically-oriented therapeutic approaches in SSc-related secondary RP.

The European professional organization of the rheumatologists – EULAR (European League Against Rheumatism) recommends standardised therapeutic approach for management of SSc-related RP based on the results of randomized clinical trials and experts' opinion. It includes administration of dihydropyridine-type CCBs, phosphodiesterase type 5 (PDE-5) inhibitors, intravenous iloprost and fluoxetine. In severe RP with digital ulcers, EULAR recommends administration of intravenous iloprost and PDE-5 inhibitors for treatment of digital ulcers, and the endothelin-receptor antagonist (ERA) – bosentan for their prevention [23] (Fig. **3**).

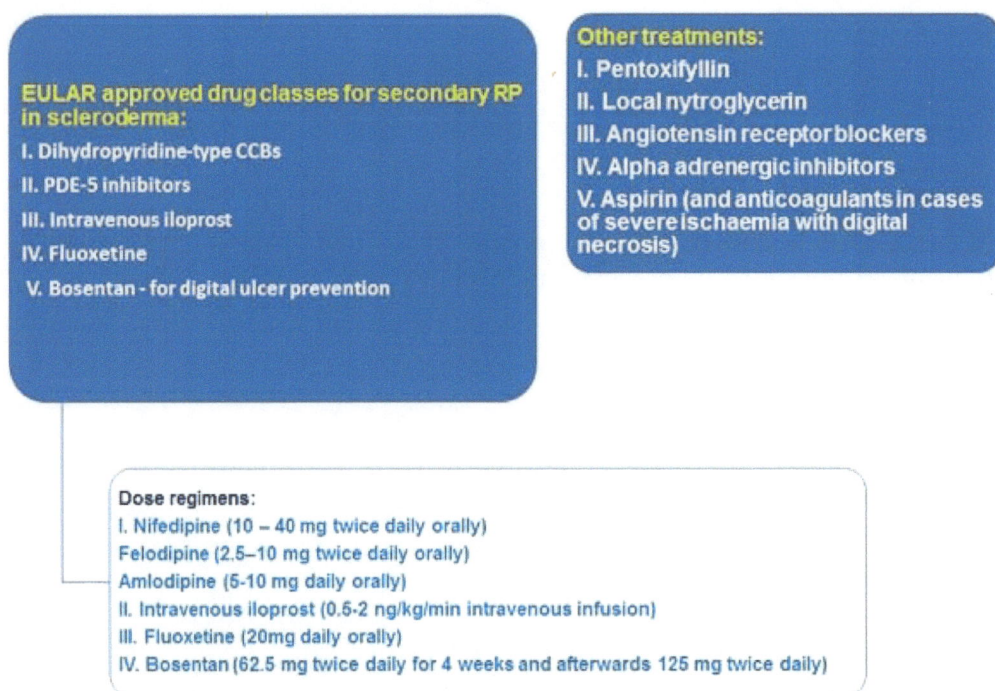

EULAR approved drug classes for secondary RP in scleroderma:

I. Dihydropyridine-type CCBs

II. PDE-5 inhibitors

III. Intravenous iloprost

IV. Fluoxetine

V. Bosentan - for digital ulcer prevention

Other treatments:

I. Pentoxifyllin

II. Local nytroglycerin

III. Angiotensin receptor blockers

IV. Alpha adrenergic inhibitors

V. Aspirin (and anticoagulants in cases of severe ischaemia with digital necrosis)

Dose regimens:

I. Nifedipine (10 – 40 mg twice daily orally)

Felodipine (2.5–10 mg twice daily orally)

Amlodipine (5-10 mg daily orally)

II. Intravenous iloprost (0.5-2 ng/kg/min intravenous infusion)

III. Fluoxetine (20mg daily orally)

IV. Bosentan (62.5 mg twice daily for 4 weeks and afterwards 125 mg twice daily)

Fig. (3). The main drug classes used in secondary RP in scleroderma.

Calcium Channel Blockers

Pharmacology

Currently, dihydropyridine-type CCBs are usually the treatment of choice for patients with both primary and secondary RP. Dihydropiridine class CCBs are potent arterial vasodilators that possess direct effects on vascular smooth muscles of coronary and peripheral vessels. They are indicated for the treatment of arterial hypertension, stable angina and in some cases for vasospastic angina [24]. In contractile cells, voltage-gated Ca^{2+} channels are of crucial importance because influx of extracellular Ca^{2+} is essential for muscle contraction and maintenance of tension. In vascular smooth muscle calcium influx affects arterial vasoconstriction and vasorelaxation and Ca^{2+} channel activity is a key determinant of vascular smooth muscle contractile state. L-type Ca^{2+} channels are the target of CCBs [25].

In vivo CCBs act mainly on the arterial vascular bed and don't modify venous tone. Thus, they do not cause orthostatic hypotension. CCBs reduce vascular resistance and afterload and decrease blood pressure. Of note, it has been observed that administration of nifedipine at therapeutic dosage induces blood pressure reduction in hypertensive patients but not in normotensive subjects [24]. In RP patients, dihydropyridine-type CCBs have been used off-label for many years.

It has been hypothesized that the action of CCBs is more complex and is not limited to vasodilation as selective calcium ion movement is involved in almost every cellular function. Of note, antiplatelet effect of nifedipine in therapeutic dose with evidence for enhanced thrombolysis has been demonstrated. Increased deformability of red blood cells induced by nifedipine has been also observed. Thus, it has been hypothesized that these additional mechanisms could contribute to the increased blood flow in RP [26]. Nifedipine (10 – 40 mg twice daily orally) is the best studied drug from the group. Other dihydropyridines commonly used in RP patients are felodipine (2.5–10 mg twice daily orally), and amlodipine (5-10 mg daily) [1, 10]. Diltiazem (benzothiazepine class CCBs) could also be used in RP at the dose of 30–120 mg three times daily orally especially in case of intolerance to dihydropyridines. Verapamil (diphenylalkylamine class of CCBs) does not possess therapeutic effect in RP patients [27 - 30].

Clinical Data

In a meta-analysis of 18 randomized controlled trials, it has been found that CCBs significantly reduce severity and frequency of attacks in primary RP and the efficacy is small. The mean frequency of vasospastic attacks per week in primary RP patients may be approximately 10.8. It has been found that in primary RP patients treated with CCBs the mean decrease of attacks per week was 2.8 to 5.0, while their severity was reduced by 33%. It has been suggested that the effect size may have been small because of the low dosing in the studies [28].

In a meta-analysis that included 8 randomized controlled trials (7 with nifedipine and 1 with nicardipine) with 109 SSc patients, it has been concluded that dihydropyridine-type CCBs reduce both frequency and severity of vasospastic attacks in SSc-related RP as their efficacy is moderate. The average decrease of frequency was 8.3 RP attacks in a 2-week period and improvement in the severity of attacks was 35% in comparison with placebo [29]. Of note, the efficacy of nifedipine in healing of SSc-related digital ulcers has been demonstrated in a double-blind, placebo-controlled, randomized trial that compared the therapeutic effect of nifedipine with those of intravenous iloprost. Both treatments have been beneficial for secondary RP in SSc in terms of reduction in the number, duration, and severity of attacks of RP and both led to healing of digital ulcers. The study included 23 patients with SSc-related RP. Twelve patients received intravenous infusions of iloprost (at the dose ranging between 0.5 and 2 ng/kg/min with gradual increase by 0 5 ng/kg/min every 15 minutes for eight hours on three consecutive days), a further single infusion at week 8 and placebo capsules. Eleven patients received nifedipine at an initial dose of 30 mg daily with gradual increase up to 60 mg daily after four weeks for another 12 weeks and placebo infusions in the conditions as those with iloprost [31].

Safety Profile

Adverse effects during treatment with dihydropyridine-type CCBs include hypotension, headache, tachycardia, flushing, dizziness, ankle edema, constipation, *etc.* Long-acting forms with slow release are better tolerated and most commonly used in clinical practice [1, 4].

Pentoxifyllin

Pharmacology

Pentoxifylline is a methylxanthine that represents an active haemorheological agent used for treatment of peripheral vascular disease, cerebrovascular disease and a number of other conditions with defective regional microcirculation [32]. Pentoxifylline is a non-selective phosphodiesterase inhibitor, whose primary actions include increase in red blood cell deformability, reduction of blood viscosity, inhibition of platelet potential for aggregation and thrombus formation [32, 33]. Blood viscosity and its flow in capillaries are mainly influenced by red cell deformability and aggregation, haematocrit, and plasma viscosity. Normally, erythrocytes are flexible that allows easy passage through capillaries. Contrary, blood cell rigidity compromises blood flow in microcirculation and increases blood viscosity. Erythrocyte deformability depends on the viscoelastic properties of the membrane, the viscosity of the intracellular fluid and on the cellular shape. Factors that determine the viscoelastic properties of the cell membrane are intracellular adenosine triphosphate (ATP) and calcium ion concentrations. ATP level depletion and calcium accumulation results in decreased cell flexibility. Pentoxifylline causes increased red blood cell deformability *via* increased erythrocyte ATP and other cyclic nucleotide levels [32].

The underlying pathogenic mechanisms that support such a therapeutic approach is the occurence of reduced red cell filterability and alterations in blood viscosity in acroischaemic syndromes especially after cold exposure [34, 35]. Altered behaviour of red blood cells in SSc has been observed. Decreased deformability, lower electrophoretic velocity as well as increased adherence to cultured endothelial cells have been found [36].

In addition, pentoxifyllin is considered to possess antithrombotic effect that is thought to be the result of the induced decrease in plasma fibrinogen concentration and inhibition of spontaneous and induced platelet aggregation [32, 37]. Pentoxifyllin suppresses membrane-bound phosphodiesterase of the platelets and leads to increase in intracellular cyclic adenosine monophosphate (cAMP) level. This activates a protein kinase, which itself catalyses the phosphorylation of membrane proteins by ATP and leads to inhibition of platelet aggregation potential. Moreover, pentoxifylline is suggested to stimulate prostacyclin synthesis and release, to inhibit thromboxane synthesis and to increase leucocyte filterability. Of note, the evidence for a direct vasodilatory effect of oral pentoxifyllin is limited and the administration of the drug usually does not cause change in blood pressure and heart rate [32]. Hypotension and decreased vascular tone have been reported after intravenous administration of pentoxifyllin in animals [32, 38]. It has been speculated that pentoxifyllin also produces effects on vascular tone [38 - 40] in a cyclic AMP-mediated mechanism [39, 40].

The maximal daily dose of pentoxifyllin is 1200 mg. It could be divided into three doses from 400mg, or two doses from 600 mg daily orally with meals. A combination between oral intake and venous infusions (ampules 100mg) could also be used [1, 32].

Clinical Data

The use of pentoxifyllin in RP is based on the results of small studies [34, 41, 42]. Administration of oral pentoxifylline at a dose of 400 mg three times daily in 11 female patients with primary RP for 60 days has led to a distinct improvement of peripheral blood flow and of RP symptoms in 7 among 11 patients under basal conditions and after exposure to cold. Of note, significantly improved red cell filtration has been found [34].

Pentoxifyllin is usually not recommended in severe RP [1]. However, there are case reports for beneficial effects of pentoxifyllin in RP with severe clinical course. Digital ulcer healing has been observed in a case of severe RP in systemic lupus erythematosus [43]. In two patients with peripheral gangrene due to SSc, intravenous pentoxifyllin has led to stabilisation of clinical situation without further development of ischaemic lesions and with demarcation of the gangrenous areas [39]. Considering its properties to improve haemorheology, pentoxifylline could be used in combination with other drugs in secondary SSc-related RP [44].

Safety Profile

Currently used slow-release tablets are well-tolerated and gastrointestinal symptoms (nausea, vomiting, dyspepsia, meteorism/flatus/bloating/belching, abdominal discomfort, diarrhoea) are the most common adverse events. In placebo-controlled trials in patients with peripheral vascular disorders, gastrointestinal side effects (about 3%) were the most common complaints, although the frequency of those and other adverse effects did not differ significantly in patients on pentoxifyllin or placebo. Cardiovascular (angina, arrhythmias/palpitations, flushing) and neurological (nervousness, dizziness, headache, insomnia, tremor, blurred vision) adverse events occur rarely. Discontinuation due to side effects was registered in 3.1 and 0% of patients receiving pentoxifylline and placebo. In patients with cerebrovascular diseases, administration of pentoxifylline 300 to 600 mg daily was associated again most commonly with gastrointestinal adverse events while side effects from other organ systems *i.e.*, cardiovascular, psychological/neurological, hepatic or dermatological effects each occurred in less than 0.25% [32].

Nitric Oxide Pathway

Phosphodiesterase-5 Enzyme Inhibitors

Pharmacology

Targeting the NO pathway is a key therapeutic strategy in the management of digital vascular disease in SSc. It includes administration of PDE-5 inhibitors and topical application of glyceryl trinitrate (GTN), the latter being a donor for NO [45, 46].

NO is the main endothelium-derived vasodilator that acts also as an inhibitor of platelet activation and vascular smooth muscle proliferation. Its synthesis is regulated by a family of NO synthases. NO exerts its effects *via* cyclic guanosine-5-monophosphate (cGMP), which is quickly degraded *in vivo* under the action of enzymes phosphodiesterases [46, 47]. As cGMP is mainly hydrolyzed by phosphodiesterase-5A, its inhibition by PDE-5 inhibitors decreases cGMP metabolism and thus preserves and potentiates NO effects that include vasodilation and improved perfusion [47].

Clinical Data

Currently, three PDE-5 inhibitors (sildenafil, tadalafil and vardenafil) are available. Their primary approved indication is erectile dysfunction. Subsequently, sildenafil and tadalafil have been approved for the treatment of pulmonary hypertension. Treatment of RP patients with PDE-5 inhibitors has gained increased attention in the last years [46] and currently, they are recommended by EULAR in SSc patients with severe RP and/or those, who do not show satisfactory response to CCBs [23]. In a meta-analysis that included 6 randomized controlled trials (2 with sildenafil, 3 with tadalafil and 1 with vardenafil) it has been concluded that PDE-5 inhibitors significantly improve frequency and duration of RP attacks. There is also evidence for their efficacy in healing of digital ulcers. PDE-5 inhibitors were used in the following dosages *i.e.*, sildenafil 50mg bid or as a single daily dose of sildenafil with modified-release 200 mg; tadalafil 20 mg once daily or 20 mg on alternate days; vardenafil 10 mg bid. The choice of the dosage regimen is associated with the half-lives of the different drugs that are 3–5 h for sildenafil and vardenafil and about 18 h for tadalafil [47].

The effect of PDE-5 enzyme inhibitor sildenafil (20mg three times daily for 12 weeks) on healing of digital ulcers in SSc patients has been evaluated in a randomized, double-blind study (SEDUCE study). The primary end point, that was the time to digital ulcer healing, was not reached, partly because of an unexpectedly high healing rate in the placebo group. The time to digital ulcer healing was determined for each digital ulcer present at entry as the delay between week 0 and the first visit on which healing was observed. However, a significant decrease in the number of digital ulcers at weeks 8 and 12 was observed in sildenafil *vs* placebo group that confirms a sildenafil benefit [48]. Of note, administration of single doses sildenafil on demand did not show clinically relevant efficacy [49]. According to the current EULAR recommendations, PDE-5 inhibitors should be considered as second-line treatment for severe SSc-related RP and/or cases with insufficient therapeutic effect from the treatment with CCBs, the latter being an established treatment with good safety profile [23].

Safety Profile

Side effects during treatment with PDE-5 inhibitors are common and include different forms of vasomotor reactions, flushing, erythema, night sweats, headache, insomnia, anxiety, fluid retention, pain in the extremities, myalgias, back pain, allergic reaction, chest pain, dyspepsia, diarrhoea, dry mouth, gastritis, gastro-esophageal reflux disease, bloating, haemorrhoids, epistaxis, nasal stuffiness, cough, visual abnormalities (blurred vision, ocular irritation and hyperaemia), anaemia.

Topical Glyceryl Trinitrate

Pharmacology

Treatment of peripheral vascular syndrome with a topical drug without significant systemic effects is a tempting option. GTN serves as NO donor and its local application is an approach that could induce vasodilation in an endothelial independent manner [50 - 52]. Thus, this therapeutic strategy could be efficacious also in SSc patients in whom endothelial injury is an well-recognized pathology [51].

Clinical Trials and Safety Profile

Clinical efficacy and safety profile of sustained-release GTN patches (0.2 mg/h) in RP patients have been assessed in a randomized, double-blind, placebo-controlled study that included both primary RP patients (n = 21) and patients with secondary RP in SSc (n = 21). The application of GTN patches demonstrated clinical efficacy and significantly reduced the number and severity of RP attacks (p < 0.05) in patients with both primary and SSc-related secondary RP. However, the examination by infrared thermography did not demonstrate a significant improvement in patients treated with GTN patches. Headache, refractory to treatment, was the reason for withdrawal of eight patients from the study and appeared also in approximately 80% of the remaining patients (Teh *et al.*, 1995) [52].

Anderson *et al.* (2002) investigated the effect of the local application of 2% GTN ointment on blood flow in 10 patients with primary RP, 13 patients with secondary RP in limited cutaneous SSc and 10 controls using laser Doppler imaging. After the initial evaluation of the blood flow of the dorsum of the index, middle and ring fingers of the non-dominant hand, 2% GTN ointment was applied on the dorsum of one finger for 1 min; placebo ointment - on the dorsum of a second finger for 1 min, and the third finger remained untreated. The effect on the digital blood flow of these three fingers was evaluated *via* laser Doppler scanning immediately after the application and after 10 and 20 min. The increase in blood flow response was significantly higher for GTN as compared with placebo. Adverse events were not observed among the participants in the study [51].

A novel formulation of GTN - MQX-503 has been evaluated in a multicentre, randomized, placebo-controlled trial that included 69 patients with primary RP and 150 patients with secondary RP (131 of whom had SSc). MQX-503 represents a microemulsion formulation of topical nitroglycerin gel with a proprietary surfactant system that is designed for rapid, nonirritating, local delivery of the active substance. The induced mean change in the Raynaud's Condition Score *vs* baseline was significantly greater in patients treated with MQX-503 as compared with placebo. Changes in the frequency and duration of RP episodes and the subjective assessments did not differ significantly between the treatment and the placebo group. Of note, MQX-503 had a good safety profile similar to that of placebo [53]. In a recent meta-analysis (Curtiss *et al.*, 2018), that included 7 placebo-controlled trials with 346 patients, the effect of local topical nitrate preparation in primary and secondary RP was evaluated. Four of the studies used nitroglycerin ointments, two - the nitroglycerin gel vehicle MQX-503, and one used compounded nitrite. It has been concluded that the therapeutic effect of the topical nitrates is moderate-to-large. The subgroup analysis demonstrated a large treatment effect in secondary RP and moderate effect in the primary forms [50].

In their meta-analysis Curtiss *et al.* (2018) have found that the side effects during treatment with topical nitrates were mild but greater in studies, in which the participants used large quantities of nitroglycerin ointment applied on the entire hand. The most common adverse event was headache that was often reported up to 2 hours after administration of the nitrates that suggests a delayed onset of systemic effects. In some cases headache during treatment with topical nitrates is severe and may limit compliance. Suggested approaches to avoid this adverse event is use of nitroglycerin ointment in a lower concentration (1% rather than 2%), variable individual dosing with titration by the patient. Of note, the authors have proposed as a well-tolerated option the use of 1% nitroglycerin applied to the distal phalanges of selected fingers. MQX-503 represents an alternative nitroglycerin gel vehicle that has been designed to improve safety profile and shows side effect rates similar to placebo. Nitrite compounded with mild acids is an alternative option that rapidly releases NO without development of systemic side effects. Serious adverse reactions during treatment with topical nitrates were not registered. Of note, concomitant administration of topical nitrates with PDE-5 inhibitors has not been evaluated as the latter are contraindicated to be used in combination with systemic nitrates because of the risk of pronounced hypotension [50].

Prostacyclin Pathway

Impaired prostacyclin/PgI$_2$ synthesis is a well-known consequence of the endothelial damage in SSc [54]. Prostacyclin is synthesized from arachidonic acid in the healthy vascular endothelium [55]. Currently, intravenous prostanoid therapy is the "gold standard" for management of severe SSc-related RP with digital ulcers. The most commonly prescribed agent is *intravenous iloprost* [54].

Iloprost

Pharmacology

Iloprost is a synthetic analogue of the endogenous prostacyclin. It is more stable with a longer elimination half-life. Iloprost is completely metabolised by β-oxidation and is mainly excreted *via* the renal system (70%). Faecal excretion is approximately 12 to 17%. Elimination of iloprost is biphasic with an initial half-life of distribution of 4 min and elimination half-life of approximately 20-30 min. Iloprost is an arterial vasodilator and inhibitor of platelet aggregation. The ratio of antiaggregatory to vasodilatory potency *in vivo* is 2-7:1. The suggested mechanism of its antiaggregatory effect involves platelet receptor-mediated activation of adenyl cyclase that increases the level of cAMP, thus influencing phospholipase activity and cytosolic calcium levels. It has been suggested that drugs, which interfere with thromboxane A2 synthesis such as aspirin, appear to increase the antiaggregatory effect of iloprost that should be taken into account in cases of concomitant administration. Similarly to its effects in platelets, it has been suggested that the effect of iloprost on blood vessels may involve an increase in smooth muscle cAMP secondary to receptor activation. In human and animal artery specimens, iloprost inhibits contraction induced by arachidonic acid, thromboxane A2 analogue, angiotensin II, *etc*. In humans, iloprost causes decrease in peripheral vascular resistance and mean arterial blood pressure with a slight increase in heart rate and cardiac index. In addition, iloprost enhances renal blood flow and has a natriuretic effect, but the latter is independent of the haemodynarnic changes. Regarding the other components of haemostasis, iloprost is suggested to have some fibrinolytic activity. In addition, iloprost is thought to inhibit neutrophil adhesion and chemotaxis, but evidence for a significant effect on blood viscosity is weak [55].

Clinical Data

Intravenous iloprost possesses a proven efficacy for reduction the frequency and severity of attacks of SSc-related RP and for healing of ischaemic digital ulcers that is observed in double-blind controlled studies [30, 56 - 59]. It is approved for the treatment of severe RP at the dose of 0.5-2 ng/kg/min depending on the individual tolerance. The dose in the first 30 minutes is 0.5ng/kg/min and afterwards it could be increased with 0.5ng/kg/min at 30-minute intervals. In patients with chronic renal failure indicated for dyalisis and liver cirrhosis the dose should be reduced half of the recommended because of the decreased elimination. The duration of the infusion is 6 hours and monitoring of heart rate and blood pressure prior to the infusion and after every increase in the infusion rate should be performed. The therapeutic course recommended by the manufacturer is up to 4 weeks. The usual duration of intravenous iloprost infusions in secondary RP in SSc is 3-5 days. A recent expert consensus suggested a 1-3 days monthly infusions with iloprost to be used for treatment of RP and digital ulcers and a single monthly infusion to be given for digital ulcers prevention. A validation of these suggestions have been proposed as they are thought to be a possible way for personalization of treatment with intravenous iloprost according to patients' needs [60].

The need for hospitalization, the prolonged intravenous infusion, side effects and high price are limiting factors for the use of iloprost. Considering costs and feasibility intravenous iloprost is recommended by EULAR for SSc-related RP after failure of oral therapies (CCBs and PDE-5 inhibitors) [23].

Interestingly, it has been demonstrated that short term infusions of iloprost provide long-lasting symptom relief in SSc-related RP in a study that compared the effect of nifedipin and intravenous iloprost in secondary RP in SSc (12 patients on iloprost). Iloprost infusions for three consecutive days induced increases in microcirculatory blood flow at week 4 that reached maximum at week 8. The effect was maintained for another four weeks by a single infusion at week 8 and was no longer evident at week 16. These results suggest that a process of continuous recovery take place for a longer period that is distinct from the immediate vasodilative response during iloprost infusion. The underlying mechanisms for the long-term benefits of intravenous iloprost are suggested to be related to the improvement of endothelial structure and function [31].

The complex effects of iloprost on microvascular endothelium as well as the observed long beneficial clinical effect despite its short half-life raise the question about its potential disease-modifying properties. It has been suggested that iloprost downregulates the expression of adhesion molecules on phagocytes and endothelial cells [61]. A significant reduction of the soluble forms of the adhesion molecules *i.e*, P-selectin, vascular cell adhesion molecule -1/VCAM-1 as well as decrease in ET-1 level has been registered after treatment with intravenous iloprost [62]. Significantly lower production of inteleukin-1β/IL-1β has been detected in 19 SSc patients after treatment with iloprost (a 5-day course of iloprost, at a dose of 2.0 ng/kg per minute followed by a 1-day infusion every 6 weeks) as compared with SSc patients treated with nifedipine (n=12, 20 mg twice daily) [63]. Of note, in a longer observational study of Bettoni *et al.* (2002) that included 30 SSc patients (17 patients with diffuse cutaneous SSc and 13 with limited cutaneous form of the disease), a significant decrease in skin score was registered only in patients with diffuse cutaneous involvement. The patients were treated with iloprost infusions for 5 consecutive days and afterwards a maintenance infusion was given every 3 weeks. The median follow-up was 36 months [61]. Improvement in the skin score has been also observed by other authors in a longer follow-up after 1 year of intermittent treatment with intravenous iloprost [63, 64].

Safety Profile

Adverse events during intravenous iloprost therapy include headache, nausea, vomiting, diarrhoea, myalgia, arthralgia, chills, fever, arrhythmia, hypotension including orthostatic hypotension, chest pain (especially in patients with coronary heart disease), erythema and pain at the infusion site [58, 59, 61]. Contra-indications for treatment with intravenous iloprost are pregnancy, breastfeeding, conditions, in which the effect of the intravenous iloprost on platelets may increase the risk of haemorrhage (acute peptic ulcer, intracranial haemorrhage, trauma), severe coronary heart disease, unstable angina, myocardial infarction in the last 6 months, acute or chronic heart failure from II to IV New York Heart Asso-ciation/NYHA functional classes, severe arrhythmia, and suspicion of pulmonary congestion. Risk of haemorrhage is increased in patients, who receive therapy with antiplatelet drugs, heparin or indirect anticoagulants.

Of note, ischaemic vascular complications, *i.e.*, myocardial infarction and stroke, were recorded in a significantly higher number of patients, who have received prostanoid treatment (iloprost and alprostadil) *vs* controls. Thus, careful risk assessment should be performed prior to prostanoid therapy [65].

Epoprostenol

Pharmacology

Another available prostanoid is *epoprostenol* that has been the first prostacyclin agent approved by the US Food and Drug Administration/FDA in 1995. The drug is not available in all European countries. It is indicated for patients with pulmonary arterial hypertension (PAH). There are also reports for its off-label administration in RP. Epoprostenol is a very potent but short-lived compound whose elimination half-life is 6 minutes, and the hemodynamic changes that it induces reverse within 10 minutes of infusion discontinuation. Epoprostenol acts as a vasodilator of pulmonary and systemic arterial blood vessels and as an inhibitor of platelet aggregation [55, 66].

Intravenous epoprostenol should only be considered in the therapeutic armamentarium in patients with severe RP after failure of or intolerance to oral therapies. Hospitalization of the patients as well as monitoring for haemodynamic changes and adverse effects are necessary as with other intravenous prostanoids. If possible, the infusion of epoprostenol should be performed through a central intravenous line, but a peripheral line may also be used for temporary access. The initial dose of intravenous epoprostenol for treatment of refractory RP with or without digital ulcers should be no greater than 2 ng/kg/min and the rate of increase could be 1 ng/kg/min every 15 minutes. For limiting drug exposure and adverse reactions, intermittent infusions with duration 5 to 6 hours could be used initially, but continuous infusions for up to 72 hours in patients unresponsive to intermittent treatment could also be considered. The clinical effects in RP patients may only be transient. Whether there is a sustained effect after discontinuation of epoprostenol therapy is not clear [66].

Safety Profile

Side effects of epoprostenol include catheter-associated infections of the infusion site, low platelet count, haemorrhages, nervousness, headache, tachy- and bradycardia, flushing, hypotonia, nausea, vomiting, diarrhoea, abdominal colic or discomfort, skin rash, jaw pain, arthralgia, pain at the infusion site, chest pain, pulmonary oedema [66].

Prostaglandin E$_1$ (Alprostadil)

Prostaglandin E$_1$ (alprostadil) is a potent vasodilator that has also demonstrated a beneficial effect on severity and frequency of vasospastic attacks and on digital ulcer healing in SSc-related RP [67]. However, in a double-blind, placebo-controlled trial that included 55 patients with RP (both primary and secondary SSc-related RP), the treatment with prostaglandin E$_1$ was not superior to placebo. Prostaglandin E$_1$ was administered intravenously at a dose 10 ng/kg/min for 72 hours *via* a central venous catheter and placebo was administered in the same manner [68]. The data about the use of this prostanoid in RP are scarce [66].

Treprostinil

Treprostinil is a synthetic prostacyclin analogue approved for treatment of PAH. It is administered preferably by subcutaneous infusion or *via* intravenous infusion if subcutaneous infusion is not tolerated. Healing of digital ulcers in severe SSc-related RP under treatment with continuous subcutaneous treprostinil was reported [69, 70]. However, there is limited experience with parenteral treprostinil in RP patients. The mode of its administration *via* continuous infusion may be another limiting factor for its use. Moreover, high rate of severe injection site reactions has been reported (41.7%, 5/12) that lead to drug discontinuation [70]. Of note, inhaled formulations of prostanoids (treprostinil, iloprost) are available for treatment of PAH but they are not studied as therapeutic options in RP [71].

Oral Prostanoids

Oral prostanoids are less effective for the treatment of RP patients in comparison with intravenous iloprost, although some beneficial effects could be seen [23, 72]. Currently, they are not approved for this indication [66, 73].

Oral Iloprost

Pharmacology

Given orally, iloprost is absorbed very quickly and maximum plasma concentration is reached within 10 minutes. However, it undergoes extensive biotransformation in the liver and gut wall and just < 20% of the drug reaches the systemic circulation [55]. A study on the pharmacokinetics of oral iloprost (50µg twice daily for 8 days with dosing interval of 5 hours) in SSc patient has demonstrated that there is no evidence for delayed drug absorption in SSc patients, despite the fact that nine out of 10 patients had gastrointestinal complaints. Plasma levels were evaluated for 10 hours on days 1 and 8 (11 samples at 1-hour intervals, starting immediately before the first capsule). Moreover, SSc patients had higher systemic iloprost exposure after both daily doses and on both monitored study days that could not be explained with impaired renal function, but probably are associated with altered metabolic clearance of iloprost [74].

Clinical Data

In a multicenter, randomized, parallel-group, placebo-controlled double-blind study that included 308 scleroderma patients treated with oral iloprost (n=157, at a dose of 50µg twice daily) or placebo (n=151), the mean reduction in the average duration and daily frequency of vasospastic attacks from baseline to week 5-6 was not significant between the two groups. The duration of treatment was 6 weeks with further 6 weeks of post-treatment follow-up. After 6-week treatment period there was not a significant difference in the Raynaud's condition score between patients treated with iloprost and placebo. Considering a variety of factors *i.e.,* use of other vasodilators, disease duration, subtype of cutaneous skin involvement (limited or diffuse), the number of digital ulcers at baseline did not change the lack of significant difference between the treatment groups. Thus, it has been concluded that oral iloprost (at a dose of 50 *µg* twice daily) is not superior to placebo in SSc-related RP during 6-week treatment period or during post-treatment follow-up [75]. Another multicentre, randomized, parallel-group study compared the effect of two different doses of oral iloprost and placebo given for 6 weeks with additional 6 weeks of follow-up. It included 103 patients with secondary SSc-related RP (35 – received placebo, 33 were on iloprost 50 µg twice daily, 35 – on iloprost 100 µg twice daily). At the end of the treatment (6 weeks), a significant decrease in duration of attacks was observed but not in their severity and frequency. At the end of the follow-up (12 weeks), a significant decrease in the total daily duration of attacks and their severity was registered, but not in their frequency. The treatment was discontinued prematurely in 9% of patients on placebo, in 30% of those treated with iloprost 50 µg twice daily and in 51% of patients, who received the higher dose of 100 µg twice daily and the discontinuation was due to adverse effects in 6, 27 and 51% respectively for the three patient groups. The study results suggest that both daily dosages of oral iloprost (50 and 100 µg oral twice daily) may be effective in secondary RP in SSc, but the lower dosage is better tolerated [76].

Safety Profile

Most commonly observed side effects during treatment with oral iloprost include headache, flushing, nausea, dizziness, diarrhoea [75].

Oral Treprostinil

Treprostinil diolamine is a salt of the prostacyclin analogue treprostinil developed for oral administration as an extended-release tablet. It is approved for PAH World Health Organisation/WHO functional class I, including secondary PAH in the context of SSc. In a recent double-blind, placebo-controlled trial, administration of oral treprostinil demonstrated small and statistically insignificant reduction in net ulcer burden. The net ulcer burden was defined as the sum between all baseline "active" ulcers (unless graded "healed") and all new ulcers (unless graded "healed") *vs* placebo. 148 SSc patients were included in the study: 72 – on treprostinil, and 76 – on placebo. The initial dose of oral treprostinil in the study was 0.25 mg twice daily titrated gradually to a maximum dose of 16 mg twice daily. Initially, the dose was increased with 0.25 mg twice daily every 48-72 hours and upon reaching a dose of 5 mg twice daily, the titration of the dose was allowed to be with 0.5 mg twice daily at the same interval within the physician's decision. At week 20, mean net ulcer burden was reduced - 0.43 in patients on treprostinil (1.80 *vs* 1.37), and -0.10 ulcers (1.61 *vs* 1.51) in those receiving placebo, but the difference was not statistically significant (p=0.20) [77]. In a subsequent multicenter, retrospective study, digital ulcer burden was evaluated in 51 patients in the year after withdrawal of oral treprostinil. Of note, digital ulcer burden increased significantly at 3-6 and 6-12 months after treprostinil discontinuation. These data provide evidence for a beneficial effect of oral treprostinil for the vascular complications of SSc and suggest the necessity from future studies [78].

Prostacyclin Receptor Agonist

Another approach to influence the prostacyclin pathway is *via* administration of oral, selective prostacyclin receptor agonist selexipag. It has been recently approved for the long-term treatment of PAH in adults (WHO functional classes II and III). A randomized, placebo-controlled, phase 2 study evaluated the efficacy of selexipag in secondary SSc-related RP (38 patients - on placebo and 36 - on selexipag). Selexipag was administered at an initial daily dose of 200 µg twice daily and was increased every 3 days in increments of 200 µg until the appearance of unmanageable side effects such as headache and diarrhoea. The maximum allowed daily dosage was 1600 µg. In cases of adverse events, the dose was either continued or reduced by 200 µg and this dose was considered to be the individual highest tolerated dosage. The results of the study demonstrated that selexipag did not reduce the number of RP attacks in comparison with placebo [79].

Serotonin Inhibition – Fluoxetine

Pharmacology

Fluoxetine is a serotonin-specific reuptake inhibitor and antidepressant. Despite the relatively low quality of published evidence, in the EULAR recommendations (2017), fluoxetine is suggested as a therapeutic option in SSc-related RP, especially in patients, who do not tolerate or do not respond to vasodilators [23].

Serotonin/5-hydroxytryptamine (5-HT) is a signaling molecule in diverse systems in the brain and in the peripheral tissues [80]. It is produced in the central nervous system where it serves as a neurotransmitter and does not cross the blood-brain barrier [80, 81]. The quantity of serotonin in the brain is small, while most of the serotonin in the body (about 95%) is produced in the gut by the enterochromaffin subtype of enteroendocrine cells and by serotonergic neurons of the myenteric plexus. Enterochromaffin cells contain the rate-limiting enzyme in serotonin's biosynthesis, tryptophan hydroxylase-1, while enteric and central serotonergic neurons contain another type 2 isoform of the enzyme. Enterochromaffin cells synthesize far more serotonin as compared with central and peripheral serotonergic neurons. Serotonin derived from the enterochromaffin cells overflows to reach the gastrointestinal lumen and blood. It is caught by the platelets and stored in them. Platelets are a rich and sole source of serotonin in blood, but they lack tryptophan hydroxylase and thus cannot synthesize it [80]. The platelets take up serotonin from the plasma *via* a serotonin transporter [82]. In normal conditions, the circulating serotonin levels are low. However, platelet activation raises plasma serotonin levels as a result of its release by the platelet dense granules [82, 83]. Serotonin promotes platelet aggregation and vasoconstriction of surrounding blood vessels, thus facilitating haemostasis [82]. Acting as a serotonin reuptake inhibitor, fluoxetine suppresses the uptake of serotonin into platelets and in this way decreases its release during platelet activation and aggregation [83]. Thus, it has been suggested that selective serotonin reuptake inhibitors could increase also bleeding time [82]. The mechanism of action of fluoxetine in RP patients is thought to be a result of the reduction of the circulating levels of the selective vasoconstrictor serotonin [83]. Platelet serotonin depletion induced by fluoxetine reaches 95% [84]. Healthy endothelium does not contain any stimuli necessary for platelet activation and *via* the produced substances prostacyclin and NO, the platelets are kept in an inactive state [81]. Enhanced platelet activation and aggregation has been found in SSc patients [85, 86] with increased release of the granule components such as beta-thromboglobulin [85]. Of note, it has been also suggested that serotonin links vascular damage, platelet activation and tissue fibrosis *via* transforming growth factor/TGF-β-mediated activation of 5-HT(2B) receptors that strongly induces extracellular matrix synthesis in interstitial fibroblasts [87].

Clinical Data and Safety Profile

The effect of fluoxetine (20 mg daily) has been evaluated in a small study that included 26 primary RP patients and 27 cases with SSc-related RP. Of note, a superior efficacy *vs* nifedipine (40 mg daily) has been observed regarding the frequency and severity of RP attacks that were reduced in both groups but statistical significance was present in fluoxetine group only. The drugs were administered for 6 weeks, and after a 2-week washout period each group was crossed over to the other treatment arm. The patients were not formally assessed for presence of depression and although the eventual improvement of psychological state could also influence the responses in self-reported diaries, the authors suggested that such an association is not present. Subgroup analysis revealed that the greatest response was observed in females and in cases with primary RP. Moreover, a significant improvement in the thermographic response to cold challenge was also observed in the same patient groups *i.e.,* females and primary RP patients. Administration of fluoxetine was associated with adverse events such as apathy, lethargy and impaired concentration [83].

Endothelin Pathway and Endothelin-Receptor Antagonists

Endothelin Pathway

ET is a 21 amino-acid peptide and was first isolated from the supernatant of cultured porcine aortic endothelial cells by Yanagisawa *et al.* (1988). It acts as one of the most potent vasoconstrictors [88]. In fact, the endothelins are a family of three vasoactive 21-amino-acid peptides with three isoforms (ET-1, ET-2 and

ET-3). ET-1 is the most abundant isoform and is produced primarily by endothelial cells, but also by a variety of other cell types *i.e.,* mesenchymal cells (smooth muscle cells, fibroblasts). The three isoforms of ET bind to two ET receptors – ET receptor subtype A (ET-A) and subtype B (ET-B). Their affinity for ET-B is equal, while for ET-A receptors, it differs being highest for ET-1, followed by ET-2 and ET-3 [89, 90]. The ET-A receptor subtype is the predominant form in vascular smooth muscle cells and its activation causes vasoconstriction in both large and small blood vessels. It is also the major subtype in the heart structures. The ET-B receptors are present on both endothelial and vascular smooth muscle cells. They are predominantly found in brain, lung, kidney, and aorta. The ET-B receptors on endothelial cells mediate vasodilation in response to ET-1 through the production of NO and prostacyclin and promote ET-1 clearance [91, 92]. ET-1 is produced as a pre-pro polypeptide of 212 amino acids, which is processed to proET-1 or big ET-1 by a series of converting enzymes. The big ET-1 is a large, relatively inactive ET molecule that exhibits approximately 1% of the activity of the fully functional 21-amino-acid peptide. The membrane-bound ET-converting enzyme-1 acts on the big ET-1 and leads to formation of the functionally active, 21-aminoacid form ET-1. Under the action of the membrane-bound enzyme ET-converting enzyme-1. Finally, ET-1 is the molecule that binds to the specific ET receptors expressed by different cell types [90, 93].

ET-1 acts as a potent vasoconstrictor, mitogen for smooth muscle cells, pro-fibrotic and pro-inflammatory mediator [92, 94]. It is suggested that ET-1 is able to activate and re-program the functional phenotypes of different cell types *i.e.,* vascular smooth muscle cells, microvascular pericytes and tissue fibroblasts into pro-fibrogenic cells with myofibroblasts-like activity that are major offenders of tissue fibrosis [94]. ET-1 acts in a paracrine and autocrine manner. ET-1 production is controlled by a number of soluble factors, including the profibrotic factor - TGF-β [90].

The ET receptors are members of the G-protein–coupled receptors that has been exploited successfully as targets for the development of new drugs. Thus, ERA have been successfully established in clinical practice for the treatment of PAH (idiopathic and secondary to scleroderma) that is associated with increased ET levels in plasma and tissues and activation of ET pathways. Currently, three nonpeptide ERAs are used in clinical practice *i.e.,* bosentan, ambrisentan and macitentan [95]. Concerns about hepatic safety led to the withdrawal of sitaxsentan (a selective ET-A receptor antagonist) from global markets in 2010 [96].

Clinical Data

Bosentan

The first approved ERA has been bosentan, which is a dual receptor antagonist of ET-A and ET-B receptors. Bosentan is approved for treatment of idiopathic and SSc-related PAH. It is also the only ERA approved for prevention of appearance of new digital ulcers in SSc. Bosentan has no proven efficacy in the treatment of active SSc-related digital ulcers. However, in two high quality randomized controlled trials (the RAPIDS-1 and -2), it has been observed that bosentan prevents appearance of new digital ulcers in SSc patients, particularly in those with multiple digital ulcers [97]. Bosentan is administered initially at a dose of 62.5 mg twice daily for 4 weeks, and afterwards the dose is increased up to 125 mg twice daily [97 - 99].

Macitentan

The effect of bosentan on the prevention of new digital ulcers in SSc has not been proved for other ERAs in large randomized trials (DUAL-1 and DUAL-2 study for macitentan) [23, 100]. *Macitentan* is a novel dual ERA of ET-A and ET-B receptors that is approved for treatment of SSc-related PAH. It is administered as a single daily dose of 10 mg [101]. Macitentan is suggested to differ with better efficacy and safety profile *vs* bosentan. Compared with bosentan, macitentan has greater potency and longer receptor occupancy (17 minutes *vs* 70seconds for bosentan), probably as a result of interaction with different amino acid residues in the ET receptors. In addition, macitentan differs with better safety profile for liver toxicity. Hepatic injury caused by bosentan is thought to occur independently from ET receptors and to be associated with inhibition of the bile salt export pump that leads to accumulation of cytotoxic bile salts and hepatocellular damage. Macitentan is thought to enter the liver *via* passive diffusion and not by active uptake. Macitentan has also reduced edema fluid retention compared with bosentan. Of note, macitentan also differs with fewer interactions with other drugs, without requirements for adjustment the doses in patients with renal or hepatic dysfunction [95]. Of note, a case report of swift and complete treatment of digital ulcers in a SSc patient treated with macitentan has been reported. Macitentan was administered at a dose of 10 mg, without concomitant drugs in a patient who developed hepatotoxicity with elevated transaminases during treatment with bosentan. Digital ulcer healing has been observed at the 3rd month. Moreover, the safety profile was good and transaminases level returned to normal [102].

Ambrisentan

Ambrisentan is a potent and selective inhibitor of ET-A receptors (ET-A:ET-B - 4000:1) used for treatment of PAH. Its longer half-life (9–15 hours) allows once-daily dosing (5–10 mg per day). Ambrisentan (at a dose of up to 10 mg daily as tolerated) has been evaluated in a prospective, 24-week open-label study that included 20 SSc patients, of whom 16 patients completed 24 weeks. Fourteen patients (88%) experienced complete healing of all digital ulcers during the study. The mean number of new digital ulcers that developed 4 weeks before week 24 was not different from the number that developed before baseline, but they were small. The total number of digital ulcers per patient significantly decreased at week 24 as well as the mean maximum diameter of the lesions. Ambrisentan did not prevent the development of new digital ulcers over a 4-week time period after 24 weeks. Thus, it has been concluded that larger, placebo-controlled studies are necessary for further evaluation of the efficacy of ambrisentan in SSc-related digital ulcers [103].

Safety Profile

The risk of liver damage and teratogenicity are the two major concerns related to the use of ERAs [23]. ERAs are contraindicated during pregnancy and in women at child-bearing age, who do not use effective contraception, the latter being indicated also one month after discontinuation of the therapy. Monthly pregnancy tests are recommended in the course of treatment with ERAs. Increase in hepatic aminotransferases occurred in approximately 10% of patients who received treatment with bosentan in a dose-dependent manner being reversible after dose reduction or drug discontinuation [104]. Ambrisentan has been associated with lower liver toxicity as compared with bosentan [105, 106]. The frequency of spontaneous reports of possible hepatic injury induced by ambrisentan during a post marketing observation was 2.87% [96]. Different safety profile of ERAs is suggested to be associated with different chemical structure. Bosentan and sitaxsentan have both sulfonamide-based structure, whereas ambrisentan is propanoic acid–based. The different chemical structure leads to diverse effect on hepatocytes. *In vitro* analysis demonstrated that both bosentan and sitaxsentan, but not ambrisentan inhibit human hepatic transporters, which could explain the different hepatic safety profile observed clinically [107]. Monthly check of liver transaminases as well as 2 weeks after every increase in the dose is recommended during treatment with bosentan, while for ambrisentan this mandatory requirement is removed by FDA in 2011 although it remains advisable [96]. In cases of drug-induced elevation of aminotransferases more than 8 times of the upper limit or in case of appearance of clinical symptoms of hepatic injury *i.e.,* nausea, vomiting, fever, abdominal pain, jaundice, extreme fatigue, flu-like syndrome (arthralgia, myalgia, fever), or if there is accompanying increases in bilirubin level more than 2 times, the treatment with bosentan should be discontinued and reintroduction of the drug is not allowed. If increase in transaminases level is between 3 and 5 times, the treatment should be temporarily discontinued and liver enzymes monitored every two weeks. In cases of transaminases elevation between 5 and 8 times, the treatment is discontinued, follow-up is performed at 2-week interval and if liver enzymes return to normal, re-administration of the drug could be discussed. Monitoring of the aminotransferases is recommended within 3 days after re-initiation of treatment with ERAs. In addition, haemoglobin control is recommended monthly during the first 4 months of treatment with ERAs and every three months afterwards as dose-dependent decrease of haemoglobin level is possible. Other adverse effects of ERAs are headache, anaemia, palpitations, chest pain, nasal congestion, peripheral oedema [97, 99, 105, 108, 109].

Renin-Angiotensin System

Angiotensin II Receptor Blocker – Losartan

Pharmacology

Blocking the action of the vasoconstrictor angiotensin II using angiotensin II receptor antagonist has been also tried as a therapeutic option in RP. Of note, experimental data suggest more complex action of angiotensin II including stimulation of ET-1 secretion. *In vivo*, intravenous administration of angiotensin II in 23 patients with essential hypertension and 8 control subjects did not change plasma or urine ET-1 levels. However, *in vitro* experiments with cultured human vascular endothelial cells derived from umbilical cord veins demonstrated that angiotensin II stimulates ET-1 secretion in a time- and dose-dependent manner. Moreover, this *in vitro* effect of angiotensin II was abolished by candesartan - an inhibitor of the membrane-bound angiotensin II receptor type 1. These results suggest that angiotensin II regulates ET-1 release from cultured endothelial cells through an angiotensin II receptor type 1-dependent pathway, while circulating levels of ET-1 are not affected [110]. In *in vitro* studies, it has been also demonstrated that angiotensin II stimulates expression of pre-pro-ET mRNA [111] and simulates ET-1 release from different cell types including cultured endothelial cells [112] and vascular smooth muscle cells [113]. The interaction between angiotensin II and ET pathway has been also confirmed in animal models. It has been demonstrated that in the aortas of rats with angiotensin II - induced hypertension, tissue ET-1 content was increased threefold and contractions to ET-1 were impaired. The angiotensin type 1 receptor blocker losartan prevented the angiotensin II – induced increase in local aortic ET-1 concentrations [114].

Clinical Data

In a randomized, parallel-group, controlled trial with 15 weeks duration the effect of losartan (50 mg/daily) and nifedipine (40 mg/daily) administered for 12 weeks was compared in 25 patients with primary RP and 27 patients with SSc-related RP (Dziadzio *et al.*, 1999). Losartan demonstrated superior efficacy in comparison with nifedipine. The reduction in the severity episodes *vs* baseline was significant only in patients treated with losartan ($p<0.05$) and decrease in the frequency of the vasospastic episodes was found only in the losartan group ($p < 0.01$). In addition, a significant reduction in the level of soluble VCAM-1 and procollagen type I N-terminal propeptide ($p<0.01$) was registered mainly in SSc patients, while the clinical efficacy was greater in the primary RP group [115]. In a small group of primary RP patients (n=15) treated with losartan (12.5 mg once daily), a statistically significant reduction in the number and severity of vasospastic attacks has been also observed [116].

Safety Profile

In the comparative study of Dziadzio *et al.*, adverse events were significantly more common in patients taking nifedipine (39%, 10/26 patients) as compared with those taking losartan (12%, 3/26), ($p<0.005$). 12% of the patients from the losartan group (3/26) reported about occasional dizziness [115].

Angiotensin-Converting enzyme Inhibitors

Inhibition of the renin-angiotensin system using angiotensin-converting enzyme (ACE) inhibitors has been also tried in RP patients. In a placebo-controlled trial that included 15 primary RP patients treated with 25 mg captopril three times daily or placebo for 6 weeks, a significant improvement in cutaneous blood flow has been observed in patients treated with captopril, but frequency and severity of vasospastic attacks were not changed [117]. The effect of enalapril was also assessed in 17 RP patients (9 with primary RP and 8 with scleroderma-related RP) in a prospective, double-blind trial. Each patient was treated with 20 mg enalapril daily and placebo for 3 weeks with a 2-week washout period between the treatment courses. A reduction in the frequency of RP attacks *vs* placebo was observed especially in primary RP patients without effect on the cold challenge test. Thus, it has been concluded that enalapril, could be beneficial for RP symptoms especially in primary forms [118]. The therapeutic effect of prolonged administration of quinapril was evaluated in 210 patients with secondary RP in SSc with limited cutaneous involvement in a multicenter, randomized, double-blind, placebo-controlled study. The duration of treatment was 2–3 years at a dose of 80 mg daily or the maximum tolerated dosage. Effect on the appearance of digital ulcers at the hands or the frequency and severity of RP episodes was not observed. Treatment with quinapril did not alter the treatments that were prescribed for infected ulcers or severe RP symptoms. The number of patients, who received intravenous iloprost, antibiotics for digital ulcers, and who required changes in vasodilator dosages were similar in the quinapril and placebo group. Quinapril was not tolerated by one-fifth of the patients, with dry cough being the most frequent side effect. Based on the study results, it has been concluded that long-term treatment with quinapril for up to 3 years did not reduce the occurrence of digital ulcers and did not improve RP symptoms [119]. Thus, current evidence does not support the use of ACE-inhibitors for the treatment of RP or its complications in scleroderma patients [4].

Alpha-Adrenergic Blockers

Prazosin

Pharmacology

Postjunctional alpha-adrenoceptors mediate vasoconstriction and play a major role in the nervous control of vascular tone ana in the regulation of skin temperature. They may be of alpha-1 and alpha-2 subtype and the two subtypes may co-exist in the same vascular region. Adrenoceptors in the skin vessels of human fingers are of both alpha-1 and alpha-2 subtype. Prazosin and doxazosine inhibit the alpha-1 postsynaptic adrenoreceptor and thus mediate peripheral vasodilation [120,121]. After local administration of vasoactive substances into the finger skin by iontophoresis and subsequent evaluation of the blood flow *via* laser Doppler, it has been demonstrated that doxazosine diminished the blood flow reduction induced by the alpha-1 selective agonist, phenylephrine, but not that caused by the alpha-2 selective agonist [120].

Clinical Data

Prazosin is approved for treatment of essential and secondary arterial hypertension, as well as for primary and secondary RP. In arterial hypertension the daily therapeutic dose of prazosin is higher, varying usually between 6 and 15 mg daily (tablets 2mg). The initial dose is 1 mg with gradual increase to 2 and 3 mg (twice and three times daily) at interval of 3-7 days. Afterwards, the dose is adjusted according to the patient's needs and therapeutic response. In RP, the recommended daily dosage is lower *i.e.,* 1-2 mg twice daily. The initial dose is 1 mg for a period of 3-7 days. The dose is adjusted according to the therapeutic effect. To avoid the immediate hypotensive effect and sudden collapse, the first intake of the medication as well as every increase in the dose should be done at bedtime. In a meta-analysis that included two placebo-controlled trials with a total of 40 patients, it has been concluded that prazosin (3 or 4 mg daily) is more effective than placebo in the treatment of RP secondary to scleroderma, but the effect is modest [122].

Safety Profile

Prazosin is associated with a number of side effects such as hypotension including orthostatic hypotension, nausea, dizziness, headache, blurred vision, vertigo, palpitations, collapse, anxiety, depression, dyspnea, nasal congestion, dry mouth, constipation or diarrhoea, skin rashes, oedema, frequent urination. The side effects of prazosin and considerable influence on haemodynamics limit its use and currently it is not commonly chosen in patients with RP. However, it could be considered in patients with concomitant arterial hypertension.

Alpha-2c Adrenergic Receptor Antagonists

The alpha-2c adrenergic receptors are suggested to be involved in cold-induced vasoconstriction [123, 124]. They are not active at room temperature and are activated during cold exposure as a result from translocation from the Golgi complex to the cellular membrane [125, 126]. The effect of a single dose of the selective alpha-adrenergic antagonist with preferential binding to the alpha-2c adrenergic receptors (OPC28326) was evaluated in a double-blind, placebo-controlled, randomized crossover study in patients with RP secondary to scleroderma. Thirteen patients were enrolled and 12 of them completed the study. It has been demonstrated that OPC-28326 improves recovery after a cold challenge in a dose-dependent manner. A significantly shorter mean time to recover 50% and 75% of the pretreatment digital skin temperature was observed in a patient group that was on 40 mg OPC-28326 as compared with the placebo group. In the 10 mg OPC-28326 group, these recovery times tended to be also shorter, but the difference *vs* placebo was not significant [127]. However, administration of the high-potency alpha-2c adrenoceptor antagonist (ORM-12741) in a phase IIa, randomized, double-blind, single-dose, placebo-controlled study in 12 patients with secondary SSc-related RP did not expedite recovery from a cold challenge in the fingers [128]. These contradictory results require further clarification of the use of alpha-2c receptor antagonists in RP. Currently, these drugs are not available for use in routine clinical practice.

Statins

Pharmacology

Apart from their lipid-lowering effect, statins have various other activities the so-called pleiotropic effects that include improvement of vascular function, inhibition of smooth muscle proliferation and inflammation [129]. Statins inhibit the rate-limiting step of cholesterol synthesis by inhibiting 3-hydroxy-3-methylglutaryl coenzyme A reductase that leads to a decrease of mevalonate. Mevalonate is a substrate for synthesis not only of cholesterol, but also of several biologically important lipid intermediates *i.e.,* farnesyl pyrophosphate and geranylgeranyl pyrophosphate that regulate the post-translational modification (prenylation) of a variety of proteins such as guanosine triphosphate hydrolases/GTPases, influencing in this way their proper localization and activation. Two major GTPases are Rho and Ras family proteins, which regulate a number of cellular pathways, including those involving mitogen-activated protein kinase, c-Jun N-terminal kinase, extracellular signal-regulated kinase, phosphatidylinositol-3 kinase, and peroxisome proliferators-activated receptor. The statins inhibit Rho and Ras prenylation and their inactive forms are accumulated in the cytoplasm that is suggested explanation of the pleiotropic effects of statins [130].

It has been suggested that statins reduce ET-1 levels and it has been evaluated in a meta-analysis of 15 randomized controlled trials. The studies included total number of 810 participants (421 – on statin therapy and 389 controls). The following statins were assessed *i.e.,* 10 to 80 mg atorvastatin, 10 to 40 mg pravastatin, 40 mg simvastatin and fluvastatin, and 0.15 mg cerivastatin with duration of the therapy ranging between 2 weeks and 12 months. A significant reduction of ET-1 level has been observed under treatment with lipophilic statins (atorvastatin, simvastatin, fluvastatin, and cerivastatin) but not with a hydrophilic statin (pravastatin) [131].

Of note, additional benefit for vascular recovery induced by statins has been proposed to be associated with increase in the level of endothelial progenitor cells [132 - 135]. It has been demonstrated that atorvastatin can increase bone marrow–derived circulating endothelial precursors and may lead to improvement of symptoms of RP with significant reduction in Raynaud's condition score [133]. During a longer period of follow-up, it has been demonstrated that beneficial effects of atorvastatin treatment persisted for a long period, at least for 24 months of treatment. The reduction in Raynaud's condition score and patient assessment by visual analogue scale/VAS was significant at month 3 and became more pronounced at months 12 and 24, indicating that the effects of the statins were persistent and cumulative. However, the atorvastatin induced 1.2 to 6.1-fold increase in endothelial progenitor cells number at 1 month from baseline, but it was transient and gradually decreased thereafter. Thus, it has been concluded that the observed long-term therapeutic effect of statins on peripheral vascular syndrome in SSc is a result from a mechanism independent of the endothelial progenitor cells although in the early response their transient mobilization may play a role [134]. Interestingly, Del Papa *et al.* (2008) have observed that simvastatin treatment significantly increased the level of endothelial progenitor cells in the hypercholesterolemic group, but not in SSc patients [135].

Clinical Data

Based on the knowledge about pleiotropic effects of statins to improve vascular function, their efficacy for the treatment of peripheral vasculopathy in SSc has been evaluated. A significant reduction in a number of digital ulcers in SSc patients has been observed in patients treated with atorvastatin 40 mg daily for 4 months in a randomized, double-blind, placebo-controlled clinical trial that included 84 SSc patients (56 - on statin and 28 – on placebo). In addition, a significant improvement in disability scores and functional status as well as a decrease in endothelial markers of activation was registered [136]. Overall, evidence for the therapeutic efficacy of statins in peripheral vascular ischaemia in SSc is limited and requires further research to confirm their efficacy as an adjunctive therapy in scleroderma patients.

Safety Profile

The safety profile of statins in SSc patients has been reported to be reasonable [132]. Known side effects during therapy with statins include headache, abdominal pain, increase of liver transaminases and creatine kinase, rarely myopathy or rhabdomyolisis, slightly increased risk of new-onset diabetes and of haemorrhagic stroke. Asymptomatic increases in liver transaminases does not seem to be harmful and statins are suggested to be a safe therapy in patients with elevated transaminases from nonalcoholic fatty liver disease or stable viral hepatitis B and C [137].

Antiplatelet Therapy and Anticoagulants

Prevention of thrombus formation is a major function of the healthy endothelium. The profound endothelial damage in SSc determines the prothrombotic state with increased platelet activation and aggregation. Different substances derived from platelets are found to be increased in SSc such as circulating levels of thromboxane A2, β- thromboglobulin, platelet factor 4, serotonin [10, 138]. Expression of platelet activation markers (P-selectin, GPIIbIIIa, CD40L) in SSc patients were found to correlate with disease activity and severity [139]. Circulating platelet aggregates and plasma beta-thromboglobulin are parameters that reflect the degree of platelet activation. Their levels were found to be significantly higher in 38 scleroderma patients as compared with 18 controls. Of note, treatment with dipyridamole and aspirin led to their significant reduction in

10 patients [85]. The crucial role of platelets in the pathogenesis of SSc is suggested to be related to the following mechanisms *i.e.,* i) contribution to tissue ischaemia *via* formation of vascular microthrombi; ii) interaction with leukocytes that leads to the subsequent inflammatory response; iii) at sites with vascular injury - release of potent mitogens such as TGF-β, platelet-derived growth factor; iiii) release of serotonin that stimulates fibroblasts sensitivity and contributes to the development of fibrosis [140].

In addition, it has been suggested that inhibition of *fibrinolysis* occurs in secondary RP in SSc [10]. A disturbed release of the tissue-plasminoge--activator/t-PA has been reported in SSc as well as increased levels of its inhibitor/t-PAI [141]. The chronic inhibition of NO synthesis has been suggested to induce the expression of t-PAI and ACE in vascular tissues. Angiotensin II also has been proposed to induce t-PAI in vascular endothelial cells [142].

Despite the evidence for involvement of activated platelets and coagulation disturbances in pathogenesis of SSc, data about the role of antiplatelet drugs (aspirin) and anticoagulants (heparin) in scleroderma-related RP are scarce [142, 143, 144, 145]. Denton *et al.* (2000) evaluated the effect of long-term therapy with low-molecular weight heparin in a prospective, parallel group study that compared heparin with conventional treatment for a period of 24 weeks. The study included 30 patients (19 with scleroderma-related RP, of whom 14 were with limited and 5 with diffuse cutaneous involvement; and 11 primary RP patients). Sixteen patients received low molecular weight heparin and 14 were included in the control group. A significant improvement in the severity of RP attacks was registered after 4 weeks, and was maximal by 20 weeks. Various mechanisms have been suggested to be associated with the action of heparin in RP patients. The authors underline that the relevance of intravascular microthrombi or emboli to RP is uncertain, and heparin may produce beneficial effect as a result of improved endothelial function. Of note, serum levels of adhesion molecules intercellular adhesion molecule-1/ICAM-1, VCAM-1 and E-selectin were lower after completion of heparin therapy, but the changes were not statistically significant. Thus, further evaluation of the role of heparin in the management of RP is necessary [143].

In an own study that evaluated retrospectively frequency, subtype distribution, therapeutic approach and clinical outcome of digital ulcers in 60 SSc patients, it has been found that all patients with digital ulcers had been treated with antiplatelet drug (mainly low-dose aspirin (80 – 100 mg per day) and clopidogrel in one patient). Patients with digital gangrene (n = 3) were treated with subcutaneous low molecular weight heparin for 1 month and after achievement of clinical improvement they were switched to low-dose aspirin. A positive clinical outcome was found in the majority of the patients. The healing of digital ulcers occurred for an average period of 3.4 months (range 2-12 months) in 95% of cases (20/21). Development of osteomyelitis with subsequent amputation of the distal phalanx was registered in a single case [145].

Based on the current experience and knowledge about the pathogenic process of peripheral vasculopathy in SSc, it could be concluded that low-dose aspirin (80-100 mg daily) should be included in the therapeutic protocol of all SSc patients with digital ulcers [44, 144, 145]. Regarding anticoagulation, it is not currently recommended to be used routinely in the management of RP and should be regarded as a treatment of second choice [44]. In severe scleroderma-related vasculopathy with presence of digital gangrene, treatment with subcutaneous low molecular weight heparin is beneficial and should be included in the therapeutic armamentarium for a short period (for example 1-month therapeutic course) until achievement of clinical improvement with subsequent switch to low- dose aspirin [145]. Short-term treatment with low molecular weight heparin (for a period from 1 week to 1 month) could be also considered in cases with SSc-related ischaemic digital ulcers that are larger in area and resistant to treatment.

Treatment of Digital Ulcers in Severe RP in SSc

In severe scleroderma-related RP complicated with digital ulcers, EULAR recommendations suggest administration of *intravenous iloprost* and *PDE-5 inhibitors* for treatment of digital ulcers and *ERA - bosentan* for their prevention [23]. Ischaemic digital ulcers in SSc require a complex approach that includes administration of increased doses of vasodilators as well as use of combinations of drugs with different mechanism of action, antiplatelet drugs or anticoagulants, antibiotics, local treatment, analgesics. In an own retrospective study, therapeutic strategies in the management of SSc-related digital ulcers were evaluated. All SSc patients (n=21) with digital ulcers received a vasodilator – CCB (nifedipine, felodipine, amlodipine) that was given as monotherapy in 5 patients, while in 16 cases it was administered in combination with either an intravenous pentoxifyllin (n = 7) or with intravenous iloprost in 10-day courses (n = 9). All SSc patients with digital ulcers received an antiplatelet drug that was aspirin in all cases except a single patient who was on therapy with clopidogrel. As mentioned above, patients with digital gangrene (n = 3) received a 1-month therapy with subcutaneous low molecular weight heparin until clinical improvement had been observed with subsequent continuation with low-dose aspirin. Thirty-eight percent (8/21) of the patients with digital ulcers – those with digital gangrene and with ulcers with local and systemic signs of inflammation received antibiotic treatment [145]. Overall, chronic ulcers, ulcers with signs of inflammation and digital gangrene are indicated for antibiotic treatment [145, 146]. Appropriate antibiotics in these cases are penicillins, cephalosporins, quinolones [146]. Treatment modification according the antibiotic sensitivity test may be required. In cases of infections with anaerobes, clindamycin and metronidazole could be used [145]. Systemic rather than topical administration of antibiotics is preferred. The route of administration of antibiotics is oral, or parenteral in more severe cases. Infection of digital ulcers usually responds well to antibiotics. However, higher dosage and prolonged courses may be indicated considering the poor skin perfusion that may cause impaired penetration of the antibiotics and lower tissue level. Development of osteomyelitis due to the spread of infection into the underlying bone is a rare finding [146].

Additional measures in the management of SSc patients with digital ulcers include appropriate protection of the hands by using gloves during daily activities to avoid wetting or bacterial contamination. Immunosuppressive treatment should be discontinued if possible until digital ulcer healing in order to facilitate the recovery and to avoid infections. Local treatment with antiseptics should also be a mandatory part of the complex care for patients with scleroderma-related digital ulcers. Antiseptic dressings with jod povidone (solution or ointment) or with silver-coated medications are recommended and are also beneficial for healing of digital ulcer as well as for their prevention [145, 147]. Local application of vitamin E containing gel (acetic ester of alpha-tocopherol) has also demonstrated improved clinical outcome with reduced time of healing and faster resolution of pain in scleroderma-related digital ulcers [148]. Debridement and surgery are reserved for resistant and complicated cases [144, 145, 147]. Surgical treatment include arterial bypass, digital arterial reconstruction, sympathectomies could be considered in patients with refractory nonhealing digital ulcers or within tractable pain [147]. The selective digital sympathectomy is a well established surgical technique for treatment of single ischaemic digits. The technique represents dissection and stripping of the adventitia from the digital arteries at the base of a digit that may lead to improved arterial pulsatile flow. It has been suggested that cervical sympathectomy should be considered only in cases with risk of major tissue loss, because the effects are, in general, not long lasting and in addition long-term side effects may occur. More proximal surgery *i.e.,* ulnar artery bypass or ulnar and radial artery adventectomy, could also be advocated in selected cases [146].

Combination Therapy in Severe Peripheral Vascular Syndrome with Digital Ulcers in SSc

As underlined above, in the everyday practice, it is a common approach to administer combination therapy during periods of worsening of RP in SSc and in the presence of digital ulcers *i.e.,* intravenous iloprost or intravenous pentoxyphillin together with the continuing supportive treatment with CCB as was observed in an own retrospective study [145]. Increases in the dosage of the administered drugs in the periods of clinical deterioration (most commonly CCBs) could also be considered. The efficacy of combination vasoactive therapies for digital ulcers in SSc has not been evaluated in randomized controlled trials [149]. In a randomized, placebo-controlled trial that evaluated the effect of sildenafil on ischaemic digital ulcer healing in SSc (SEDUCE study), the patient subgroup, which received concomitant treatment of sildenafil and bosentan, demonstrated significantly shorter time to healing *vs* the group on bosentan plus placebo. These results suggest that the combination therapy of sildenafil and bosentan leads to additive beneficial effects [48]. Successful healing of SSc-related digital ulcers has been reported in clinical cases treated with bosentan and sildenafil [150] including in a low-dose regimen [151]. Thus, treatment of severe RP in SSc by a combination of drugs that target different pathogenic pathways of the peripheral vascular pathology *i.e.,* endothelin (ERA) and NO-mediated pathway (phosphodiesterase inhibitors) is reasonable and should be used in the individualized therapeutic approaches. Other combination therapies could also be considered in order to influence the different pathogenic mechanisms of RP using different combinations of CCBs, angiotensin receptor blocker, topical nitroglycerin ointment and the haemorheologic agent - pentoxifylline [146].

Other Treatments

Botulinum Toxin

Botulinum toxin represents a polypeptide produced by the bacterium Clostridium botulinum and contains a protease that inhibits acetylcholine release at the neuromuscular junction and the eccrine sweat glands. Among seven known serotypes of botulinum toxin (A–G), type A has been extensively studied and used in clinical practice [152]. Injections with botulinum toxin have been approved by the US FDA for a number of pathological conditions *i.e.,* blepharospasm, cervical dystonia, moderate to severe glabellar lines, hyperhidrosis, ocular strabismus, torticollis. In addition, various off-label uses of botulinum toxin have been reported such as chronic headaches, migraines, poststroke spasticity, piriformis syndrome, facial wrinkles, incontinence, *etc* [153].

Local injections of botulinum toxin A in the fingers and hands have been tried for the treatment of RP including secondary scleroderma-related forms. Beneficial effects have been reported [152 - 156] including successful healing of digital ulcers in cases with intractable ischaemia [152, 156]. In a case series study that included 10 SSc patients with secondary RP, the beneficial effect of the injection of 10 U of botulinum toxin A into the hand was registered in the absence of systemic or local adverse events. Treatment with botulinum toxin resulted in decreased Raynaud's score and pain assessed by VAS and the effect continued 16 weeks after the injection. Skin temperature recovery after cold water stimulation evaluated by thermography significantly improved 4 weeks after treatment *vs* baseline. Five of the patients had intractable digital ulcers and all ulcers in five patients healed within 12 weeks after injection [152].

Improvement in blood flow and in RP symptoms could be associated with botulinum-induced acetylcholine-mediated vascular smooth muscle paralysis that suppresses vascular spasm and contraction. In addition, it has been suggested that botulinum toxin A can block the release of norepinephrine and inhibit the expression of adrenergic receptors in the vessel walls that leads to decreased vasoconstriction and pain alleviation. Of note, surface expression of adrenergic receptors could be stimulated by reactive oxygen species produced in smooth muscle cells in response to cooling. In *in vitro* studies, using human umbilical vein endothelial cells, it has been demonstrated that botulinum toxin A significantly prevented the oxidant-induced intracellular accumulation of reactive oxygen species in vascular endothelial cells [157]. Currently, the role of botulinum toxin A injections among other therapeutic strategies for treatment of RP as well as the appropriate dosing and therapeutic regimen remain to be determined [154]. Thus, the effect of this therapeutic approach in RP patients should be evaluated in future randomized, controlled studies.

Rho-Kinase Inhibitors

As mentioned above, the alpha-2c adrenergic receptors that are inactive at standard temperature are translocated and activated during cold exposure [125, 126]. Rho-kinase is involved in cold-induced translocation of the alpha2c-adrenoreceptors to the plasma membrane and in addition is a key mediator of pleiotropic effects of statins [121]. Rho is a member of the Ras family of small GTP-binding proteins that cycles between a guanosine diphosphate/GDP-bound inactive state and a GTP-bound active state [158]. Rho and its downstream effector, Rho kinase play a crucial role in regulating the actin cytoskeleton and in different processes such as intracellular transport, gene transcription, messenger RNA expression. Direct inhibition of Rho-Rho kinase is anti-atherogenic as a result of increased endothelial NO synthesis, decreased vascular smooth muscle cell contraction and proliferation, inhibited cytokine formation, inflammatory cell trafficking and proliferation, and reduced thrombogenic endothelial potential [159, 160]. The effect of a single dose fasudil, that is an inhibitor of Rho/Rho-kinase pathway, has been evaluated in a single-center, double-blind, placebo-controlled, randomized study. Fasudil (oral dose 40 mg or 80 mg) and placebo were administered 2 hours before a standardised cold challenge. The primary outcome measures were the fall in skin temperature after a cold provocation and time for recovery 50% and 70% of initial pre-challenge digital skin temperature. However, significant benefit regarding skin temperature recovery time and digital blood flow after cold challenge was not observed [161].

CONCLUSION

In conclusion, choosing an appropriate therapeutic approach in RP patients requires individualization of the treatment according to the severity of the symptoms. In the practice of the rheumatologists, primary RP patients require consultation, whose major aim is exclusion of underlying disorder and reassurance of the patient about the benign course of the condition. Of note, RP may be an initial symptom of systemic rheumatic disease, thus, the patients should be informed about the necessity for regular follow-up. Being mainly a functional disorder, primary RP has mild clinical course and excellent prognosis. Endothelial damage is absent and trophic changes are not observed. Thus, primary RP patients could be managed with non-pharmacological measures and if the results are not satisfactory, oral well-tolerated drugs are administered. Among rheumatic diseases, RP is most frequent in SSc. Here, the profound endothelial injury is expressed with severe course of RP and often is complicated with development of digital ulcers. Resistant cases of secondary SSc-related RP with digital ulcers require complex personalized treatment based on the knowledge about the complex underlying pathogenesis including administration of drugs with different mechanisms of action in different combinations.

CONFLICT OF INTEREST

The author confirms that she has no conflict of interest to declare for this publication.

ACKNOWLEDGEMENTS

Declared none.

REFERENCES

[1]   Wigley FM. Clinical practice. Raynaud's Phenomenon. N Engl J Med 2002; 347(13): 1001-8.
        [http://dx.doi.org/10.1056/NEJMcp013013] [PMID: 12324557]

[2]   Cortes S, Cutolo M. Capillaroscopic patterns in rheumatic diseases. Acta Reumatol Port 2007; 32(1): 29-36.
        [PMID: 17450762]

[3]   Ho M, Belch JJF. Raynaud's phenomenon: state of the art 1998. Scand J Rheumatol 1998; 27(5): 319-22.
        [http://dx.doi.org/10.1080/030097498550154311] [PMID: 9808392]

[4]   Wigley FM, Flavahan NA. Raynaud's Phenomenon. N Engl J Med 2016; 375(6): 556-65.

[http://dx.doi.org/10.1056/NEJMra1507638] [PMID: 27509103]

[5]   Planchon B, Pistorius MA, Beurrier P, De Faucal P. Primary Raynaud's phenomenon. Age of onset and pathogenesis in a prospective study of 424 patients. Angiology 1994; 45(8): 677-86.
        [http://dx.doi.org/10.1177/000331979404500802] [PMID: 8048777]

[6]   Garner R, Kumari R, Lanyon P, Doherty M, Zhang W. Prevalence, risk factors and associations of primary Raynaud's phenomenon: systematic review and meta-analysis of observational studies. BMJ Open 2015; 5(3): e006389.
        [http://dx.doi.org/10.1136/bmjopen-2014-006389] [PMID: 25776043]

[7]   LeRoy EC, Medsger TA Jr. Raynaud's phenomenon: a proposal for classification. Clin Exp Rheumatol 1992; 10(5): 485-8.
        [PMID: 1458701]

[8]   Khan F. Vascular abnormalities in Raynaud's phenomenon. Scott Med J 1999; 44(1): 4-6.
        [http://dx.doi.org/10.1177/003693309904400102] [PMID: 10218222]

[9]   Chikura B, Moore T, Manning J, Vail A, Herrick AL. Thumb involvement in Raynaud's phenomenon as an indicator of underlying connective tissue disease. J Rheumatol 2010; 37(4): 783-6.
        [http://dx.doi.org/10.3899/jrheum.091117] [PMID: 20194444]

[10]   Block JA, Sequeira W. Raynaud's phenomenon. Lancet 2001; 357(9273): 2042-8.
        [http://dx.doi.org/10.1016/S0140-6736(00)05118-7] [PMID: 11438158]

[11]   Herrick AL. The pathogenesis, diagnosis and treatment of Raynaud phenomenon. Nat Rev Rheumatol 2012; 8(8): 469-79.
        [http://dx.doi.org/10.1038/nrrheum.2012.96] [PMID: 22782008]

[12]   Müller-Ladner U. Raynaud's phenomenon and peripheral ischemic syndromes. 1st ed. Bremen: UNI-MED Verlag AG 2008; pp. 18-30.

[13]   Husein-Elahmed H, Callejas-Rubio JL, Ortega Del Olmo R, Ríos-Fernandez R, Ortego-Centeno N. Severe Raynaud syndrome induced by adjuvant interferon alfa in metastatic melanoma. Curr Oncol 2010; 17(4): 122-3.
        [http://dx.doi.org/10.3747/co.v17i4.519] [PMID: 20697523]

[14]   Lapossy E, Gasser P, Hrycaj P, Dubler B, Samborski W, Muller W. Cold-induced vasospasm in patients with fibromyalgia and chronic low back pain in comparison to healthy subjects. Clin Rheumatol 1994; 13(3): 442-5.
        [http://dx.doi.org/10.1007/BF02242940] [PMID: 7835007]

[15]   Steven AO. Raynaud's phenomenon.Secrets of rheumatology. Moscow: Binom 2001; pp. 614-9.

[16]   Muir AH, Robb R, McLaren M, Daly F, Belch JJ. The use of Ginkgo biloba in Raynaud's disease: a double-blind placebo-controlled trial. Vasc Med 2002; 7(4): 265-7.
        [http://dx.doi.org/10.1191/1358863x02vm455oa] [PMID: 12710841]

[17]   Bredie SJ, Jong MC. No significant effect of ginkgo biloba special extract EGb 761 in the treatment of primary Raynaud phenomenon: a randomized controlled trial. J Cardiovasc Pharmacol 2012; 59(3): 215-21.
        [http://dx.doi.org/10.1097/FJC.0b013e31823c0bed] [PMID: 22030896]

[18]   Triggle CR, Samuel SM, Ravishankar S, Marei I, Arunachalam G, Ding H. The endothelium: influencing vascular smooth muscle in many ways. Can J Physiol Pharmacol 2012; 90(6): 713-38.
        [http://dx.doi.org/10.1139/y2012-073] [PMID: 22625870]

[19]   Müller-Ladner U, Lambova S. Editorial: Vascular damage in systemic sclerosis. Curr Rheumatol Rev 2013; 9(4): 233-6.
        [http://dx.doi.org/10.2174/1573397109041404171237728] [PMID: 26932286]

[20]   Rajagopalan S, Pfenninger D, Kehrer C, *et al.* Increased asymmetric dimethylarginine and endothelin 1 levels in secondary Raynaud's phenomenon: implications for vascular dysfunction and progression

of disease. Arthritis Rheum 2003; 48(7): 1992-2000.
[http://dx.doi.org/10.1002/art.11060] [PMID: 12847693]

[21]   Vancheeswaran R, Azam A, Black C, Dashwood MR. Localization of endothelin-1 and its binding
        sites in scleroderma skin. J Rheumatol 1994; 21(7): 1268-76.
        [PMID: 7525957]

[22]   Zamora MR, O'Brien RF, Rutherford RB, Weil JV. Serum endothelin-1 concentrations and cold
        provocation in primary Raynaud's phenomenon. Lancet 1990; 336(8724): 1144-7.
        [http://dx.doi.org/10.1016/0140-6736(90)92766-B] [PMID: 1978025]

[23]   Kowal-Bielecka O, Fransen J, Avouac J, *et al.* Update of EULAR recommendations for the treatment
        of systemic sclerosis. Ann Rheum Dis 2017; 76(8): 1327-39.
        [http://dx.doi.org/10.1136/annrheumdis-2016-209909] [PMID: 27941129]

[24]   Godfraind T. Discovery and development of calcium channel blockers. Front Pharmacol 2017; 8: 286.
        [http://dx.doi.org/10.3389/fphar.2017.00286]

[25]   Cribbs LL. Vascular smooth muscle calcium channels: could "T" be a target? Circ Res 2001; 89(7):
        560-2.
        [http://dx.doi.org/10.1161/res.89.7.560] [PMID: 11577019]

[26]   Rademaker M, Meyrick-Thomas RH, Kirby JD, Kovacs IB. Altered *in vitro* hemostasis, clotting, and
        thrombolysis after oral nifedipine in normal volunteers. Angiology 1988; 39(8): 747-51.
        [http://dx.doi.org/10.1177/000331978803900807] [PMID: 3421508]

[27]   Rirash F, Tingey PC, Harding SE, *et al.* Calcium channel blockers for primary and secondary
        Raynaud's phenomenon. Cochrane Database Syst Rev 2017; 12: CD000467.
        [http://dx.doi.org/10.1002/14651858.CD000467.pub2] [PMID: 29237099]

[28]   Thompson AE, Pope JE. Calcium channel blockers for primary Raynaud's phenomenon: a meta-
        analysis. Rheumatology (Oxford) 2005; 44(2): 145-50.
        [http://dx.doi.org/10.1093/rheumatology/keh390] [PMID: 15546967]

[29]   Thompson AE, Shea B, Welch V, Fenlon D, Pope JE. Calcium-channel blockers for Raynaud's
        phenomenon in systemic sclerosis. Arthritis Rheum 2001; 44(8): 1841-7.
        [http://dx.doi.org/10.1002/1529-0131(200108)44:8<1841::AID-ART322>3.0.CO;2-8]   [PMID:
        11508437]

[30]   Smith CR, Rodeheffer RJ. Treatment of Raynaud's phenomenon with calcium channel blockers. Am J
        Med 1985; 78(2B): 39-42.
        [http://dx.doi.org/10.1016/0002-9343(85)90168-8] [PMID: 3976694]

[31]   Rademaker M, Cooke ED, Almond NE, *et al.* Comparison of intravenous infusions of iloprost and oral
        nifedipine in treatment of Raynaud's phenomenon in patients with systemic sclerosis: a double blind
        randomised study. BMJ 1989; 298(6673): 561-4.
        [http://dx.doi.org/10.1136/bmj.298.6673.561] [PMID: 2467711]

[32]   Ward A, Clissold SP. Pentoxifylline. A review of its pharmacodynamic and pharmacokinetic
        properties, and its therapeutic efficacy. Drugs 1987; 34(1): 50-97.
        [http://dx.doi.org/10.2165/00003495-198734010-00003] [PMID: 3308412]

[33]   Linnemann B, Erbe M. Raynaud's phenomenon and digital ischaemia--pharmacologic approach and
        alternative treatment options. Vasa 2016; 45(3): 201-12.
        [http://dx.doi.org/10.1024/0301-1526/a000526] [PMID: 27129065]

[34]   Neirotti M, Longo F, Molaschi M, Macchione C, Pernigotti L. Functional vascular disorders: treatment
        with pentoxifylline. Angiology 1987; 38(8): 575-80.
        [http://dx.doi.org/10.1177/000331978703800801] [PMID: 3631642]

[35]   Tietjen GW, Chien S, Leroy EC, Gavras I, Gavras H, Gump FE. Blood viscosity, plasma proteins, and
        Raynaud syndrome. Arch Surg 1975; 110(11): 1343-6.
        [http://dx.doi.org/10.1001/archsurg.1975.01360170083011] [PMID: 53042]

[36] Kovacs IB, Sowemimo-Coker SO, Kirby JD, Turner P. Altered behaviour of erythrocytes in scleroderma. Clin Sci (Lond) 1983; 65(5): 515-9.
[http://dx.doi.org/10.1042/cs0650515] [PMID: 6617097]

[37] Schröer RH. Antithrombotic potential of pentoxifylline. A hemorheologically active drug. Angiology 1985; 36(6): 387-98.
[http://dx.doi.org/10.1177/000331978503600608] [PMID: 3927788]

[38] Sonkin PL, Chen LE, Seaber AV, Hatchell DL. Vasodilator action of pentoxifylline on microcirculation of rat cremaster muscle. Angiology 1992; 43(6): 462-9.
[http://dx.doi.org/10.1177/000331979204300602] [PMID: 1595940]

[39] Goodfield MJ, Rowell NR. Treatment of peripheral gangrene due to systemic sclerosis with intravenous pentoxifylline. Clin Exp Dermatol 1989; 14(2): 161-2.
[http://dx.doi.org/10.1111/j.1365-2230.1989.tb00917.x] [PMID: 2598492]

[40] Cowley AJ, Heptinstall S, Mitchell JR. Similarity between platelet and blood-vessel reactivity. Lancet 1985; 2(8447): 154-5.
[http://dx.doi.org/10.1016/S0140-6736(85)90256-9] [PMID: 2862343]

[41] Belch JJ, Ho M. Pharmacotherapy of Raynaud's phenomenon. Drugs 1996; 52(5): 682-95.
[http://dx.doi.org/10.2165/00003495-199652050-00006] [PMID: 9118818]

[42] Arosio E, Montesi G, Zannoni M, Paluani F, Lechi A. Comparative efficacy of ketanserin and pentoxiphylline in treatment of Raynaud's phenomenon. Angiology 1989; 40(7): 633-8.
[http://dx.doi.org/10.1177/000331978904000705] [PMID: 2662829]

[43] Goldberg J, Dlesk A. Successful treatment of Raynaud's phenomenon with pentoxifylline. Arthritis Rheum 1986; 29(8): 1055-6.
[http://dx.doi.org/10.1002/art.1780290822] [PMID: 3741520]

[44] García-Carrasco M, Jiménez-Hernández M, Escárcega RO, *et al.* Treatment of Raynaud's phenomenon. Autoimmun Rev 2008; 8(1): 62-8.
[http://dx.doi.org/10.1016/j.autrev.2008.07.002] [PMID: 18692160]

[45] Hughes M, Moore T, Manning J, *et al.* Reduced perfusion in systemic sclerosis digital ulcers (both fingertip and extensor) can be increased by topical application of glyceryl trinitrate. Microvasc Res 2017; 111: 32-6.
[http://dx.doi.org/10.1016/j.mvr.2016.12.008] [PMID: 28027937]

[46] Kumana CR, Cheung GTY, Lau CS. Severe digital ischaemia treated with phosphodiesterase inhibitors. Ann Rheum Dis 2004; 63(11): 1522-4.
[http://dx.doi.org/10.1136/ard.2003.015677] [PMID: 15479910]

[47] Roustit M, Blaise S, Allanore Y, Carpentier PH, Caglayan E, Cracowski JL. Phosphodiesterase-5 inhibitors for the treatment of secondary Raynaud's phenomenon: systematic review and meta-analysis of randomised trials. Ann Rheum Dis 2013; 72(10): 1696-9.
[http://dx.doi.org/10.1136/annrheumdis-2012-202836] [PMID: 23426043]

[48] Hachulla E, Hatron PY, Carpentier P, *et al.* Efficacy of sildenafil on ischaemic digital ulcer healing in systemic sclerosis: the placebo-controlled SEDUCE study. Ann Rheum Dis 2016; 75(6): 1009-15.
[http://dx.doi.org/10.1136/annrheumdis-2014-207001] [PMID: 25995322]

[49] Roustit M, Giai J, Gaget O, *et al.* On-demand sildenafil as a treatment for Raynaud Phenomenon: a series of n-of-1 trials. Ann Intern Med 2018; 169(10): 694-703.
[http://dx.doi.org/10.7326/M18-0517] [PMID: 30383134]

[50] Curtiss P, Schwager Z, Cobos G, Lo Sicco K, Franks AG Jr. A systematic review and meta-analysis of the effects of topical nitrates in the treatment of primary and secondary Raynaud's phenomenon. J Am Acad Dermatol 2018; 78(6): 1110-1118.e3.
[http://dx.doi.org/10.1016/j.jaad.2018.01.043] [PMID: 29408338]

[51]   Anderson ME, Moore TL, Hollis S, Jayson MI, King TA, Herrick AL. Digital vascular response to topical glyceryl trinitrate, as measured by laser Doppler imaging, in primary Raynaud's phenomenon and systemic sclerosis. Rheumatology (Oxford) 2002; 41(3): 324-8.
[http://dx.doi.org/10.1093/rheumatology/41.3.324] [PMID: 11934971]

[52]   Teh LS, Manning J, Moore T, Tully MP, O'Reilly D, Jayson MI. Sustained-release transdermal glyceryl trinitrate patches as a treatment for primary and secondary Raynaud's phenomenon. Br J Rheumatol 1995; 34(7): 636-41.
[http://dx.doi.org/10.1093/rheumatology/34.7.636] [PMID: 7670782]

[53]   Chung L, Shapiro L, Fiorentino D, *et al.* MQX-503, a novel formulation of nitroglycerin, improves the severity of Raynaud's phenomenon: a randomized, controlled trial. Arthritis Rheum 2009; 60(3): 870-7.
[http://dx.doi.org/10.1002/art.24351] [PMID: 19248104]

[54]   Wigley FM, Herrick AL. Management of Raynaud's phenomenon and digital ulcers. Curr Treatm Opt Rheumatol 2015; 1(1): 68-81.
[http://dx.doi.org/10.1007/s40674-014-0006-z]

[55]   Grant SM, Goa KL. Iloprost. A review of its pharmacodynamic and pharmacokinetic properties, and therapeutic potential in peripheral vascular disease, myocardial ischaemia and extracorporeal circulation procedures. Drugs 1992; 43(6): 889-924.
[http://dx.doi.org/10.2165/00003495-199243060-00008] [PMID: 1379160]

[56]   McHugh NJ, Csuka M, Watson H, *et al.* Infusion of iloprost, a prostacyclin analogue, for treatment of Raynaud's phenomenon in systemic sclerosis. Ann Rheum Dis 1988; 47(1): 43-7.
[http://dx.doi.org/10.1136/ard.47.1.43] [PMID: 2449871]

[57]   Torley HI, Madhok R, Capell HA, *et al.* A double blind, randomised, multicentre comparison of two doses of intravenous iloprost in the treatment of Raynaud's phenomenon secondary to connective tissue diseases. Ann Rheum Dis 1991; 50(11): 800-4.
[http://dx.doi.org/10.1136/ard.50.11.800] [PMID: 1722967]

[58]   Wigley FM, Wise RA, Seibold JR, *et al.* Intravenous iloprost infusion in patients with Raynaud phenomenon secondary to systemic sclerosis. A multicenter, placebo-controlled, double-blind study. Ann Intern Med 1994; 120(3): 199-206.
[http://dx.doi.org/10.7326/0003-4819-120-3-199402010-00004] [PMID: 7506013]

[59]   Wigley FM, Seibold JR, Wise RA, McCloskey DA, Dole WP. Intravenous iloprost treatment of Raynaud's phenomenon and ischemic ulcers secondary to systemic sclerosis. J Rheumatol 1992; 19(9): 1407-14.
[PMID: 1279170]

[60]   Ingegnoli F, Schioppo T, Allanore Y, *et al.* Practical suggestions on intravenous iloprost in Raynaud's phenomenon and digital ulcer secondary to systemic sclerosis: Systematic literature review and expert consensus. Semin Arthritis Rheum 2018 Apr 4; pii(S0049-0172(18)): 30013-1.

[61]   Bettoni L, Geri A, Airò P, *et al.* Systemic sclerosis therapy with iloprost: a prospective observational study of 30 patients treated for a median of 3 years. Clin Rheumatol 2002; 21(3): 244-50.
[http://dx.doi.org/10.1007/PL00011223] [PMID: 12111631]

[62]   Rehberger P, Beckheinrich-Mrowka P, Haustein UF, Sticherling M. Prostacyclin analogue iloprost influences endothelial cell-associated soluble adhesion molecules and growth factors in patients with systemic sclerosis: a time course study of serum concentrations. Acta Derm Venereol 2009; 89(3): 245-9.
[http://dx.doi.org/10.2340/00015555-0632] [PMID: 19479119]

[63]   Della Bella S, Molteni M, Mascagni B, Zulian C, Compasso S, Scorza R. Cytokine production in scleroderma patients: effects of therapy with either iloprost or nifedipine. Clin Exp Rheumatol 1997; 15(2): 135-41.
[PMID: 9196864]

[64]   Biasi D, Carletto A, Caramaschi P, *et al.* Iloprost as cyclic five-day infusions in the treatment of scleroderma. An open pilot study in 20 patients treated for one year. Rev Rhum Engl Ed 1998; 65(12): 745-50.
[PMID: 9923042]

[65]   Colaci M, Sebastiani M, Giuggioli D, *et al.* Cardiovascular risk and prostanoids in systemic sclerosis. Clin Exp Rheumatol 2008; 26(2): 333-6.
[PMID: 18565257]

[66]   Cruz JE, Ward A, Anthony S, Chang S, Bae HB, Hermes-DeSantis ER. Evidence for the Use of Epoprostenol to Treat Raynaud's Phenomenon With or Without Digital Ulcers. Ann Pharmacother 2016; 50(12): 1060-7.
[http://dx.doi.org/10.1177/1060028016660324] [PMID: 27465880]

[67]   Martin MF, Tooke JE. Effects of prostaglandin E1 on microvascular haemodynamics in progressive systemic sclerosis. Br Med J (Clin Res Ed) 1982; 285(6356): 1688-90.
[http://dx.doi.org/10.1136/bmj.285.6356.1688] [PMID: 6816332]

[68]   Mohrland JS, Porter JM, Smith EA, Belch J, Simms MH. A multiclinic, placebo-controlled, double-blind study of prostaglandin E1 in Raynaud's syndrome. Ann Rheum Dis 1985; 44(11): 754-60.
[http://dx.doi.org/10.1136/ard.44.11.754] [PMID: 3904643]

[69]   Engel G, Rockson SG. Treprostinil for the treatment of severe digital necrosis in systemic sclerosis. Vasc Med 2005; 10(1): 29-32.
[http://dx.doi.org/10.1191/1358863x05vm579cr] [PMID: 15920997]

[70]   Chung L, Fiorentino D. A pilot trial of treprostinil for the treatment and prevention of digital ulcers in patients with systemic sclerosis. J Am Acad Dermatol 2006; 54(5): 880-2.
[http://dx.doi.org/10.1016/j.jaad.2006.02.004] [PMID: 16635673]

[71]   McMahan ZH, Wigley FM. Raynaud's phenomenon and digital ischemia: a practical approach to risk stratification, diagnosis and management. Int J Clin Rheumatol 2010; 5(3): 355-70.
[http://dx.doi.org/10.2217/ijr.10.17] [PMID: 26523153]

[72]   Pope J, Fenlon D, Thompson A, *et al.* Iloprost and cisaprost for Raynaud's phenomenon in progressive systemic sclerosis. Cochrane Database Syst Rev 2000; (2): : CD000953.
[PMID: 10796395]

[73]   Herrick AL. Evidence-based management of Raynaud's phenomenon. Ther Adv Musculoskelet Dis 2017; 9(12): 317-29.
[http://dx.doi.org/10.1177/1759720X17740074] [PMID: 29201156]

[74]   Janssena MC, Wollersheim H, Kraus C, Hildebrand M, Watson HR, Thien T. Pharmacokinetics of oral iloprost in patients with Raynaud's phenomenon secondary to systemic sclerosis. Prostaglandins Other Lipid Mediat 2000; 60(4-6): 153-60.
[http://dx.doi.org/10.1016/S0090-6980(99)00060-X] [PMID: 10751645]

[75]   Wigley FM, Korn JH, Csuka ME, *et al.* Oral iloprost treatment in patients with Raynaud's phenomenon secondary to systemic sclerosis: a multicenter, placebo-controlled, double-blind study. Arthritis Rheum 1998; 41(4): 670-7.
[http://dx.doi.org/10.1002/1529-0131(199804)41:4<670::AID-ART14>3.0.CO;2-I] [PMID: 9550476]

[76]   Black CM, Halkier-Sørensen L, Belch JJ, *et al.* Oral iloprost in Raynaud's phenomenon secondary to systemic sclerosis: a multicentre, placebo-controlled, dose-comparison study. Br J Rheumatol 1998; 37(9): 952-60.
[http://dx.doi.org/10.1093/rheumatology/37.9.952] [PMID: 9783759]

[77]   Seibold JR, Wigley FM, Schiopu E, *et al.* Digital ulcers in SSc treated with oral treprostinil: a randomized, double-blind, placebo-controlled study with open-label follow-up. J Scleroderma Relat Disord 2017; 2: 42-9.
[http://dx.doi.org/10.5301/jsrd.5000232]

[78]   Shah AA, Schiopu E, Chatterjee S, *et al.* The recurrence of digital ulcers in patients with systemic sclerosis after discontinuation of oral treprostinil. J Rheumatol 2016; 43(9): 1665-71.
[http://dx.doi.org/10.3899/jrheum.151437] [PMID: 27307535]

[79]   Denton CP, Hachulla É, Riemekasten G, *et al.* Efficacy and safety of selexipag in adults with Raynaud's phenomenon secondary to systemic sclerosis: a randomized, placebo-controlled, phase II study. Arthritis Rheumatol 2017; 69(12): 2370-9.
[http://dx.doi.org/10.1002/art.40242] [PMID: 29193819]

[80]   Gershon MD, Tack J. The serotonin signaling system: from basic understanding to drug development for functional GI disorders. Gastroenterology 2007; 132(1): 397-414.
[http://dx.doi.org/10.1053/j.gastro.2006.11.002] [PMID: 17241888]

[81]   Ntelis K, Solomou EE, Sakkas L, Liossis SN, Daoussis D. The role of platelets in autoimmunity, vasculopathy, and fibrosis: Implications for systemic sclerosis. Semin Arthritis Rheum 2017; 47(3): 409-17.
[http://dx.doi.org/10.1016/j.semarthrit.2017.05.004] [PMID: 28602360]

[82]   Berger M, Gray JA, Roth BL. The expanded biology of serotonin. Annu Rev Med 2009; 60: 355-66.
[http://dx.doi.org/10.1146/annurev.med.60.042307.110802] [PMID: 19630576]

[83]   Coleiro B, Marshall SE, Denton CP, *et al.* Treatment of Raynaud's phenomenon with the selective serotonin reuptake inhibitor fluoxetine. Rheumatology (Oxford) 2001; 40(9): 1038-43.
[http://dx.doi.org/10.1093/rheumatology/40.9.1038] [PMID: 11561116]

[84]   Pigott TA, Pato MT, Bernstein SE, *et al.* Controlled comparisons of clomipramine and fluoxetine in the treatment of obsessive-compulsive disorder. Behavioral and biological results. Arch Gen Psychiatry 1990; 47(10): 926-32.
[http://dx.doi.org/10.1001/archpsyc.1990.01810220042005] [PMID: 2222131]

[85]   Kahaleh MB, Osborn I, Leroy EC. Elevated levels of circulating platelet aggregates and beta-thromboglobulin in scleroderma. Ann Intern Med 1982; 96(5): 610-3.
[http://dx.doi.org/10.7326/0003-4819-96-5-610] [PMID: 6176160]

[86]   Goodfield MJ, Orchard MA, Rowell NR. Whole blood platelet aggregation and coagulation factors in patients with systemic sclerosis. Br J Haematol 1993; 84(4): 675-80.
[http://dx.doi.org/10.1111/j.1365-2141.1993.tb03145.x] [PMID: 8217827]

[87]   Dees C, Akhmetshina A, Zerr P, *et al.* Platelet-derived serotonin links vascular disease and tissue fibrosis. J Exp Med 2011; 208(5): 961-72.
[http://dx.doi.org/10.1084/jem.20101629] [PMID: 21518801]

[88]   Yanagisawa M, Kurihara H, Kimura S, *et al.* A novel potent vasoconstrictor peptide produced by vascular endothelial cells. Nature 1988; 332(6163): 411-5.
[http://dx.doi.org/10.1038/332411a0] [PMID: 2451132]

[89]   Fagan KA, McMurtry IF, Rodman DM. Role of endothelin-1 in lung disease. Respir Res 2001; 2(2): 90-101.
[http://dx.doi.org/10.1186/rr44] [PMID: 11686871]

[90]   Abraham D, Distler O. How does endothelial cell injury start? The role of endothelin in systemic sclerosis. Arthritis Res Ther 2007; 9 (Suppl. 2): S2.
[http://dx.doi.org/10.1186/ar2186] [PMID: 17767740]

[91]   Das S, Mishra TK, Satpathy C, Routray SN. Endothelins and endothelin receptor antagonists. JIACM 2004; 5(1): 55-9.

[92]   Galié N, Manes A, Branzi A. The endothelin system in pulmonary arterial hypertension. Cardiovasc Res 2004; 61(2): 227-37.
[http://dx.doi.org/10.1016/j.cardiores.2003.11.026] [PMID: 14736539]

[93]   La M, Reid JJ. Endothelin-1 and the regulation of vascular tone. Clin Exp Pharmacol Physiol 1995;

22(5): 315-23.
[http://dx.doi.org/10.1111/j.1440-1681.1995.tb02008.x] [PMID: 7554421]

[94]   Shiwen X, Leask A, Abraham DJ, Fonseca C. Endothelin receptor selectivity: evidence from *in vitro* and pre-clinical models of scleroderma. Eur J Clin Invest 2009; 39 (Suppl. 2): 19-26.
[http://dx.doi.org/10.1111/j.1365-2362.2009.02117.x] [PMID: 19335743]

[95]   Maguire JJ, Davenport AP. Endothelin receptors and their antagonists. Semin Nephrol 2015; 35(2): 125-36.
[http://dx.doi.org/10.1016/j.semnephrol.2015.02.002] [PMID: 25966344]

[96]   Ben-Yehuda O, Pizzuti D, Brown A, *et al.* Long-term hepatic safety of ambrisentan in patients with pulmonary arterial hypertension. J Am Coll Cardiol 2012; 60(1): 80-1.
[http://dx.doi.org/10.1016/j.jacc.2012.03.025] [PMID: 22578922]

[97]   Korn JH, Mayes M, Matucci Cerinic M, *et al.* Digital ulcers in systemic sclerosis: prevention by treatment with bosentan, an oral endothelin receptor antagonist. Arthritis Rheum 2004; 50(12): 3985-93.
[http://dx.doi.org/10.1002/art.20676] [PMID: 15593188]

[98]   McLaughlin VV, Archer SL, Badesch DB, *et al.* ACCF/AHA 2009 Expert Consensus Document on Pulmonary Hypertension A Report of the American College of Cardiology Foundation Task Force on Expert Consensus Documents and the American Heart Association. J Am Coll Cardiol 2009; 53: 1573-619.
[http://dx.doi.org/10.1016/j.jacc.2009.01.004] [PMID: 19389575]

[99]   Rubin LJ, Badesch DB, Barst RJ, *et al.* Bosentan therapy for pulmonary arterial hypertension. N Engl J Med 2002; 346(12): 896-903.
[http://dx.doi.org/10.1056/NEJMoa012212] [PMID: 11907289]

[100] Khanna D, Denton CP, Merkel PA, *et al.* Effect of macitentan on the development of new ischemic digital ulcers in patients with systemic sclerosis: DUAL-1 and DUAL-2 randomized clinical trials. JAMA 2016; 315(18): 1975-88.
[http://dx.doi.org/10.1001/jama.2016.5258] [PMID: 27163986]

[101] Patel T, McKeage K. Macitentan: first global approval. Drugs 2014; 74(1): 127-33.
[http://dx.doi.org/10.1007/s40265-013-0156-6] [PMID: 24297706]

[102] Giner Serret E. Swift and complete healing of digital ulcers after macitentan treatment. Case Rep Rheumatol 2016; 2016: 1718309.
[http://dx.doi.org/10.1155/2016/1718309] [PMID: 27994906]

[103] Chung L, Ball K, Yaqub A, Lingala B, Fiorentino D. Effect of the endothelin type A-selective endothelin receptor antagonist ambrisentan on digital ulcers in patients with systemic sclerosis: results of a prospective pilot study. J Am Acad Dermatol 2014; 71(2): 400-1.
[http://dx.doi.org/10.1016/j.jaad.2014.04.028] [PMID: 25037794]

[104] Galiè N, Humbert M, Vachiery JL, *et al.* 2015 ESC/ERS Guidelines for the diagnosis and treatment of pulmonary hypertension: The Joint Task Force for the Diagnosis and Treatment of Pulmonary Hypertension of the European Society of Cardiology (ESC) and the European Respiratory Society (ERS): Endorsed by: Association for European Paediatric and Congenital Cardiology (AEPC), International Society for Heart and Lung Transplantation (ISHLT). Eur Respir J 2015; 46(4): 903-75.
[http://dx.doi.org/10.1183/13993003.01032-2015] [PMID: 26318161]

[105] Galiè N, Olschewski H, Oudiz RJ, *et al.* Ambrisentan for the treatment of pulmonary arterial hypertension: results of the ambrisentan in pulmonary arterial hypertension, randomized, double-blind, placebo-controlled, multicenter, efficacy (ARIES) study 1 and 2. Circulation 2008; 117(23): 3010-9.
[http://dx.doi.org/10.1161/CIRCULATIONAHA.107.742510] [PMID: 18506008]

[106] McGoon MD, Frost AE, Oudiz RJ, *et al.* Ambrisentan therapy in patients with pulmonary arterial hypertension who discontinued bosentan or sitaxsentan due to liver function test abnormalities. Chest 2009; 135(1): 122-9.

[http://dx.doi.org/10.1378/chest.08-1028] [PMID: 18812445]

[107] Hartman JC, Brouwer K, Mandagere A, Melvin L, Gorczynski R. Evaluation of the endothelin receptor antagonists ambrisentan, darusentan, bosentan, and sitaxsentan as substrates and inhibitors of hepatobiliary transporters in sandwich-cultured human hepatocytes. Can J Physiol Pharmacol 2010; 88(6): 682-91.
[http://dx.doi.org/10.1139/Y10-060] [PMID: 20628435]

[108] Denton CP, Humbert M, Rubin L, Black CM. Bosentan treatment for pulmonary arterial hypertension related to connective tissue disease: a subgroup analysis of the pivotal clinical trials and their open-label extensions. Ann Rheum Dis 2006; 65(10): 1336-40.
[http://dx.doi.org/10.1136/ard.2005.048967] [PMID: 16793845]

[109] Galiè N, Rubin Lj, Hoeper M, *et al.* Treatment of patients with mildly symptomatic pulmonary arterial hypertension with bosentan (EARLY study): a double-blind, randomised controlled trial. Lancet 2008; 371(9630): 2093-100.
[http://dx.doi.org/10.1016/S0140-6736(08)60919-8] [PMID: 18572079]

[110] Ferri C, Desideri G, Baldoncini R, *et al.* Angiotensin II increases the release of endothelin-1 from human cultured endothelial cells but does not regulate its circulating levels. Clin Sci (Lond) 1999; 96(3): 261-70.
[PMID: 10029562]

[111] Imai T, Hirata Y, Emori T, Yanagisawa M, Masaki T, Marumo F. Induction of endothelin-1 gene by angiotensin and vasopressin in endothelial cells. Hypertension 1992; 19(6 Pt 2): 753-7.
[http://dx.doi.org/10.1161/01.HYP.19.6.753] [PMID: 1592477]

[112] Emori T, Hirata Y, Ohta K, *et al.* Cellular mechanism of endothelin-1 release by angiotensin and vasopressin. Hypertension 1991; 18(2): 165-70.
[http://dx.doi.org/10.1161/01.HYP.18.2.165] [PMID: 1909304]

[113] Sung CP, Arleth AJ, Storer BL, Ohlstein EH. Angiotensin type 1 receptors mediate smooth muscle proliferation and endothelin biosynthesis in rat vascular smooth muscle. J Pharmacol Exp Ther 1994; 271(1): 429-37.
[PMID: 7965744]

[114] d'Uscio LV, Shaw S, Barton M, Lüscher TF. Losartan but not verapamil inhibits angiotensin II-induced tissue endothelin-1 increase: role of blood pressure and endothelial function. Hypertension 1998; 31(6): 1305-10.
[http://dx.doi.org/10.1161/01.HYP.31.6.1305] [PMID: 9622146]

[115] Dziadzio M, Denton CP, Smith R, *et al.* Losartan therapy for Raynaud's phenomenon and scleroderma: clinical and biochemical findings in a fifteen-week, randomized, parallel-group, controlled trial. Arthritis Rheum 1999; 42(12): 2646-55.
[http://dx.doi.org/10.1002/1529-0131(199912)42:12<2646::AID-ANR21>3.0.CO;2-T]   [PMID: 10616013]

[116] Pancera P, Sansone S, Secchi S, Covi G, Lechi A. The effects of thromboxane A2 inhibition (picotamide) and angiotensin II receptor blockade (losartan) in primary Raynaud's phenomenon. J Intern Med 1997; 242(5): 373-6.
[http://dx.doi.org/10.1046/j.1365-2796.1997.00219.x] [PMID: 9408065]

[117] Rustin MH, Almond NE, Beacham JA, *et al.* The effect of captopril on cutaneous blood flow in patients with primary Raynaud's phenomenon. Br J Dermatol 1987; 117(6): 751-8.
[http://dx.doi.org/10.1111/j.1365-2133.1987.tb07356.x] [PMID: 3322358]

[118] Janini SD, Scott DG, Coppock JS, Bacon PA, Kendall MJ. Enalapril in Raynaud's phenomenon. J Clin Pharm Ther 1988; 13(2): 145-50.
[http://dx.doi.org/10.1111/j.1365-2710.1988.tb00171.x] [PMID: 2839529]

[119] Gliddon AE, Doré CJ, Black CM, *et al.* Prevention of vascular damage in scleroderma and autoimmune Raynaud's phenomenon: a multicenter, randomized, double-blind, placebo-controlled

trial of the angiotensin-converting enzyme inhibitor quinapril. Arthritis Rheum 2007; 56(11): 3837-46.
[http://dx.doi.org/10.1002/art.22965] [PMID: 17968938]

[120] Lindblad LE, Ekenvall L. Alpha-adrenoceptors in the vessels of human finger skin. Acta Physiol Scand 1986; 128(2): 219-22.
[http://dx.doi.org/10.1111/j.1748-1716.1986.tb07969.x] [PMID: 2877542]

[121] Baumhäkel M, Böhm M. Recent achievements in the management of Raynaud's phenomenon. Vasc Health Risk Manag 2010; 6: 207-14.
[http://dx.doi.org/10.2147/VHRM.S5255] [PMID: 20407628]

[122] Pope J, Fenlon D, Thompson A, *et al.* Prazosin for Raynaud's phenomenon in progressive systemic sclerosis. Cochrane Database Syst Rev 2000; (2): : CD000956.
[PMID: 10796398]

[123] Coffman JD, Cohen RA. Role of alpha-adrenoceptor subtypes mediating sympathetic vasoconstriction in human digits. Eur J Clin Invest 1988; 18(3): 309-13.
[http://dx.doi.org/10.1111/j.1365-2362.1988.tb01264.x] [PMID: 2843379]

[124] Flavahan NA, Cooke JP, Shepherd JT, Vanhoutte PM. Human postjunctional alpha-1 and alpha-2 adrenoceptors: differential distribution in arteries of the limbs. J Pharmacol Exp Ther 1987; 241(2): 361-5.
[PMID: 3033211]

[125] Chotani MA, Flavahan S, Mitra S, Daunt D, Flavahan NA. Silent alpha(2C)-adrenergic receptors enable cold-induced vasoconstriction in cutaneous arteries. Am J Physiol Heart Circ Physiol 2000; 278(4): H1075-83.
[http://dx.doi.org/10.1152/ajpheart.2000.278.4.H1075] [PMID: 10749700]

[126] Jeyaraj SC, Chotani MA, Mitra S, Gregg HE, Flavahan NA, Morrison KJ. Cooling evokes redistribution of α2C-adrenoceptors from Golgi to plasma membrane in transfected human embryonic kidney 293 cells. Mol Pharmacol 2001; 60(6): 1195-200.
[http://dx.doi.org/10.1124/mol.60.6.1195] [PMID: 11723226]

[127] Wise RA, Wigley FM, White B, *et al.* Efficacy and tolerability of a selective alpha(2C)-adrenergic receptor blocker in recovery from cold-induced vasospasm in scleroderma patients: a single-center, double-blind, placebo-controlled, randomized crossover study. Arthritis Rheum 2004; 50(12): 3994-4001.
[http://dx.doi.org/10.1002/art.20665] [PMID: 15593189]

[128] Herrick AL, Murray AK, Ruck A, *et al.* A double-blind, randomized, placebo-controlled crossover trial of the α2C-adrenoceptor antagonist ORM-12741 for prevention of cold-induced vasospasm in patients with systemic sclerosis. Rheumatology (Oxford) 2014; 53(5): 948-52.
[http://dx.doi.org/10.1093/rheumatology/ket421] [PMID: 24489014]

[129] Almuti K, Rimawi R, Spevack D, Ostfeld RJ. Effects of statins beyond lipid lowering: potential for clinical benefits. Int J Cardiol 2006; 109(1): 7-15.
[http://dx.doi.org/10.1016/j.ijcard.2005.05.056] [PMID: 16054715]

[130] Kuwana M. Potential benefit of statins for vascular disease in systemic sclerosis. Curr Opin Rheumatol 2006; 18(6): 594-600.
[http://dx.doi.org/10.1097/01.bor.0000245720.02512.3e] [PMID: 17053504]

[131] Sahebkar A, Kotani K, Serban C, *et al.* Statin therapy reduces plasma endothelin-1 concentrations: A meta-analysis of 15 randomized controlled trials. Atherosclerosis 2015; 241(2): 433-42.
[http://dx.doi.org/10.1016/j.atherosclerosis.2015.05.022] [PMID: 26074317]

[132] Ladak K, Pope JE. A review of the effects of statins in systemic sclerosis. Semin Arthritis Rheum 2016; 45(6): 698-705.
[http://dx.doi.org/10.1016/j.semarthrit.2015.10.013] [PMID: 26639033]

[133] Kuwana M, Kaburaki J, Okazaki Y, Yasuoka H, Kawakami Y, Ikeda Y. Increase in circulating

endothelial precursors by atorvastatin in patients with systemic sclerosis. Arthritis Rheum 2006; 54(6): 1946-51.
[http://dx.doi.org/10.1002/art.21899] [PMID: 16729283]

[134] Kuwana M, Okazaki Y, Kaburaki J. Long-term beneficial effects of statins on vascular manifestations in patients with systemic sclerosis. Mod Rheumatol 2009; 19(5): 530-5.
[http://dx.doi.org/10.3109/s10165-009-0199-4] [PMID: 19590932]

[135] Del Papa N, Cortiana M, Vitali C, *et al.* Simvastatin reduces endothelial activation and damage but is partially ineffective in inducing endothelial repair in systemic sclerosis. J Rheumatol 2008; 35(7): 1323-8.
[PMID: 18528965]

[136] Abou-Raya A, Abou-Raya S, Helmii M. Statins: potentially useful in therapy of systemic sclerosis-related Raynaud's phenomenon and digital ulcers. J Rheumatol 2008; 35(9): 1801-8.
[PMID: 18709692]

[137] Hu M, Cheung BM, Tomlinson B. Safety of statins: an update. Ther Adv Drug Saf 2012; 3(3): 133-44.
[http://dx.doi.org/10.1177/2042098612439884] [PMID: 25083232]

[138] Kahaleh B, Meyer O, Scorza R. Assessment of vascular involvement. Clin Exp Rheumatol 2003; 21(3) (Suppl. 29): S9-S14.
[PMID: 12889215]

[139] Agache I, Rădoi M, Duca L. Platelet activation in patients with systemic scleroderma--pattern and significance. Rom J Intern Med 2007; 45(2): 183-91.
[PMID: 18333373]

[140] Ramirez GA, Franchini S, Rovere-Querini P, *et al.* The role of platelets in the pathogenesis of systemic sclerosis. Front Immunol 2012 Jun 18; 3: 160.
[http://dx.doi.org/10.3389/fimmu.2012.00160]

[141] Ames PR, Lupoli S, Alves J, *et al.* The coagulation/fibrinolysis balance in systemic sclerosis: evidence for a haematological stress syndrome. Br J Rheumatol 1997; 36(10): 1045-50.
[http://dx.doi.org/10.1093/rheumatology/36.10.1045] [PMID: 9374919]

[142] Triggle CR, Samuel SM, Ravishankar S, Marei I, Arunachalam G, Ding H. The endothelium: influencing vascular smooth muscle in many ways. Can J Physiol Pharmacol 2012; 90(6): 713-38.
[http://dx.doi.org/10.1139/y2012-073] [PMID: 22625870]

[143] Denton CP, Howell K, Stratton RJ, Black CM. Long-term low molecular weight heparin therapy for severe Raynaud's phenomenon: a pilot study. Clin Exp Rheumatol 2000; 18(4): 499-502.
[PMID: 10949727]

[144] Lambova S, Batalov A, Dobrev H, Sapundzhiev L, Müller-Ladner U. Digital ulcers in systemic sclerosis - how to manage in 2013? Curr Rheumatol Rev 2013; 9(4): 274-8.
[http://dx.doi.org/10.2174/1573397109044140417125803] [PMID: 26932293]

[145] Lambova S, Batalov A, Sapundzhiev L, Müller-Ladner U. Digital ulcers in systemic sclerosis - frequency, subtype distribution and clinical outcome. Curr Rheumatol Rev 2013; 9(4): 268-73.
[http://dx.doi.org/10.2174/1573397109044140417125627] [PMID: 26932292]

[146] Denton C, Korn J. Digital ulceration and critical digital ischemia in scleroderma. Scleroderma Care Res 2003; 1: 12-6.

[147] Galluccio F, Matucci-Cerinic M. Two faces of the same coin: Raynaud phenomenon and digital ulcers in systemic sclerosis. Autoimmun Rev 2011; 10(5): 241-3.
[http://dx.doi.org/10.1016/j.autrev.2010.09.008] [PMID: 20863907]

[148] Fiori G, Galluccio F, Braschi F, *et al.* Vitamin E gel reduces time of healing of digital ulcers in systemic sclerosis. Clin Exp Rheumatol 2009; 27(3) (Suppl. 54): 51-4.
[PMID: 19796562]

[149] Hughes M, Herrick AL. Digital ulcers in systemic sclerosis. Rheumatology (Oxford) 2017; 56(1): 14-25.
[http://dx.doi.org/10.1093/rheumatology/kew047] [PMID: 27094599]

[150] Moinzadeh P, Hunzelmann N, Krieg T. Combination therapy with an endothelin-1 receptor antagonist (bosentan) and a phosphodiesterase V inhibitor (sildenafil) for the management of severe digital ulcerations in systemic sclerosis. J Am Acad Dermatol 2011; 65(3): e102-4.
[http://dx.doi.org/10.1016/j.jaad.2011.04.029] [PMID: 21839301]

[151] Ambach A, Seo W, Bonnekoh B, Gollnick H. Low-dose combination therapy of severe digital ulcers in diffuse progressive systemic sclerosis with the endothelin-1 receptor antagonist bosentan and the phosphodiesterase V inhibitor sildenafil. J Dtsch Dermatol Ges 2009; 7(10): 888-91.
[http://dx.doi.org/10.1111/j.1610-0387.2009.07057.x] [PMID: 19302565]

[152] Motegi S, Yamada K, Toki S, et al. Beneficial effect of botulinum toxin A on Raynaud's phenomenon in Japanese patients with systemic sclerosis: A prospective, case series study. J Dermatol 2016; 43(1): 56-62.
[http://dx.doi.org/10.1111/1346-8138.13030] [PMID: 26173902]

[153] Neumeister MW, Chambers CB, Herron MS, et al. Botox therapy for ischemic digits. Plast Reconstr Surg 2009; 124(1): 191-201.
[http://dx.doi.org/10.1097/PRS.0b013e3181a80576] [PMID: 19568080]

[154] Iorio ML, Masden DL, Higgins JP. Botulinum toxin A treatment of Raynaud's phenomenon: a review. Semin Arthritis Rheum 2012; 41(4): 599-603.
[http://dx.doi.org/10.1016/j.semarthrit.2011.07.006] [PMID: 21868066]

[155] Uppal L, Dhaliwal K, Butler PE. A prospective study of the use of botulinum toxin injections in the treatment of Raynaud's syndrome associated with scleroderma. J Hand Surg Eur Vol 2014; 39(8): 876-80.
[http://dx.doi.org/10.1177/1753193413516242] [PMID: 24369360]

[156] Van Beek AL, Lim PK, Gear AJ, Pritzker MR. Management of vasospastic disorders with botulinum toxin A. Plast Reconstr Surg 2007; 119(1): 217-26.
[http://dx.doi.org/10.1097/01.prs.0000244860.00674.57] [PMID: 17255677]

[157] Uchiyama A, Yamada K, Perera B, et al. Protective effect of botulinum toxin A after cutaneous ischemia-reperfusion injury. Sci Rep 2015; 5: 9072.
[http://dx.doi.org/10.1038/srep09072] [PMID: 25766279]

[158] Bailey SR, Eid AH, Mitra S, Flavahan S, Flavahan NA. Rho kinase mediates cold-induced constriction of cutaneous arteries: role of alpha2C-adrenoceptor translocation. Circ Res 2004; 94(10): 1367-74.
[http://dx.doi.org/10.1161/01.RES.0000128407.45014.58] [PMID: 15087420]

[159] Nohria A, Prsic A, Liu PY, et al. Statins inhibit Rho kinase activity in patients with atherosclerosis. Atherosclerosis 2009; 205(2): 517-21.
[http://dx.doi.org/10.1016/j.atherosclerosis.2008.12.023] [PMID: 19167712]

[160] Rikitake Y, Liao JK. Rho-kinase mediates hyperglycemia-induced plasminogen activator inhibitor-1 expression in vascular endothelial cells. Circulation 2005; 111(24): 3261-8.
[http://dx.doi.org/10.1161/CIRCULATIONAHA.105.534024] [PMID: 15956119]

[161] Fava A, Wung PK, Wigley FM, et al. Efficacy of Rho kinase inhibitor fasudil in secondary Raynaud's phenomenon. Arthritis Care Res (Hoboken) 2012; 64(6): 925-9.
[http://dx.doi.org/10.1002/acr.21622] [PMID: 22275160]

CHAPTER 6

Traditional Medicine Based Cardiovascular Therapeutics

Sriram Kumar, Rekha Ravindran*, **Sakthi Abbirami Gowthaman, Sujata Roy** and **Johanna Rajkumar**

Department of Biotechnology, Rajalakshmi Engineering College, Rajalakshmi Nagar, Thandalam, Chennai-602105,Tamil Nadu, India

Abstract: Cardiovascular diseases continue being the major cause of death worldwide, despite the constant and consistent efforts made towards the management and control of coronary artery diseases. These diseases are resulted by the metabolic imbalance involving elevated energy requirements and deficient oxygen supply to the cardiac myocytes, ultimately leading to myocardial necrosis. These diseases are closely associated with several changes in metabolic and signaling pathways that involve increased oxidative stress, excessive cytoplasmic and mitochondrial calcification, elevated lipid peroxidation, disturbed antioxidant homeostasis, dynamic cellular metabolism, irreversible DNA damage, and other pathophysiological alterations. The mechanism of pharmacological action demonstrated by modern western medicines usually adopt the lock-and-key model that involves the action of a principle therapeutic agent onto a specific and selective target to regulate a prime metabolic and signaling pathway, therefore becoming unsuitable to treat the disorders mediated by multiple molecular pathways. The side-effects associated with the use of such synthetic drugs are also an alarming health concern. The traditional system of medicine applies multiple natural ingredients that contain several active metabolites, therefore imparting a holistic pharmacological effect on multiple targets that orchestrate multiple pathways, without eliciting significant side-effects. This book chapter reviews various Indian and Chinese polyherbal formulations designed and developed according to the traditional system of medicine, which have been appropriately formulated and adequately characterized *in-vitro*, *in-vivo*, and *in-silico* following the stipulated scientific standards and medical regulations. Significant emphasis is also laid to review the informatic branches and cellular models available to evaluate and assess the pharmacology and toxicology of such polyherbal formulations.

Keywords: Ayurveda, Cardiovascular Diseases, Chinese Therapeutics, Cell Lines, Herboinformatics, Indian Therapeutics, *in-vitro*, Polyherbal Formulations, Pharmacoinformatics, Traditional Medicine, Toxicoinformaics.

* **Corresponding Author Dr. Rekha Ravindran:** Department of Biotechnology, Rajalakshmi Engineering College, Rajalakshmi Nagar, Thandalam, Chennai-602105, Tamil Nadu, India; Email: rekha.ravendran@rajalakshmi.edu.in

Atta-ur-Rahman & M. Iqbal Choudhary (Eds.)

INTRODUCTION

Cardiovascular Diseases

Cardiovascular disease is a general term for all types of diseases that affect the heart or blood vessels including numerous problems, many of which are related to a process called atherosclerosis. It is the major threat and cause of heart disease [1]. It is a condition that develops when a substance such as plaque builds up in the walls of the arteries. The build-up generally narrows the arteries making it harder for the blood to flow through. If a clot forms, it can also block the blood flow. Sometimes, this may even lead to a heart attack or stroke. CVD is generally associated with the build-up of fatty deposits inside the arteries and also associated with damage to arteries in an organ such as the brain, heart, kidneys, and eyes. Cardiovascular disease (CVD) is one of the leading causes of disability and death in the world. It is also regarded as the leading cause of mortality and morbidity in both men and women [2].

CVD is a class of diseases that involves heart and blood vessels. It also includes coronary artery diseases (CAD) such as myocardial infarction, commonly known as stroke and angina. Apart from this, other diseases that are associated with CVD are congenital heart disease, venous thrombosis, heart arrhythmia, rheumatic heart, heart failure, cardiomyopathy, stroke, hypertensive heart disease, valvular heart disease, and so on. Atherosclerosis is one of the main causes of CVD that includes the risk factor such as hypertension, hypercholesterolaemia and cigarette smoking, obesity, poor diet, and excessive alcohol consumption [3]. In the United States, 43% of the death rate is due to Cardiovascular disease [4]. In 1990, the death rate due to CVD was estimated to be 12.3 million (25.8%), while the death rate reached as high as 17.9 million (32.1%) in 2015 [5]. The death rate has been more in developing countries while the rate declined in most of the developed countries. Generally, older people are more affected by CVD.

Pathophysiology of CVD

Studies show that atherosclerosis and diabetes are the major precursors for cardiovascular disease (CVD). Apart from this obesity, diabetes mellitus, hypercholesterolaemia, and chronic kidney disease are also often linked with cardiovascular disease [6]. Diabetes is the primary risk factor for CVD. It also affects the heart muscles leading to diastolic and systolic heart failure. Atherosclerosis is a major threat to people with macrovasculature even with or without diabetes [7].

Different Types of CVD

There are many cardiovascular diseases involved in the heart and blood vessels. The type of CVD involved with the blood vessels (arteries, veins or capillaries) is known as vascular disease. They include diseases such as Aneurysm, Buerger's disease, Raynaud's disease or phenomenon, Atherosclerosis, Peripheral artery disease, Renal artery disease, Cerebrovascular disease (stroke), Peripheral venous disease, and other blood clotting disorders. The cardiovascular diseases associated with heart or cardiac are Arrhythmia (irregular heartbeat or rhythm), Angina (for both cardiac and vascular disease), Dilated cardiomyopathy, Heart attack, Congenital heart disease, Mitral valve prolapse, Mitral regurgitation, Pulmonary stenosis, Hypertrophic cardiomyopathy, and Rheumatic heart disease (a complication of strep throat) [6, 7].

INDIAN CARDIOVASCULAR THERAPEUTICS

Following are some of the important Indian cardiovascular therapeutics that have attracted significant research interests:

Ambrex

Ambrex is a licensed polyherbal formulation consisting of five Indian herbs: Withania somnifera, Cycas circirnalis, Orchis mascula, Shorea, robusta, and amber (a resin from Pinus succinifera) that are "Generally safe" are blended together in accordance to the Siddha system of medicine. In a study, FTIR characterization of Ambrex demonstrated C=O stretching in carbonyl compounds contributed by the presence of high content of terpenoids and flavanoids [8], while the GC-MS analysis revealed Methyl-Commate-A as the key metabolite in its volatile-fraction [9]. An *in-vivo* study revealed that pre-treatment with Ambrex increases the ISPH-stimulated down-regulation of TCA-cycle enzymes (ICDH, SDH and α-KGDH) and decreases the ISPH-induced up-regulation of apoptotic genes (p53, bax and caspase-3) and anti-apoptotic gene (bcl-2) to their normal levels [8]. Another study characterized the morphology of Ambrex formulation by SEM and assessed its cardioprotective activity against ISPH-induced myocardial necrosis in rats, by quantifying its effects on different oxidative stress markers and cardiac biomarkers through biochemical and histopathological evaluations. Ambrex serves as a unique metal-deficient to the best of our knowledge in siddha medicine based polyherbal nano-formulation characterized and evaluated in India. Pretreatment with Ambrex significantly maintained the tissue levels of oxidative stress markers and serum levels of cardiac biomarkers at their respective normals. It also attenuated the magnitude of ISPH-induced oxidative stress, ROS generation and LPO as reflected by biochemical evaluations, and ameliorated the degree of ISPH-induced myocardial necrosis and membrane damage as reflected by histopathological evaluations. The prospective protein-targets of Ambrex and the signalling pathway that mediates this activity through a molecular docking approach suggested that Ambrex exhibits cardioprotective activity by maintaining the intracellular antioxidant homeostasis and myocardial membrane architecture probably through the inhibition of PKCβ protein [10].

Abana

Abana is an Indian ayurvedic herbomineral (medicinal plants and mineral complexes) preparation [11]. It involves many ingredients that significantly protect it against hypertension and ischaemia (restriction in blood supply to tissues) and are also involved in the treatment of cardiovascular disease. It possesses anti-hypercholesterolemic, anti-arrhythmic, and anti-thrombotic properties. Some of the important ingredients of the abana are Terminalia arjuna, Withania somnifera, Nardostachys jatamansi, Tinosporia cordifolia, Boerhaavia diffusa, Terminalia chebula, Glycyrrhiza glabra, *etc* [12]. Clinical studies have shown that this preparation possesses the down-regulation of beta-adrenergic receptors property [13]. Some ingredients like Terminalia arjuna, Nardostachys jatamansi, and Glycyrrhiza glabra that are used in the preparation of abana are used in the prevention of cardiovascular disorders [14]. Abana has brought a significant improvement in the case of hypertension, angina pectoris, and heart disease. It is used along with lipistat and arogyavardhini vati in the treatment of Hyperlipidemia (elevated lipid level) and Dyslipidemia (abnormal lipid level). It also regulates high blood pressure and mild blood pressure [15].

Arjunarishta

Arjunarishta is an ancient liquid oral formulation prescribed in Ayurveda for cardiovascular disorders [16]. It is popularly used as an herbal heart tonic. It regulates the blood pressure and cholesterol by promoting and strengthening the cardiac and heart muscles. It is also known as Parthadyarishta and is prepared using natural fermentation. The major ingredients used in this formulation are *Terminalia arjuna*, *Madhuca indica*, *Vitis vinifera*, and *Woodfordia fruticose*. The formulation is prepared by making a decoction of three plants in a specified amount. Crushed jaggery and the flowers of *Woodfordia fruticosa* are then added and preparation is kept for a specified period after which it undergoes fermentation and generates alcohol that helps in the extraction of active principles and also serves as a preservative. Ashavas and arishtas are very popular in India, due to their medicinal uses, taste, alcoholic and physiological content [17].

One of the major ingredients of this formulation, *Terminalia arjuna* is a native plant used as a cardioprotective agent found in India and Southeast Asia [18]. It is commonly administered as arishta, ghrita (medicated ghee), or as a powder. The plant contains triterpenoids, glycosides, flavonoids, and tannins. *In vivo* and *In vitro* of this plant have shown a positive result for cardiovascular disease so far. It also improved the symptoms of refractory chronic congestive heart failure. The bark of this plant is used in the prevention of ischemic-reperfusion injury induced oxidative stress and tissue injury of the heart in rabbits [19]. Since Arjunarishta is prepared by decoction, it is likely that non-polar constituents are not present in the formulation and the cardioprotective activities may be due to the polar constituents of *Terminalia arjuna* [16]. Some of the health benefits of arjunarishta are it minimizes Counter Cardiac Arrhythmia, Chest pain, fights Ischemic cardiomyopathy, treats Mitral regurgitation, prevents heart attack, and helps in Chronic Respiratory Disease.

Arogh

Arogh is an ayurvedic formulation and has been studied for its antioxidant property. It is composed of nine active plant ingredients namely, *Nelumbo nucifera, Hibiscus rosasinensis, Hemidesmus indicus, Rosa damascena, Zingiber officinale, Eclipta alba, Terminalia chebula, Glycyrrhiza glabra,* and *Quercus infectoria*. The combined effect of these plant extract in Arogh protects the cell against the threats of superoxide and peroxides generated by isoproterenol and is considered as a useful drug for Myocardial Infarction. Arogh prevents Atherosclerosis and reduces the risk of Coronary Heart Disease by increasing TC/HDL ratio and HDL level [20]. Arogh protects the myocardium by preventing the lipid peroxidation of membrane bound polyunsaturated fatty acids thereby ensuring myocardial membrane structural integrity and function. It has shown an effective treatment in hypercholesteremia. It also reduced the level of Cholesterol, Triglycerides, and LDL in patients with Angina and Hypertension [21, 22].

BHUx

BHUx is a patented polyherbal formulation targeting oxidative stress and inflammation [23]. It consists of a water-soluble extract of five medicinal plants namely, *Commiphora mukul, Balsamodendron mukul, Terminalia arjuna, Semecarpus anacardium,* and *Strychnos nux vomica* at a particular ratio. BHUx is capable of reducing the progress of atherosclerosis by its calcium channel-modulatory, anti-inflammatory, and antioxidant property. It was developed to simultaneously target inflammation, hyperlipidemia, endothelial dysfunction, and instability of plaque [24]. The PCT application was filed in 2003 and the US patent was approved in 2006. Based on scientific observations, BHUx is suggested as a novel polyherbal formulation with multi-targeted action. It acts as an antioxidant, anti-inflammatory, hypolipidemic and as an atheroma stabilizer [25].

Lipistat

Lipistat is an Indian ayurvedic and herbal medicine used to reduce the level of cholesterol in the blood. It is manufactured by Dabur. It reduces the LDL (Low Density Lipoprotein) and enhances the HDL (High Density Lipoprotein) level in the blood thereby promoting proper blood circulation in the body. Lipistat offers a potent combination of ayurvedic herbs that work on Hyperlipidaemia and maintains the cardiac function. It also brings down the level of high cholesterol and triglycerides. The key ingredients of lipistat are *Terminalia arjuna, Inula racemose,* and *Commiphora mukul* in equal proportions [26]. *Terminalia arjuna* has a remarkable cardioprotective, heart muscle strengthening, and Cardiac stimulant properties [27]. *Inula racemose* has a potent beneficial effect on the Cardiovascular system. It also has beta-blocking and anti-anginal activity [28]. *Commiphora mukul* has thrombosis, hyperlipidemic, and fibrinolytic activity [29]. Lipistat provides partial effectiveness in the prevention of myocardial necrosis. It is also effective in the treatment and the management of ischemic heart disease [30].

Liposem

Liposem is a polyherbal formulation containing 17 medicinal plants of therapeutic importance against hypercholesterolaemia and cholesterol management. It provides support to those affected from metabolic disorders leading to cardiac problems such as atherosclerosis, hypercholesterolaemia, and hyperlipidaemia. It generally acts by normalizing the lipid profile. The cardiovascular effect of liposem is possible related to its antioxidant property since the lipid peroxidation of LDL plays a major role in the development of atherosclerosis. It also demonstrates strong hypolipidemic impacts in conjunction with the potent antioxidant property that provides additional benefits in the inhibition of oxidative stress and in the prevention and treatment of atherosclerosis [31].

Marutham

Marutham is an Indian polyherbal formulation containing eight plant constituents. The active constituents of Marutham are known to possess cardioprotective, anti-hyperlipidaemic, and antioxidant properties. The eight important constituents of marutham are *Allium sativum, Withania somnifera, Glycyrrhiza glabra, Wedelia calendulaceae, Nelumbium speciosum, Tinospora cordifolia, Emblica officinalis,* and *Terminalia arjuna*. Marutham exhibits cardioprotective activity and protects the myocardium against isoproterenol-induced myocardial infarction [32].

Triglize

Triglize is a polyherbal formulation used in the treatment of High cholesterol, hypertension, myocardial necrosis, coronary atherosclerosis, hypercholesterol, ischemic heart diseases, hypertension, and obesity. It is formulated using the aqueous extracts of *Terminalia arjuna, Cissus quadrangularis, Boerhaavia diffusa, Commiphora mukul, Phyllanthus embilica, Terminalia bellirica, Terminalia chebula, Tribulus terrestris, Allium sativum, and Trigonella foenumgraecum* as active ingredients. Triglize exhibits radical scavenging property, antioxidant property, and diuretic activity. Diuretics play a key role in the management of congestive heart failure and hypertension. Since it exhibits diuretic activity, it is useful in the management of cardiovascular diseases. It is currently approved for use in humans as ayurvedic medicine in the treatment of cardiovascular diseases such as hypertension and cardiac failure [33].

TRADITIONAL CHINESE MEDICINE

Bushen Kangle

Bushen Knagle is a Chinese therapeutic medicine which has the following key ingredients: Epimedium Herb (35.1%), Prepared Fleece-flower Root (2.1%), peanut kernel (6.3%), Turtle Shell (Burned) (0.75%), Asiatic Cornelian Cherry Fruit (Prepared) (2.7%), Cassia Bark (0.38%), Barbary wolfberry Fruit (2.1%), dog kidney (Prepared) (7.5%), Prepared Rehmannia Root (1.5%), Amur Cork-tree bark (Prepared) (5.1%), Himalayan Teasel Root (0.45%), Chinese Magnoliavine Fruit (2.4%), Sea-horse (1.5%), Human Placenta (24.9%), Eucommia Bark (2.0%), Ginseng (4.5%), Fructus Alpiniae Oxyphyllae (Prepared) (0.75%). It is generally available in a capsule form with yellow-brown powder inside and tastes slightly salty and bitter. It is regarded as a pure Chinese medicine made by modern science and technology according to good manufacturing practice (GMP). It shows a good effect in treating sexual function decline, lumbar, leg pain, insomnia, forgetfulness. The capsule is mainly used for strengthening Yang, tonifying kidney, nourishing Qi and blood, promote the production of the vital essence and marrow, improving body and brain. The most important raw material Epimedium herb is a superior medicine for strengthening Yang of the kidney, improving body and dispelling rheumatism [34].

Dang Gui Long Hui Wan

Dang Gui Long Hui Wan has been widely used as a traditional Chinese medicine for the treatment of chronic myelogenous leukemia (CML). It has a potent growth inhibitory effects in the tumor cells of human [35]. It is made of 11 kinds of traditional Chinese medical herbs: A. sinensis (Oliv) Diels, Aloe vera L., Gennana scaber L., Saussurea lappa Clarke, Scutellaria baicalensis Georgi, Phillodendron chinensis Schneid, Coptis chinensis Franch, Gardenia jasminoides Ellis, Rheum palmarus L., Indigofera tinctoria L., and Moschus moschiferus [36]. The compound pill recipe is a mixture of 11 ingredients such as Da huang, Dang gui, Huang bai, Huang lian, Huang qin, Long dan, Lu hui, Mu xiang, Qing dai, She xiang, and Zhi zi. Of these, Qing Dai was found to be the most effective component, Indirubin extracted from Qing dai, an anti-tumor component is used in the treatment of chronic disease and is effective against CML

Er Chen Wan

Er Chen Wan is a Chinese herbal medicine with the key ingredients: ginger (fresh rhizome), poria (sclerotium) and tangerine (dried rind). It is a yellowish-brown pill used to remove phlegm damp and regulate the stomach function. It is used to treat cough with copious expectoration, stuffy sensation in the chest and epigastrium, nausea and vomiting due to the stagnation of damp-phlegm. The classic herbal formulation consists of Radix Glycyrrhizae, Pericarpium Citri Reticulate, Rhizoma Pinelliae and Poria [37].

Fu Fang Dan Shen

It is an herbal preparation consisting of Notoginseng (Radix and rhizome of Panax notoginseng (Burk.), Salvia miltiorrhiza (Radix and rhizome of Salvia miltiorrhiza Bge.) and Borneolum Syntheticum. It is widely used to improve cardiac angina, coronary heart disease, circulation problem and atherosclerosis [38, 39]. It is also used for menstrual disorders, high blood pressure during pregnancy, chronic liver disease, inflamed pancreas and diabetes. Dan Shen appears to thin the blood by preventing platelet and blood clotting. It widens the blood vessels thereby increasing circulation. It is also used in the treatment of hyperlipidemia, angina pectoris and acute ischemic stroke [40]. It is also used for reducing weight, relieving bruises and wound healing.

Fu Fang Ge Qing

It is a Chinese traditional medicine with the herbal formulation of Gan chan, Huang chi, Bai guo, Zi wan, Ku xing ren, Qian hu, Fu zi, Wu wein zi, Hu jia. It is a Phlegm expelling medicine available in tablet form and is used for retaining the phlegm turbidity in the lung [37].

Jiang Zhi Ling

Traditional Chinese Medicine (TCM) have been used in the prevention and treatment of atherosclerosis and lower lipid for thousands of years. Jiang-Zh-

-Ning (JZN), a widely used Chinese medicine, is composed of nuciferine (from HeYe, folium nelumbinis), stilbene glycoside (from ShouWu, fleeceflower root), hyperin (from ShanZha, fructus crataegi), and chrysophanol (from JueMingZi, semen cassiae). The four main herbs Folium Nelumbinis, Fleeceflower Root, Fructus Crataegi, and Semen Cassiae have been used in clinic on obesity for centuries as in "QianJinFang" (Prescriptions Worth Thousands Gold). It significantly reduces or lowers serum cholesterol levels in the body [41].

Jin Kui Shen Qi Wan

Jin Kui Shen Qi Wan is one of the most ancient Chinese herbal formulations. It is commonly used as a tonic to nourish the yang of the Yin-Yang. It is available in pill or capsule form. It is widely prescribed for hypertensive patients with kidney *yang* deficiency syndrome in China and is used in the treatment of hypertension [42].

Ke Chuan

Ke Chuan Wan is a natural Chinese herbal supplement specially formulated to help open the airways and for breathing smoothly. It includes six main herbs namely Jie Geng, Jing Jie, Bai Bu, Fang Feng, Bei Mu and Bai Qian [43]. The meta-analysis of Zhi sou san, a popular herbal remedy for cough, concluded that this medicine offers significant benefits. Compared with that of western medicine, it is effective in the pulmonary function in terms of FEV1 [44].

Qing Nao Jiang Ya

It is a natural Chinese herbal supplement that helps in calming the liver and subdues the yang to help maintain healthy blood pressure. It is composed of 11 herbs that act together in calming the liver, subduing the yang, enriching the yin, and support healthy blood [45]. It is available in tablet form sold under the name HypertenSure™. It also aids in maintaining visual equilibrium, healthy brain function and circulation.

Sheng Mai Yin

Sheng-Mai Yin (SMY), a modern Chinese formula based on Traditional Chinese Medicine, is used in the treatment of cardiovascular diseases in Eastern Asia [46]. The name Sheng mai means "to generate the pulse", indicating that the prescription is generally given to persons having a weak pulse, with the expectation that the pulse strength will improve markedly. It is widely used to treat cardiac diseases characterized by the deficiency of Qi and Yin syndrome in China. Sheng-Mai Yin based treatment is officially recorded in the Chinese

Pharmacopoeia. This formulation is used to treat people with serious illness, heart attack, congestive heart failure, or severe bronchitis, and to treat a sudden drop in blood pressure that are mainly associated with cardiogenic or septic shock. It is generally given as a liquid or a decoction or as an intravenous drip. The formula comprises of three main ingredients Ginseng, Ophiopogen and schizandra [47].

Su He Xiang Wan

The main function of this formulation is to warm and aromatically open up the orifices, transform turbidity and promote qi circulation. It is also used to treat an excess cold with dampness and turbid phlegm. The main herbal ingredient of this medicine is Su he xiang (Styrax Liquidis, Rose Maloes Resin, Styrax), Bing pian (Borneol), She xiang (Secretio Moschus, Naval Secretions of Musk Deer, Musk), Mu xiang (Radix Aucklandiae Lappae, Costus Root, Saussurea, Aucklandia), An xi xiang (Benzoinum), Tan xiang (Lignum Santali Albi, Heartwood of Sandalwood, Santalum), Chen xiang (Lignum Aquilariae, Aloeswood, Quilaria), Ding xiang (Flos Caryophylli, Clove Flower Bud), Ru xiang (Gummi Olibanum, Frankincense, Mastic), Xiang fu (Rhizoma Cyperi Rotundi, Nut Grass Rhizome, Cyperus), Bi ba (Fructus Piperis Longi, Long Pepper Fruit), Xi jiao Herba Cephalanoplos, Small Thistle), Bai zhu Rhizoma Atractyloids Macrocephaelae, White Atractylodes Rhizome), He zi (Fructus Terminaliae Chebulae, Myrobalan Fruit, Terminalia, Chebula)and Zhu sha (Cinnabaris, Cinnabar). It is one of the commonly prescribed formulae for qi stroke, cold stroke and other disorders. It is also best suited for cerebrovascular accident conditions, angina pectoris, hysteria, seizure disorders and post-concussion syndrome [37].

Tian Wang Bu Xin Dan

Tian Wang Bu Xin Dan (TWBXD), Traditional Chinese Medicine (TCM), has been used widely for treating insomnia in China [48]. Tianwang Buxin Dan (Ginseng and Zizyphus), one of the widely used patent remedies for nourishing the heart and calming the mind. The name refers to the "King of Heaven" or "Heavenly King" (*tian* = heaven; *wang* = king, ruler) and to the action of supplementing the heart (*buxin*), being prepared in the form of a large pill rolled in cinnabar (*dan*; without cinnabar, the preparation should be called simply a pill: wan). The formula was first recorded 1638 A.D in the Shesheng Mipou (Secret Investigations into Obtaining Health) written by Hong Ji just before the fall of the Ming Dynasty. There is a story explaining the formula's unusual name-that Hong Ji had a dream in which the heavenly king visited him and gave him the formula. The main ingredients of this are Ginseng, polygala, platycodon, zizyphus, Ophiopogon, asparagus, Rehmannia, scrophularia. Of these, rehmannia is the key ingredient in the recipe for Tianwang Buxin Dan ranging, comprising 31% of the total weight.

Tong Xin Luo

Tong xin luo capsule is a traditional Chinese herb used for cardiovascular diseases in China and some other Asian countries. In combination with routine angina therapy, it appears to reduce the risk of subsequent AMI, PTCA or CABG, angina attacks and severity, as well as improving symptoms and ischemic changes on the electrocardiogram (ECG) [49]. It exerts a variety of pharmacological effects including anti-hypertensive effects and improves ventricular remodelling [50]. It was extracted and freeze-dried from a mixture of red peony root, borneol, ginseng and spine date seed [51].

Xie Qing Wan

It is a herbal formulation available in pill form used for purging liver fire, drains damp-heat from the liver and gall bladder, alleviates pain, reduces swelling and harmonizes the blood. The main ingredients of this herbal formulation are Dang Gui (Angelicae Sinensis root), Long Dan Cao (Gentianae root), Zhi Zi (Liguisticum root), Da Huang (Rhei rhizome and root), Qiang Huo (Notopterygii root) and Fang Feng (Saposhnikoviae root) [37].

Xin Bao Wan

It is a Chinese herbal medicine comprising the important constituents such as Yang Jin Hua (*Datura metel L*), Ren Shen (*Panax ginseng C. A. Mey),* Lu Rong (*Pilose Antler Cornu Cervi Pantotrichum*), Rou Gui (*Cassia Bark Cortex Cinnamomi*), Fu Zi (Zhi) [*Aconite (Processed) Radix Aconiti Lateralis Preparata*], San Qi (*Notoginseng Root Radix Notoginseng),* Bing Pian (*Borneol Broneolum Syntheticum*), She Xiang (*Musk Moschus),* Chan Su (*Toad Venom Venenum Bufonis*). It is used for heart and kidney yang deficiency, heart arteries and veins and blood stasis caused by Chronic heart failure, sick sinus syndrome, and ischemic heart disease caused by angina and ischemic electrocardiographic changes, sinus node dysfunction caused by bradycardia [37].

Yang Xin Yin

It is a combined herbal formulation widely used for the treatment of arrhythmia with or without structurally abnormal heart approved by the China Food and Drug Administration in 2003 [52]. It was developed more than 2000 years; over 70% of patients in China prefer Traditional Chinese Medicine combined with Western medicine.

INFORMATICS IN CVDD

Herboinformatics in CVDD

Herboinformatics is a specialized domain under computational ethnobiology that identifies prospective bioactive compounds from herbal formulations against potential targets of biological significance, utilizing informatics platforms like hardware, software, databases, repositories, online servers, search engines, etc [53]. The singular objective of herbal informatics is to integrate diverse informatics branches (like bioinformatics, chemoinformatics, pharmacoinformatics, toxicoinformatics, etc) with conventional drug discovery pipeline, facilitating the rationale identification of potential leads through *in-silico* investigations, which can be further validated through *in-vitro* and *in-vivo* experiments. A report released by the Division of CBRN Defence, Institute of Nuclear Medicine and Allied Sciences defines the field of 'Herbal Informatics' as 'a novel systematic approach that allows focused herbal drug discovery with ease at an enhanced pace' [54]. This domain incorporates modern approaches of information technology with the traditional knowledge of ethnobiology to retrieve and record pharmacological and toxicological information of medicinal herbs and further integrates this retrieved information with clinical knowledge pertaining to potential targets and virulence factors [55].

Pharmacoinformatics in CVDD

Pharmacoinformatics is an emerging domain in biomedical informatics that integrates information and expertise in computational pharmacology and information technology to create, manage, modify, store and retrieve data on design, discovery, development and delivery of pharmaceutical agents, drugs, compounds, formulations and substances [56]. It involves tools and techniques like computational and mathematical modeling, artificial intelligence and machine learning, computational algorithms and functions, information and database management, repository and retrieval systems, data mining and integration, support vector machines and artificial neural networks for compiling and comprehending different classes of pharmaceutical agents, their mechanism of action, routes of administration, pharmacokinetic and pharmacodynamic properties [57]. The conventional pipeline of drug design, discovery, development and delivery has become time-consuming, labor-intensive and economically expensive. Pharmacoinformatics proves to be instrumental and indispensable in this process, facilitating pharmacologists and toxicologists to predict the physiochemical and chemobiological characteristics of potential lead compounds, and validate these predictions by *in-vitro* and *in-vivo* studies [58].

Although pharmacoinformatics is in its elementary phase, it is taking giant strides in cardiovascular pharmacology. A recent study reported increased expression of S100C mRNA and protein in experimental rat models of pulmonary hypertension and myocardial infarction through pharmacogenomics approaches [59]. The study also observed increased levels of taurine in hypoxic conditions, to prevent hypoxia-induced S100C expression and cardiovascular remodeling. These results qualify S100C as a potential target in hypoxic and ischemic diseases. Delayed cerebral vasospasm following aneurysmal subarachnoid hemorrhage is reported to induce cerebral ischemia and infarction [55]. Through DNA microarray experiments, the same study reported an increased expression of Heme Oxygenase-1 (HO1) and Heat Shock Protein-72 (HSP72) mRNAs in the basilar artery of an experimental rat model for cerebral vasospasm. Directed inhibition of mRNA expression through intrathecal administration of antisense HO1 and HSP72 deoxyoligos aggravated cerebral vasospasm. These results reveal that pharmacogenomics-mediated expression analysis can potentially seal the gap between *in-vitro* and *in-vivo* studies, and can provide pipelines to identify potential targets for various cardiovascular diseases.

The hERG (human ether-a-go-go-related gene) encoded potassium ion channels mediate cardiac repolarization, and drug-induced hERG-blockage causes potentially lethal ventricular tachycardia termed Torsades de Pointes [60]. Another recent study presented a pharmacoinformatics pipeline that simultaneously uses ligand-based and structure-based models for predicting hERG-inhibition potentials (IC50) of newly identified ligands in the early stages of drug discovery and development. Structure-based pharmacophore modeling and virtual screening approaches were employed, using Integrated GRid-INdependent Descriptor (GRIND) models, and Lipophilic Efficiency (LipE) cum Ligand efficiency (LE) guided template selection strategies. hERG inhibition activities (pIC50) of identified hits were subsequently predicted, and two selected hits were experimentally evaluated for hERG inhibition potentials (pIC50) through whole-cell patch-clamp assays. The resulting differences of less than ±1.6 log units between the computationally predicted and experimentally determined hERG inhibition potentials (IC50) of selected hits revealed the predictive robustness and practical reliability of the proposed pipeline in precisely ranking the potency order (from lower μM to higher nM) against hERG.

Toxicoinformatics in CVDD

Toxicoinformatics is another discipline emerging under biomedical informatics that unifies concepts and principles in information technology and computational toxicology to dissect and define biological mechanisms mediating chemical toxicity. It broadly inculcates bioinformatic and computational tools and techniques to collect and categorize comprehensive information from across the diverse biological organization (molecules, cells, tissues, organs, systems, organisms, etc) for elucidating toxicological responses towards chemical compounds [61]. It involves deploying a multiple-omics (genomics, proteomics, transcriptomics, translatomics, metabolomics, metabonomics, epigenomics, lipidomics, glycomics, microbiomics, nutriomics, cytomics, physiomics) approach in conjunction with traditional methods of bioinformatics and cheminformatics, towards a deeper understanding of the biochemical mechanisms governing molecular, cellular and systems toxicity against chemical compounds. Toxicoinformatics can also be considered as an emerging discipline under chemical informatics that specifically aims to correlate physiochemical properties and structural characteristics of chemical compounds to potential toxicity using tools and techniques of computational chemistry [62].

Several non-cardiovascular drugs are withdrawn from the pharmaceutical market as they demonstrate the potential to non-specifically inhibit hERG gene-encoded potassium ion (K+) channels, leading to undesirable side-effects like heart arrhythmia and potentially death [63]. The notorious promiscuity of K+ channels to non-specific compounds hallmarked hERG as an important anti-target for assessing the potential cardiotoxicity of a bioactive compound during the early stages of drug design [63]. Experimentally evaluating the non-specific affinity of a bioactive compound towards K+ channels through *in-vitro* and *in-vivo* assays is arduous, tedious and tiresome, and thereby calls for developing computational pipelines to reliably identify and robustly exclude potential non-specific hERG blockers [63]. Diverse QSAR (Quantitative Structure-Activity Relationship) models have been recently built, initially using a primary dataset of 4,833 compounds, and successively retrained using a larger dataset of 5,984 compounds, for evaluating hERG liability [63]. The Pred-hERG web-server incorporates these retrained QSAR models and improved validation pipelines to quickly screen large chemical libraries for potential hERG blockage and is freely available at http://labmol.farmacia.ufg.br/predherg/ [63].

The US Food and Drug Administration's Center for Food Additive Safety and Applied Nutrition presented three QSAR programs: BioEpisteme, MC4PC and Leadscope Predictive Data Miner to predict drug-induced Cardiac Adverse Effects (CAE) [64]. QSAR models were built for nine clusters affecting Purkinje nerves (arrhythmia, bradycardia, conduction disorders, electrocardiogram, palpitations, QT prolongation, rate rhythm composite, tachycardia and torsades de pointes) and five clusters affecting heart muscle (coronary artery disorders, heart failure, myocardial disorders, myocardial infarction and valve disorders) [64]. Results reflected the complementarities of the three selected programs, with predictive performances of single positive, consensus two positives and consensus three positives in the respective order: specificity of 70.7%, 91.7% and 98.0%; sensitivity of 74.7%, 47.2% and 21.0%; and chi-square (x2) values of 138.2, 206.3 and 144.2. An additional and prospective study using CAE information adopted from the US Food and Drug Administration's MedWatch Program revealed 94.3% sensitivity and 82.4% specificity, and an external evaluation of eighteen drugs with severe cardiotoxicity (not adopted for building QSAR models) revealed 88.9% sensitivity [64].

CELLULAR MODELS FOR *IN-VITRO* RESEARCH

Human Cardiac Myocytes

Human Cardiac Myocytes (HCM) are primary adherent cells isolated from human cardiac ventricles [65]. In comparison to rod-shaped freshly-isolated cardiac myocytes, cultured primary HCMs serve as better models for *in-vitro* experiments like the long-term investigation of cytokine release, mechanical strain, cell-cell interactions, etc, as they are maintained adopting a different protocol. Cultured primary HCMs initially resemble progenitor cells in being sparingly differentiated, expressing biomarkers of early-stage differentiation (like GATA-4), and having high proliferative potential. When maintained till complete confluence and subcultured for extended periods, these cells undergo further differentiation, expressing biomarkers of later-stage differentiation and forming myotube-like structures. Biomarker analysis by immunofluorescent staining revealed that these cells stain positive for sarcomeric alpha-actinin and slow muscle myosin. They serve as an essential model for *in-vitro* studies on medical conditions associated with human cardiac myocyte dysfunction (like thrombosis, atherosclerosis and hypertension) and for stent-graft biocompatibility testing.

Human Aortic Endothelial Cells

Human Aortic Endothelial Cells (HAEC) are primary adherent cells isolated from human ascending thoracic aorta and descending abdominal aorta [66]. Biomarker analysis by immunofluorescent staining revealed that these cells stain positive for CD31, von Willebrand factor and dil-LDL uptake, and stain negative for smooth muscle alpha-actin. They serve as an essential model for *in-vitro* studies on medical conditions associated with human Aortic endothelial dysfunction (such as thrombosis, atherosclerosis and hypertension) as well as for stent-graft biocompatibility testing. To mention, a recent study investigated the molecular significance of over-expressing and silencing LPP3 (Lipid Phosphate Phosphatase 3) in cultured primary HAECs using wild type and mutated cDNA constructs [67]. Silencing LPP3 increased the secretions of inflammatory cytokines, leukocyte adhesion, cell survival, cell migration and impaired angiogenesis, while over-expressing LPP3 reversed these cellular effects and stimulated apoptosis.

The study also reported that LPP3 expression is inversely correlated with vascular endothelial growth factor expression. These results reveal the protective implications of LPP3 against endothelial dysfunction (a physiological condition preceding atherosclerosis).

Human Coronary Artery Endothelial Cells

Human Coronary Artery Endothelial Cells (HCAEC) are primary adherent cells isolated from human coronary arteries (including the anterior descending and the circumflex branches) from single donors [68]. Biomarker analysis by immunofluorescent staining revealed that these cells stain positive for CD31, von Willebrand factor and dil-LDL uptake, and stain negative for smooth muscle alpha-actin. They serve as an essential model for *in-vitro* studies on medical conditions associated with human coronary artery endothelial dysfunction. For instance, a recent study evaluated protein and mRNA expression levels of chemerin adipokine in hypoxia-exposed cultured primary HCAECs at varying time points [69]. A gel shift assay suggested that hypoxia enhances the protein-DNA interaction between an SP1 transcription factor and chemerin promoter, which was further confirmed by luciferase assay. Hypoxia significantly increased tube formation and cellular migration of HCAECs, while these cellular events were significantly attenuated byPD98059 inhibitor, anti-TNF-alpha antibody and chemerin siRNA oligonucleotide. These results reveal that hypoxia up-regulates chemerin expression in HCAECs, which further is evidently mediated by TNF-alpha and partially by the ERK pathway.

Human Pulmonary Artery Endothelial Cells

Human Pulmonary Artery Endothelial Cells (HPAEC) are primary adherent cells isolated from human pulmonary arteries (main pulmonary artery, the left and the right branches) from a single donor [70]. Biomarker analysis by immunoflu-orescent staining revealed that these cells stain positive for CD31, von Willebrand factor and dil-LDL uptake, and stain negative for smooth muscle alpha-actin. They serve as an essential model for *in-vitro* studies on medical conditions associated with human pulmonary artery endothelial dysfunction. For example, a recent study characterized the molecular roles of AQP1 (aquaporin-1) in hypoxia-induced Pulmonary Hypertension (PH) using HPAECs and reported that hypoxia-induced HPAECs encompassed a significantly increased AQP1 expression [71]. The functional involvement of AQP1 in PH was further investigated using HPAECs, which demonstrated that AQP1 depletion significantly decreased proliferation and migration of HPAECs, and conversely increased cellular apoptosis. These differential cellular events were closely associated with the higher expression of the p53 tumour suppressor gene. Their results deepen our current understanding of the pathophysiology of hypoxia-induced PH and qualify AQP1 as a prospective target for PH.

Human Cardiac Microvascular Endothelial Cells

Human Cardiac Microvascular Endothelial Cells (HCMEC) are primary adherent cells isolated from human myocardium (cardiac ventricles) from a single donor [72]. Biomarker analysis by immunofluorescent staining revealed that these cells stain positive for CD31 and von Willebrand factors, and negative for smooth muscle alpha-actin. Since human myocardium encompasses specific lineages of lymphatic and blood capillaries, HCMECs comprise cardiac-derived lymphatic and blood microvascular endothelial cells. They serve as an essential model for *in-vitro* studies on medical conditions associated with human cardiac microvascular endothelial dysfunction. To mention, a recent study evaluated the potential cardiotoxicity of two anti-cancer drugs: Herceptin and Doxorubicin on non-cardiomyocytes, by quantifying tight junction formation and zona occludens-1 (ZO1) expression in HCMECs [73]. Their results reveal that these two drugs stimulate barrier perturbation and suppress barrier function in HCMECs, ultimately improving drug permeability. HCMECs also reflected detectable levels of HER2 when compared with dermal and brain HMECs, suggesting that Herceptin binding to HER2 in HCMECs may probably interfere with tight junction formation and ZO1 expression.

Human Pulmonary Microvascular Endothelial Cells

Human Pulmonary Microvascular Endothelial Cells (HPMEC) are primary adherent cells isolated from human lungs (pulmonary endothelium) from a single donor [74]. Biomarker analysis by immunofluorescent staining revealed that these cells stain positive for CD31 and von Willebrand factors, and stain negative for smooth muscle alpha-actin. Since human lungs encompass specific lineages of lymphatic and blood capillaries, HPMECs comprise lung-derived lymphatic and blood microvascular endothelial cells. They serve as an essential model for *in-vitro* studies on medical conditions associated with human pulmonary microvascular endothelial dysfunction. For instance, a recent study investigated the anti-proliferative effects of a potent BET (Bromodomain and Extra-Terminal Protein) inhibitor on primary HPMECs derived from healthy volunteers [75]. Their results reflected a significant decrease in mRNA and protein expression of IL6 and IL8s in JQ+ treated cells when compared with JQ1- (an inactive enantiomer) treated cells, with a concentration-dependent decrease in HPMEC proliferation in JQ+ treated cells. Their results suggest that BET inhibition reduces inflammation and remodeling, and hence qualifies as a prospective therapy for pulmonary arterial hypertension.

Human Dermal Microvascular Endothelial Cells

Human Dermal Microvascular Endothelial Cells (HDMEC) are primary adherent cells isolated from the human dermis (from different locations of adult skin and juvenile foreskin) from a single donor [76]. Biomarker analysis by immunofluorescent staining revealed that these cells stain positive for CD31 and von Willebrand factors, and negative for smooth muscle alpha-actin. Since human dermis encompasses specific lineages of lymphatic and blood capillaries, HDMECs comprise dermis-derived lymphatic and blood microvascular endothelial cells. They serve as an essential model for *in-vitro* studies on medical conditions associated with human dermal microvascular endothelial dysfunction. For example, a recent study explored the pathophysiological involvement of ET1 (Endothelin-1) and RhoA (a protein member of Rho GTPases) in hypertrophic scars and keloid formation using HDMECs [77]. Their results reflect that the expression level of ET1 in hypertrophic scars and keloids is comparatively higher than that in normal skin and mature scars. Their data also reveals that ET-1 secretion stimulates collagen synthesis and myofibroblast differentiation in cultured human dermal fibroblast cells through RhoA/Rho-kinase pathway, leading to hypertrophic scars and keloid formation.

CONCLUSION

Cardiovascular diseases is one of the leading causes of death worldwide. Many other complications such as diabetes, atherosclerosis, blood pressure, obesity and so on contribute to CVD. In recent times, many therapeutics formulations that are made from natural plant sources or herbal medicine contribute to the prevention and treatment of CVD. The current chapter reviews the different Indian therapeutic medicine and Chinese herbal medicine formulated for the treatment and prevention of CVD and its related diseases. It also briefly touches on the different cardiovascular cell lines used for the *in-vitro* evaluation of such natural and nature-derived therapeutics.

CONFLICT OF INTEREST

The authors declare that there is no conflict of interest.

ACKNOWLEDGEMENT

The authors acknowledge the Management of Rajalakshmi Engineering College, Chennai for their invaluable inputs.

REFERENCES

[1]   Scott J. Pathophysiology and biochemistry of cardiovascular disease. Curr Opin Genet Dev 2004; 14(3): 271-9.

[http://dx.doi.org/10.1016/j.gde.2004.04.012] [PMID: 15172670]

[2]   Yusuf S, Reddy S, Ôunpuu S, Anand S. Global burden of cardiovascular diseases: part I: general considerations, the epidemiologic transition, risk factors, and impact of urbanization. Circulation 2001; 104(22): 2746-53.
[http://dx.doi.org/10.1161/hc4601.099487] [PMID: 11723030]

[3]   Mendis S, Puska P, Norrving B. Global atlas on cardiovascular disease prevention and control. Geneva: World Health Organization 2011.

[4]   Schnall PL, Landsbergis PA, Baker D. Job strain and cardiovascular disease. Annu Rev Public Health 1994; 15(1): 381-411.
[http://dx.doi.org/10.1146/annurev.pu.15.050194.002121] [PMID: 8054091]

[5]   Moran AE, Forouzanfar MH, Roth GA, *et al.* Temporal trends in ischemic heart disease mortality in 21 world regions, 1980 to 2010: the Global Burden of Disease 2010 study. Circulation 2014; 129(14): 1483-92.
[http://dx.doi.org/10.1161/CIRCULATIONAHA.113.004042] [PMID: 24573352]

[6]   Highlander P, Shaw GP. Current pharmacotherapeutic concepts for the treatment of cardiovascular disease in diabetics. Ther Adv Cardiovasc Dis 2010; 4(1): 43-54.
[http://dx.doi.org/10.1177/1753944709354305] [PMID: 19965897]

[7]   Dokken BB. The pathophysiology of cardiovascular disease and diabetes: beyond blood pressure and lipids. Diabetes Spectr 2008; 21(3): 160-5.
[http://dx.doi.org/10.2337/diaspect.21.3.160]

[8]   Ravindran R, Sharma N, Roy S, *et al.* Interaction studies of Withania somnifera's key metabolite Withaferin A with different receptors associated with cardiovascular disease. Curr Comput Aided Drug Des 2015; 11(3): 212-21.
[http://dx.doi.org/10.2174/1573409912666151106115848] [PMID: 26548552]

[9]   Devi AJ, Ravindran R, Sankar M, Rajkumar J. Effect of ambrex (a herbal formulation) on oxidative stress in hyperlipidemic rats and differentiation of 3T3-L1 preadipocytes. Pharmacogn Mag 2014; 10(38): 165-71.
[http://dx.doi.org/10.4103/0973-1296.131030] [PMID: 24914283]

[10]   Ravindran R, Kumar S, Rajkumar J, *et al.* Inhibition of PKCβ Mediates Cardioprotective Activity of Ambrex against Isoproterenol-Induced Myocardial Necrosis: in vivo and in silico Studies. Biology and Medicine 2018 2018; 10(4): 442.
[http://dx.doi.org/10.4172/0974-8369.1000442]

[11]   Dadkar VN, Tahiliani RR, Jaguste VS, Damle VB, Dhar HL. Double blind comparative trial of Abana and methyldopa for monotherapy of hypertension in Indian patients. Jpn Heart J 1990; 31(2): 193-9.
[http://dx.doi.org/10.1536/ihj.31.193] [PMID: 2192099]

[12]   Sasikumar CS, Devi CS. Protective effect of Abana®, a poly-herbal formulation, on isoproterenol-induced myocardial infarction in rats. Indian J Pharmacol 2000; 32(3): 198-201.

[13]   Thatte MS, Doshi BS, Kulkarni RD. Effect of Abana on beta-receptors. Indian Drugs 1986; 23: 598.

[14]   Antani JA, Kulkarni RD, Antani NJ. Effect of Abana on ventricular function in ischemic heart disease. Jpn Heart J 1990; 31(6): 829-35.
[http://dx.doi.org/10.1536/ihj.31.829] [PMID: 2084279]

[15]   Dubey GP, Agrawal A, Udupa KN. Prevention and management of coronary heart disease by an indigenous compound Abana. Antiseptic 1989; 86(9): 486.

[16]   Lal U, Tripathi S, Jachak S, *et al.* HPLC analysis and standardization of Arjunarishta–an Ayurvedic Cardioprotective formulation. Sci Pharm 2009; 77(3): 605-16.
[http://dx.doi.org/10.3797/scipharm.0906-03]

[17]   Pharmacopoeial standards of Ayurvedic formulations by CCRAS Government of India, Ministry of

Health and family Planning. Revised edition. New Delhi: Department of Health 1987; pp. 1-20.

[18] Dwivedi S. Terminalia arjuna Wight & Arn.--a useful drug for cardiovascular disorders. J Ethnopharmacol 2007; 114(2): 114-29.
[http://dx.doi.org/10.1016/j.jep.2007.08.003] [PMID: 17875376]

[19] Gauthaman K, Banerjee SK, Dinda AK, Ghosh CC, Maulik SK. Terminalia arjuna (Roxb.) protects rabbit heart against ischemic-reperfusion injury: role of antioxidant enzymes and heat shock protein. J Ethnopharmacol 2005; 96(3): 403-9.
[http://dx.doi.org/10.1016/j.jep.2004.08.040] [PMID: 15619558]

[20] Suchalatha S, Thirugnanasambandam P, Maheswaran E, *et al.* Role of Arogh, a polyherbal formulation to mitigate oxidative stress in experimental myocardial infarction 2004.

[21] Suchalatha S, Shyamala Devi CS. Effect of arogh-A polyherbal formulation on the marker enzymes in isoproterenol induced myocardial injury. Indian J Clin Biochem 2004; 19(2): 184-9.
[http://dx.doi.org/10.1007/BF02894283] [PMID: 23105482]

[22] Austin A, Senthilvel G, Thirugnanasambantham P, *et al.* Clinical efficacy of a Polyherbal Instant Formulation (Arogh) in the management of Hyperlipidaemia. Cardiol 2006; 2(2): 36-8.

[23] Tripathi YB, Reddy MM, Pandey RS, *et al.* Anti-inflammatory properties of BHUx, a polyherbal formulation to prevent atherosclerosis. Inflammopharmacology 2004; 12(2): 131-52.
[http://dx.doi.org/10.1163/1568560041352301] [PMID: 15265316]

[24] Tripathi YB, Singh BK, Pandey RS, Kumar M. BHUx: a patent polyherbal formulation to prevent atherosclerosis. Evid Based Complement Alternat Med 2005; 2(2): 217-21.
[http://dx.doi.org/10.1093/ecam/neh095] [PMID: 15937563]

[25] Tripathi YB. BHUx: a patented polyherbal formulation to prevent hyperlipidemia and atherosclerosis. Recent Pat Inflamm Allergy Drug Discov 2009; 3(1): 49-57.
[http://dx.doi.org/10.2174/187221309787158443] [PMID: 19149746]

[26] Koti BC, Vishwanathswamy AH, Wagawade J, *et al.* Cardioprotective effect of lipistat against doxorubicin induced myocardial toxicity in albino rats. 2009.

[27] Singh N, Kapur KK, Singh SP, Shanker K, Sinha JN, Kohli RP. Mechanism of cardiovascular action of Terminalia arjuna. Planta Med 1982; 45(2): 102-4.
[http://dx.doi.org/10.1055/s-2007-971255] [PMID: 7111479]

[28] Tripathi YB, Tripathi P, Upadhyay BN. Assessment of the adrenergic beta-blocking activity of Inula racemosa. J Ethnopharmacol 1988; 23(1): 3-9.
[http://dx.doi.org/10.1016/0378-8741(88)90109-2] [PMID: 2901513]

[29] Satyavati GV. Guggulipid: a promising hypolipidaemic agent from gum guggul (Commiphora wightii) 1991.

[30] Seth SD, Maulik M, Katiyar CK, Maulik SK. Role of Lipistat in protection against isoproterenol induced myocardial necrosis in rats: a biochemical and histopathological study. Indian J Physiol Pharmacol 1998; 42(1): 101-6.
[PMID: 9513800]

[31] Mary NK, Shylesh BS, Babu BH, *et al.* Antioxidant and hypolipidaemic activity of a herbal formulation-Liposem. 2002.

[32] Prince PS, Suman S, Devika PT, Vaithianathan M. Cardioprotective effect of 'Marutham' a polyherbal formulation on isoproterenol induced myocardial infarction in Wistar rats. Fitoterapia 2008; 79(6): 433-8.
[http://dx.doi.org/10.1016/j.fitote.2008.01.009] [PMID: 18538507]

[33] Parasuraman S, Kumar E, Kumar A, Emerson S. Free radical scavenging property and diuretic effect of triglize, a polyherbal formulation in experimental models. J Pharmacol Pharmacother 2010; 1(1): 38-41.

[http://dx.doi.org/10.4103/0976-500X.64535] [PMID: 21808589]

[34]   http://macau.sell.everychina.com/p-94644622-bushen-kangle-capsule.html

[35]   Hoessel R, Leclerc S, Endicott JA, *et al.* Indirubin, the active constituent of a Chinese antileukaemia medicine, inhibits cyclin-dependent kinases. Nat Cell Biol 1999; 1(1): 60-7.
[http://dx.doi.org/10.1038/9035] [PMID: 10559866]

[36]   Xiao Z, Hao Y. From Danggui Longhui Wan to meisoindigo: experience in the treatment of chronic myelogenous leukemia in China. 2006.

[37]   Liu C, Huang Y. Chinese herbal medicine on cardiovascular diseases and the mechanisms of action. Front Pharmacol 2016; 7: 469.
[http://dx.doi.org/10.3389/fphar.2016.00469] [PMID: 27990122]

[38]   Wei YJ, Qi LW, Li P, Luo HW, Yi L, Sheng LH. Improved quality control method for Fufang Danshen preparations through simultaneous determination of phenolic acids, saponins and diterpenoid quinones by HPLC coupled with diode array and evaporative light scattering detectors. J Pharm Biomed Anal 2007; 45(5): 775-84.
[http://dx.doi.org/10.1016/j.jpba.2007.07.013] [PMID: 17720349]

[39]   Ren-an Q, Juan L, Chuyuan L, *et al.* Study of the protective mechanisms of Compound Danshen Tablet (Fufang Danshen Pian) against myocardial ischemia/reperfusion injury via the Akt-eNOS signaling pathway in rats. J Ethnopharmacol 2014; 156: 190-8.
[http://dx.doi.org/10.1016/j.jep.2014.08.023] [PMID: 25178948]

[40]   Zhou L, Zuo Z, Chow MS. Danshen: an overview of its chemistry, pharmacology, pharmacokinetics, and clinical use. J Clin Pharmacol 2005; 45(12): 1345-59.
[http://dx.doi.org/10.1177/0091270005282630] [PMID: 16291709]

[41]   Liu C, Huang Y. Chinese herbal medicine on cardiovascular diseases and the mechanisms of action. Front Pharmacol 2016; 7: 469.
[http://dx.doi.org/10.3389/fphar.2016.00469] [PMID: 27990122]

[42]   Xiong X, Wang P, Li X, Zhang Y. Shenqi pill, a traditional Chinese herbal formula, for the treatment of hypertension: A systematic review. Complement Ther Med 2015; 23(3): 484-93.
[http://dx.doi.org/10.1016/j.ctim.2015.04.008] [PMID: 26051584]

[43]   Wong WC, Lee A, Lam AT, *et al.* Effectiveness of a Chinese herbal medicine preparation in the treatment of cough in uncomplicated upper respiratory tract infection: a randomised double-blinded placebo-control trial. Cough 2006; 2(1): 5.
[http://dx.doi.org/10.1186/1745-9974-2-5] [PMID: 16790070]

[44]   Cheng N, Zhu J, Ding P. Clinical Effects and Safety of Zhi Sou San for Cough: A Meta-Analysis of Randomized Trials. Evidence-Based Complementary and Alternative Medicine. 2017.
[http://dx.doi.org/10.1155/2017/9436352]

[45]   Zhang B, Niu W, Xu D, *et al.* Oxymatrine prevents hypoxia- and monocrotaline-induced pulmonary hypertension in rats. Free Radic Biol Med 2014; 69: 198-207.
[http://dx.doi.org/10.1016/j.freeradbiomed.2014.01.013] [PMID: 24440469]

[46]   Ma S, Li X, Dong L, Zhu J, Zhang H, Jia Y. Protective effect of Sheng-Mai Yin, a traditional Chinese preparation, against doxorubicin-induced cardiac toxicity in rats. BMC Complement Altern Med 2016; 16(1): 61.
[http://dx.doi.org/10.1186/s12906-016-1037-9] [PMID: 26865364]

[47]   Bensky D, Barolet R. Chinese herbal medicine: formulas and strategies. Eastland Press 1990.

[48]   Yang XQ, Liu L, Ming SP, *et al.* Tian Wang Bu Xin Dan for Insomnia: A Systematic Review of Efficacy and Safety. Evidence-Based Complementary and Alternative Medicine. 2019.
[http://dx.doi.org/10.1155/2019/4260801]

[49]   Wu T, Harrison RA, Chen XY, *et al.* Tongxinluo (Tong xin luo or Tong□ xin□ luo) capsule for

unstable angina pectoris. Cochrane Database of Systematic Reviews 2006; (4):

[50]   Bu PL, Zhao XQ, Wang LL, Zhao YX, Li CB, Zhang Y. Tong-xin-luo capsule inhibits left ventricular remodeling in spontaneously hypertensive rats by enhancing PPAR-γ expression and suppressing NF-kappaB activity. Chin Med J (Engl) 2008; 121(2): 147-54.
[http://dx.doi.org/10.1097/00029330-200801020-00011] [PMID: 18272042]

[51]   Zhang L, Wu Y, Jia Z, Zhang Y, Shen HY, Wang XL. Protective effects of a compound herbal extract (Tong Xin Luo) on free fatty acid induced endothelial injury: implications of antioxidant system. BMC Complement Altern Med 2008; 8(1): 39.
[http://dx.doi.org/10.1186/1472-6882-8-39] [PMID: 18625049]

[52]   Wang X, Hu D, Dang S, *et al.* Effects of traditional Chinese medicine shensong yangxin capsules on heart rhythm and function in congestive heart failure patients with frequent ventricular premature complexes: A Randomized, double-blind, multicenter clinical trial. Chin Med J (Engl) 2017; 130(14): 1639-47.
[http://dx.doi.org/10.4103/0366-6999.209906] [PMID: 28685712]

[53]   Tanwar A, Thakur P, Chawla R, *et al.* Curative remedies for rheumatoid arthritis: herbal informatics approach for rational based selection of natural plant products. 2017.

[54]   Mashour NH, Lin GI, Frishman WH. Herbal medicine for the treatment of cardiovascular disease: clinical considerations. Arch Intern Med 1998; 158(20): 2225-34.
[http://dx.doi.org/10.1001/archinte.158.20.2225] [PMID: 9818802]

[55]   Sharma V, Sarkar IN. Bioinformatics opportunities for identification and study of medicinal plants. Brief Bioinform 2013; 14(2): 238-50.
[http://dx.doi.org/10.1093/bib/bbs021] [PMID: 22589384]

[56]   Nyola N, Jeyablan G, Kumawat M, *et al.* Pharmacoinformatics: A tool for drug discovery. Am J Pharm Tech Res. 2012; 2.(3)

[57]   Gundaram M. Pharmacoinformatics in modern drug discovery. Research and Reviews: Journal of Pharmaceutics and Nanotechnology 2016; 1-8.

[58]   Neoh CF, Zainal IN, Hameed MA, *et al.* Development and progress of pharmacoinformatics in pharmaceutical and health sciences. Journal of Young Pharmacists 2015; 7(3): 155.
[http://dx.doi.org/10.5530/jyp.2015.3.4]

[59]   Tanaka T, Oka T, Shimada Y, *et al.* Pharmacogenomics of cardiovascular pharmacology: pharmacogenomic network of cardiovascular disease models. J Pharmacol Sci 2008; 107(1): 8-14.
[http://dx.doi.org/10.1254/jphs.08R03FM] [PMID: 18490853]

[60]   Munawar S, Windley MJ, Tse EG, *et al.* Experimentally validated pharmacoinformatics approach to predict hERG inhibition potential of new chemical entities. Front Pharmacol 2018; 9: 1035.
[http://dx.doi.org/10.3389/fphar.2018.01035] [PMID: 30333745]

[61]   Welsh WJ, Tong W, Georgopoulos PG. Toxicoinformatics: An Introduction. Computational Toxicology: Risk Assessment for Pharmaceutical and Environmental Chemicals 2007; 15: 151-81.
[http://dx.doi.org/10.1002/9780470145890.ch6]

[62]   Vijay LS, Shrasti G, Priya V. Toxic Informatics: study of natural ligand for new disease era. Journal of environmental science, toxicology and food technology 2014; 8(2): 57-62.

[63]   Braga RC, Alves VM, Silva MF, *et al.* Pred-hERG: A Novel web-Accessible Computational Tool for Predicting Cardiac Toxicity. Mol Inform 2015; 34(10): 698-701.
[http://dx.doi.org/10.1002/minf.201500040] [PMID: 27490970]

[64]   Frid AA, Matthews EJ. Prediction of drug-related cardiac adverse effects in humans--B: use of QSAR programs for early detection of drug-induced cardiac toxicities. Regul Toxicol Pharmacol 2010; 56(3): 276-89.
[http://dx.doi.org/10.1016/j.yrtph.2009.11.005] [PMID: 19941924]

[65]   https://www.promocell.com/product/human-cardiac-myocytes-hcm/

[66]   https://www.promocell.com/product/human-aortic-endothelial-cells-haoec/

[67]   Touat-Hamici Z, Weidmann H, Blum Y, *et al.* Role of lipid phosphate phosphatase 3 in human aortic endothelial cell function. Cardiovasc Res 2016; 112(3): 702-13.
       [http://dx.doi.org/10.1093/cvr/cvw217] [PMID: 27694435]

[68]   https://www.promocell.com/product/human-coronary-artery-endothelial-cells-hcaec/

[69]   Chua SK, Shyu KG, Lin YF, *et al.* Tumor necrosis factor-alpha and the ERK pathway drive chemerin expression in response to hypoxia in cultured human coronary artery endothelial cells. PLoS One 2016; 11(10)e0165613
       [http://dx.doi.org/10.1371/journal.pone.0165613] [PMID: 27792771]

[70]   https://www.promocell.com/product/human-pulmonary-artery-endothelial-cells-hpaec/

[71]   Schuoler C, Haider TJ, Leuenberger C, *et al.* Aquaporin 1 controls the functional phenotype of pulmonary smooth muscle cells in hypoxia-induced pulmonary hypertension. Basic Res Cardiol 2017; 112(3): 30.
       [http://dx.doi.org/10.1007/s00395-017-0620-7] [PMID: 28409279]

[72]   https://www.promocell.com/product/human-cardiac-microvascular-endothelial-cells-hcmec/

[73]   Wilkinson EL, Sidaway JE, Cross MJ. Cardiotoxic drugs Herceptin and doxorubicin inhibit cardiac microvascular endothelial cell barrier formation resulting in increased drug permeability. Biol Open 2016; 5(10): 1362-70.
       [http://dx.doi.org/10.1242/bio.020362] [PMID: 27543060]

[74]   https://www.promocell.com/product/human-pulmonary-microvascular-endothelial-cells-hpmec/

[75]   Mumby S, Gambaryan N, Meng C, *et al.* Bromodomain and extra-terminal protein mimic JQ1 decreases inflammation in human vascular endothelial cells: Implications for pulmonary arterial hypertension. Respirology 2017; 22(1): 157-64.
       [http://dx.doi.org/10.1111/resp.12872] [PMID: 27539364]

[76]   https://www.promocell.com/product/human-dermal-microvascular-endothelial-cells-hdmec/

[77]   Kiya K, Kubo T, Kawai K, *et al.* Endothelial cell-derived endothelin-1 is involved in abnormal scar formation by dermal fibroblasts through RhoA/Rho-kinase pathway. Exp Dermatol 2017; 26(8): 705-12.
       [http://dx.doi.org/10.1111/exd.13264] [PMID: 27892645]

CHAPTER 7

Cardiovascular Disease: A Systems Biology Approach

Sujata Roy[*] and **Ashasmita S Mishra**

Department of Biotechnology, Rajalakshmi Engineering College, Rajalakshmi Nagar, Thandalam, Chennai-602105, Tamil Nadu, India

Abstract: In the post-genomic era, the main challenge is to extract meaningful and valuable information from a large pool of data generated by high throughput techniques like microarray and deep sequencing techniques. Systems biology is an emerging discipline that aids in interpreting a large amount of biological data in a meaningful way. It helps to draw significant inference from a large amount of data about the interactions of genes or proteins, by developing quantitative mathematical models. Due to its complex nature, cardiovascular diseases can be better understood using the systems biology concept. Different components of the disease like heart failure and coronary artery disease can be comprehended in a modular fashion, wherein each module consists of multiple genes and their nonlinear interactions. Another approach is population genetics or Genome-Wide Association Studies (GWAS), which has identified over two hundred chromosomal loci that modulate the risk of cardiovascular diseases. These GWAS variation data can be integrated with multi-omics data and gene network data to identify the susceptible pathways, modules and genotyping cause behind it. Identification of a hub gene in a network is one of the main approaches of research in systems biology of cardiovascular diseases. This hub gene can serve as a biomarker for early detection or therapeutic targets. Comorbidities are another cause of increased risk leading to further complications in patients with cardiovascular diseases. Analysis of association of the comorbidities, using a system biology approach, focuses on the prevention of severe vascular events. The most common comorbidities include diabetes, kidney disease, peripheral arterial disease, *etc*. Systems biology can aid in identifying special biomarkers for early diagnosis of cardiovascular comorbidities and the following careful management might lead to prolonged survival of the patient.

Keywords: Bioinformatics, Cardiovascular Diseases, Data analysis, Disease comorbidities, Genome-wide association studies, Integrated omics, Network Biology, Network Medicine, Systems Biology.

[*] **Corresponding author Sujata Roy:** Department of Biotechnology, Rajalakshmi Engineering College, Rajalakshmi Nagar, Thandalam, Chennai-602105, Tamil Nadu, India; E-mail: sujataroy@rajalakshmi.edu.in

Atta-ur-Rahman & M. Iqbal Choudhary (Eds.)

INTRODUCTION

Cardiovascular diseases (CVD) are the leading cause of death worldwide, mostly in low and middle-income countries. Despite the increasing economic and social burden of the disease, there is no proper understanding of its underlying mechanism. The Oslerian model is one of the old models in medical practice. According to this model, the presence of a given disease was identified by the anatomical abnormalities in organs and tissues. This practice has been evolved and improved over the last 100 years by methods of adopting a reductionist approach. This approach focuses on the individual analysis of the functional components of an organism. The cardiovascular disease is diversified in origin with a variety of biologically functional components. It can be defined by the presence of a cluster of cardiovascular risk factors, inflammatory changes to the vascular tissue, and development of the atherothrombotic process. The atherothrombotic process includes both atherosclerosis and its thrombotic complications. Atherosclerosis alone is a complex disease, caused by the combination of different facts like an aggregation of inflammatory cells and fibrous tissue in the wall of arteries.

Cell-based Cardiac Disease Models and Animal Models

The aim of the reductionist approach was to define the individual basic units like the genes and pathways of the entire system by eliminating the complexity of it. But at the same time, simply focusing on the individual gene or pathway is not enough in comprehending the whole biological system in disease and health condition. The integration of multigene and multi pathways is the key process in understanding the system. In this context, cell culture-based systems and animal disease models play a major role to model the pathology observed in a patient. High-throughput technologies like microarray and next-gen sequencing technologies generate multifaceted data of these model systems. There is a need for analysis of integrated genomics, transcriptomics and proteomics for those model systems.

Different types of cells that contribute to the normal functioning of the heart are cardiac fibroblasts, endothelial cells, cardiomyocytes or vascular smooth muscle cells, among which the cardiac myocytes play a major role. Isolated primary neonatal cardiomyocytes from mice and rats are considered as excellent sources for differential gene expression studies. Reprogrammed embryonic stem cells (ESC) such as induced pluripotent stem cells (iPSCs) and engineered heart tissues (EHTs)/human cardiac organoids (hCOs) are used to generate cardiomyocytes [1 - 3]. Similarly, the use of zebrafish (*Danio rerio*) and large mammalian animal models has significantly contributed to the understanding of the disease pathogenesis of cardiovascular disease in human beings. The high throughput data generated as outcomes from the high throughput experiments carried out in these model systems are the key resource of the data. Those data are analyzed using a series of bioinformatics tools or protocols which is called systems biology approach. This systems biology protocol leads to the development of diagnostic strategy and targeted therapies for human cardiovascular diseases.

Table 1. Clinical understanding of chronic cardiac diseases with reductionism (Louridas *et al.*).

Medical Applications	Reductionism's Objectives	Systems Biology Holistic Strategy
Clinical focus	Isolated clinical parameters	Interactions between components, like molecules, networks
Prevention	Isolated culprit molecular and environmental parameters	As an entity the whole range of culpable variables
Diagnosis	Isolated molecules, biomarkers, signs, symptoms	The patient as a "diseased person"
Therapy	Treating causes and symptoms	Treating the patient from a holistic perspective

Post-genomic Era and Systems Biology Concept

Before the genomic era, a biological system was comprehended using a reductionist approach, an approach that believes in understanding complex things by dissecting them into simpler constituents. The molecular biology technique facilitates the studying of the composition, structure, and interactions of essential cellular molecules such as nucleic acids and proteins. Systems biology is not only just a combination of these molecular parts it may have something greater than that. A typical system-based study comprises the following five steps.

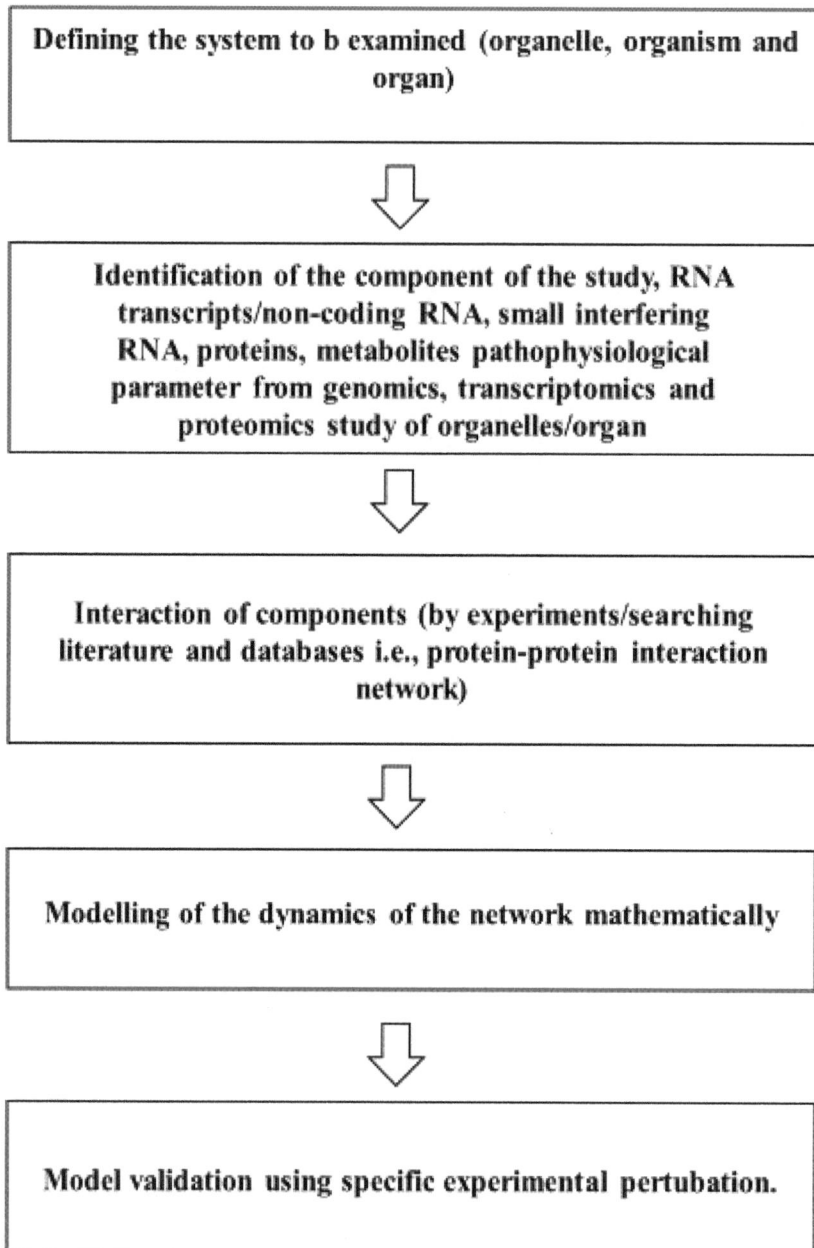

Fig. (1). Flow chart of system-based study.

The high-throughput data by advanced technical and scientific experiments is easily accessible to scientists and data analytics to understand the functioning of a cell. List of experiments that involve high-throughput technologies in biology to produce whole genome, epigenome, proteome and transcriptome data is shown in Table **2**. These integrated multi-omics data help the researcher to understand the clinical condition in both normal and diseased state of cardiovascular disease.

Table 2. List of experiments are required for system-based study (MacLellan *et al.*).

Assessed Parameter	Technique
DNA sequence/Exome sequence	NGS
DNA methylation	Microarrays, bisulfite treatment followed by NGS
Chromatin states	Chip followed by Sequencing
Transcriptome	Gene expression arrays and high throughput RNA sequencing
Levels of microRNAs	Microarrays and quantitative PCR or NGS
Protein levels	LC-MS
Protein-Protein interaction	Co-immunoprecipitation followed by LC-MS
Metabolite levels and	LC-MS NMR imaging
Microbiome (gut and others)	PCR of ribosomal RNA regions followed by NGS
Cellular process and	Imaging with a receptor system
Clinical phenotype (*in-vivo* studies)	Imaging, multiplex immunoassays

Cardiovascular disease or chronic heart failure is the outcome of several disorder states such as hypertension, ischemic heart or vascular defects. These states share several features like impaired Ca^{2+}-handling, altered energy metabolism, *etc*. Each feature reflects functional changes in specific subcellular organelles such as sarcoplasmic reticulum, sarcomeres, and mitochondria. The coordination of the features of organelles defines its physiology whereas its dis-coordination results in pathology.

Genomics and transcriptomics data produce an extensive list of differentially expressed genes that can be linked to different associated features like Ca^{2+}-handling, altered energy metabolism in diseased and normal cells. However, genes and their functions fail to explain the functional complexity of a whole organ or organism, whereas the proteomics study help in identifying the role of multiple proteins and how or whether their modifications relate to cardiac cellular phenotypes. Systems biology integrates the study of organelle genome, transcriptome, and proteome, thereby leading to the analysis of both the physiology and pathophysiological condition.

SYSTEMS BIOLOGY

What is a Network and How to Construct?

The multi-omics data finds its wide use in understanding various biological systems in a holistic manner. A systems biology approach is the construction of a network among molecular entities. The networks are made up of nodes, which represent molecular entities (such as DNA variations, RNA, proteins, and metabolites), and edges that represent the relationships between these entities. Analysis of this network helps in identifying any feedback mechanism and gene regulatory mechanism of the biological system. The topological characteristics and statistical properties, leading to the inference of functional roles played by the nodes in the network, represent the state of the molecular entities over time. Network biology captures the emergent properties of the system such as the multistability and robustness to perturbation [4 - 8].

There are two approaches in network analysis *viz.*, a) *ad hoc* network construction and b) pathway analysis. From the gene expression data, two genes are clustered/connected if the similarity between their expressions profiles is above a threshold value, the threshold is chosen by *ad hoc* manner. The pathway approach is much more straightforward to interpret but its limitation lies in the fact that it can recognize the pathways/biological processes and functions which already exist in the databases. On the other hand, the *ad hoc* approach is very challenging and has greater potential in the identification of novel pathways. Both approaches are useful for analyzing expression data applicable to a complex disease such as cardiovascular disease, although they have complementary advantages and limitations.

From Network to Modules and Models

After the construction of the gene network, it becomes the problem of graph theory. In graph theory, a clustering coefficient is a measure of the degree to which nodes in a graph tend to cluster together. Cliquishness measures the local cohesiveness of a network. If a node has k neighbors, at most $k(k-1)/2$ edges can exist between these neighbors. The clustering coefficient for a node is the fraction of the allowed number of edges that exist around the node, whereas, for a network, it is the average of the clustering coefficients of all nodes. A high clustering coefficient is the signature of a network's modularity. Modularity refers to a group of physically or functionally linked molecules (nodes) that work together to achieve a distinct function such as a transcriptional module, signaling pathway, *etc.*

A clinical phenotype correlates biochemical and genetic parameters with clinical behavioral traits. The clinical phenotype can be extrapolated to the molecular entities such as DNA, protein or to a network level. The network concept can be applied to the domain of clinical cardiology where the interacting networks can be considered as modules or phenotypes. The impact of network thinking in clinical cardiology is crucial in order to understand and describe the condition of heart failure (HF), coronary artery disease (CAD) and its progressive nature. The complexity of these diseases can be explained by this network approach where various unrelated biological/molecular entities are integrated in a hierarchical manner from networks to modules and then onto models [9, 10].

Here, we have analyzed a microarray data. A 9 week old, LDLR-/- (Low-density lipoprotein receptor (*LDLR*) deficient mouse was used for hyperlipidemia and atherosclerosis research. It was put on a sucrose-enriched high-fat diet (HFSC) for up to 20 weeks. Their respective controls were kept on a normal chow diet (NC) for up to 20 weeks. After sacrificing the gonadal white adipose tissue (GWAT) from LDLR-/-animals on NC (6 Samples) or HFSC (6 Sample) was collected. Microarray has been analyzed using platform GPL16570. In Fig. (**2**), the gene network has been analyzed for this GEO data from the GSE76812 series.

NC is the control and HFSC is the case, the co-expressed gene network in both the cases have been analyzed with the 5 candidate genes associated with cardiovascular disease like APOB, SCN5A, TGFb1, JDP2, and Oxtr. Different R packages like "geneRecommender", "minet" and "igraph" have been used to generate a co-expressed gene network and compared. The distance between the nodes indicates the betweenness centrality parameter of the nodes of the network. High betweenness has been found in the case of long non-coding RNA (lncRNA) Malat1 and a protein-coding gene hnRNPAB (heterogeneous nuclear ribonucleoprotein A/B). Li Zhang et al in 2017 have published the novel pathological role of hnRNPA1 (Heterogeneous Nuclear Ribonucleoprotein A1) in vascular smooth muscle cell function. Thus, network biology enhances our understanding of the disease condition and identifies new entity related to disease [11]. In 2019, one experimental result has been published on the role of Malat1 in cardiac fibrosis.

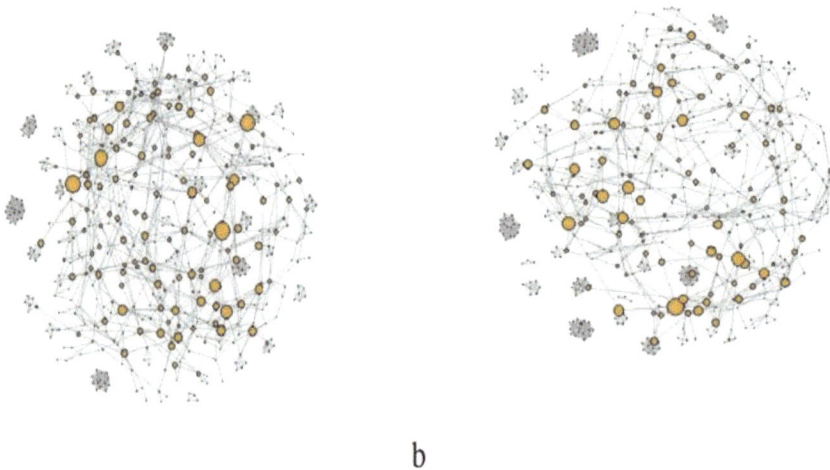

a   b

Fig. (2). A sample Gene network of GEO data, GSE76812 series. The network of co-expressed genes with five genes (APOB, SCN5A, TGFb1, JDP2 and Oxtr) associated with cardiovascular disease in a) white adipose tissue at sucrose-enriched high-fat diet. B) on a normal chow diet.

SYSTEMS GENETICS

Genomic Study and Genome-wide Association in Cardiovascular Traits

Genome-wide association study (GWAS) scans the whole genome of different individuals to see if any genetic variants are associated with the traits. Enormous studies have been conducted in understanding the genetics of cardiovascular disease. Among many thousands of variations, only a few scans contribute to disease susceptibility. The basic concept of 'systems genetics' is to establish a relation between clinical phenotype and the variations at the molecular levels (for example, mRNA, protein, or metabolite levels). The genomic regions which are associated with the expression levels/transcripts levels are termed as expression quantitative trait loci (eQTLs). In another way, it can be explained as dense single-nucleotide polymorphism (SNP) map of the DNA that explains variation in expression levels of mRNAs. For example, in several GWAS studies, it has been observed that a novel genetic locus of chromosome 1 is strongly associated with the regulation of LDL-cholesterol levels [12]. A combination of eQTL and GWAS data allows in identifying candidate causal genes. In this way through a series of studies in mice and human cohorts, the researchers have identified *SORT1* as the causal gene at the 1p13 locus which influences low-density lipoprotein cholesterol (LDL-C) and myocardial infarction (MI). In recent studies, it has been reported that *SORT1* overexpression decreased VLDL and apolipoprotein B secretion [12]. eQTL experiments require whole transcriptome profiling. The co-expressed gene network and expression module can be derived from the transcriptomic data. The gene with many network connections explains as hub genes or causal genes. The GWAS results give the picture of association of multiple genes and their variations with the disease using SNP set enrichment analysis [13-15]. The combination of GWAS results with a co-expressed gene network identifies causal genes. System genetics require further research [13-15]. The upcoming research needs to address the following questions like 1) to which extent do the interactions of specific loci contribute to the heritability of the disease, 2) which all non-coding regions elucidate molecular mechanism that affects the risk of the disease and 3) how can the treatment strategy be improved by the acquired knowledge.

SYSTEMS MEDICINE

Integrative Biology

Diseases are an interplay of genes. The crosstalk between the genes and their protein product leads to the interconnectivity between diseases and disease networks. These networks help to identify the proteins interacting with other proteins and their association with the diseases. It also helps in a better understanding of the localization, expression, and function of the associated gene. Such networks shall lead to the prediction of new disease-causing genes. A thorough analysis and evaluation of these biological/disease networks lead to the rise of the concept of network medicine. An amalgamation of integrative biology and a system-based approach would lead to the prediction of new target genes. Identification of novel modules in disease networks leads to the design of novel therapies that would have been otherwise not possible through the reductionist or molecular approach. The system-based approach is preferred over the traditional genetic approach due to the former's potential to identify novel biological disease networks [16].

Any perturbation in the biological network leads to the diseased condition and this forms the underlying concept of network medicine. Barabasi and his collaborators were the first ones to build a human disease network, wherein they used known genetic mutations as edges to link the disease nodes sharing the same mutation. This network had many interesting features and led to some unexpected findings. One of the inclusive features was that many human diseases were clustered in a single component in the network. This feature suggests that there is a common underlying mechanism of a diversified collection of diseases that involves certain abnormalities in a critical specific subset of genes. This network also suggests, unexpectedly, that most of the disease-causing genes are non-essential and do not necessarily encode hub proteins.

Network medicine has begun to penetrate and permeate the commercial field of biotechnology. In no sooner than near future, a better widespread expansion of network methodology can be seen in the field of biomedicine. For example in-network pharmacology, a study was conducted on Traditional Chinese Medicinal (TCM) formula called Compound Danshen Formula (CDF). CDF has been known to be extensively used in the treatment of CVD, but the actual underlying mechanism of function was unknown. Recently, research studies were carried out at a systemic point in order to analyze the pharmacological effect of CDF on CVDs. For the first time, Xiuxiu Li *et al.* came up with a completely new modeling system that combines oral bioavailability screening, multiple drug targets prediction and its validation, and network pharmacology to probe efficiency of the proposed TCM recipe for CVD treatment [17]. The result of this study suggested that *Radix Salvia Miltiorrhizae* (the root of *Salvia Miltiorrhizae*) is the emperor in this formula, whereas *Panax notoginseng* and *Borneolum* could serve as minister and courier drugs. This not only gives a better understanding of the mechanism of CDF but also provides significant insight into the system medicine. The traditional Indian medicine, Ayurveda, also has many medicinal formulae, that could be explored with further investigation and can be evolved by a system medicinal approach.

DISEASE COMORBITIES AND NETWORK BIOLOGY

Comorbidity is the occurrence of two or more diseases in a person at the same time. Comorbidity has been known to be associated with increased mortality rates and decreased quality of life. In order to establish an association between CVD and comorbidities, a recent study was conducted. Findings suggested strong associations of coronary artery disease and hypertension with diabetes, whereas the strongest association of CVD existed with epilepsy and arrhythmia. Thorough knowledge of the associations can lead to proper management in the primary care of the patients having both the diseases. It is evident that diseases are significantly connected than mere random comorbidities that are driven by molecular interactions. There is a need for a new drug discovery strategy to control such cases. Recently, an attempt was made by Khader Shameer *et al.* [18], in order to target the comorbidities and the disease risk of peripheral artery disease (PAD) by combining concepts of network biology and computational drug repositioning. Disciplines of network pharmacology, network biology, and systems medicine offer significant insights into the biological area to decipher interconnected molecular crosstalk to discover therapies [20]. Their analysis can be classified into four parts: i) risk factor identification and the comorbidities associated with PAD, ii) canonical disease-gene network generation, iii) functional interpretation and their analysis of the biological network and iv) repositioning of the drug using computational strategies to detect compounds capable in disrupting the molecular core sub-network.

In order to derive a disease-gene network, they selected the Gene Prospector database as the source. This database contains information regarding disease-causing genes, the risk factors involved and the relevant phenotypes. For example, a query of PAD retrieved X genes and a query using the comorbid condition chronic kidney disorder retrieved Y genes, they hypothesized that insights regarding functional cues with respect to the associated comorbidities could be derived from the functional modules and pathways enriched among the genes in the intersection of two derived gene lists (X and Y). This canonical gene list that corresponded to the molecular core module was further used to find out drugs that could showcase agonistic and antagonistic effects for any perturbations. Following, the gene list to drug matching was carried using the Chemo-Genomic Enrichment Analyses (CGEA) approach and further then, the compounds were annotated in conjunction with RepurposeDB (http://repurposedb.dudleylab.org) [19, 20]. References resource databases like RepurposeDB (http://repurpo sedb.dudleylab.org/), Connectivity Map Cmap (https://portals.broadinstitute.org/ cmap/), Genomics of Drug Sensitivity in Cancer GDSC (http://www.cancer rxgene.org/) or Cancer Cell Line Encyclopedia CCLE (https://portals. broadinstitute.org/ccle) are used to identify compounds that concordantly modulate the query signature in a direction "towards" or "away" from the query state. Then, a ranked list of candidate compounds is retrieved as an output of this analysis which may potentially be responsible to modulate a biological state of interest.

While the emergent multiple novel therapeutic strategies in the field of CVD, including loss-of-function based therapies and PCSK9 inhibitors, have made a significant contribution, the precise modulation of classical pathways and the systemic control of lipid homeostasis have ample scope in improving the optimal outcomes in patients. A network biology approach in drug repositioning strategy found already existing drugs like doxazosin, midodrine, and nadolol as top candidate drugs. The findings have been consistent with the previous therapeutic conditions associated with PAD and drugs having anti-inflammatory activities like felbinac has been ranked in the list of repurposed drugs that can modulate molecular core driven risk factors and PAD associated comorbidities. Other potential agents, capable of targeting the disease risk trajectories and comorbidities are antibacterials (ceftazidime and vancomycin), antivirals (11cyclovir), and antifungals (natamycin). This discovery opens several avenues leading to the need for the precise control of infection, inflammation and certain immune responses in the early stages of the PAD in order to potentially save patients from long-term detrimental effects. It was also noted that a subnetwork motif composed of *APOB* (gene encoding for Apolipoprotein B located in chromosome 2), *APOE* (gene encoding for Apolipoprotein E) and *LDLR (*Low-Density Lipoprotein Receptor protein-encoding gene) was a consensus sequence found across various risk factors and comorbidities. Strategies involving the development of novel molecules that could monitor and target the above genes may lead to the discovery of novel cardiovascular therapies.

TOOLS AND DATABASES

Public Data Sources, Prior Knowledge, and Data Integration

Prior knowledge resources are the basis for further analysis. The availability of the existing and newly generated data increases the scope of system medicine research. Even though data integration is a challenge, many of the algorithms and approaches mentioned below have already been proposed and/or applied in the field of cardiovascular diseases. Large consortia have collected and maintained cohorts of matching clinical patient, animal model, omics data (*TCGA; GEO,* and ArrayExpress) and of cell line profiles (CCLE, and LINCS). Available data include sequencing data for genomics and transcriptomics, microarray mRNA, miRNA data, and mass spectrometry data for proteomic analyses along with many other "omics" data types. Table **3** lists several well-known public omics data repositories.

Table 3. Overview of publicly available omics data resources (Kramer *et al.*).

Name	Description	URL
1000 Genomes project	Sequence Variation Data	http://www.1000genomes.org
Array Express	Functional Genomics Data	https://www.ebi.ac.uk/arrayexpress
GEO Gene Expression Omnibus	Functional Genomics Data and Tools for analysis	http://www.ncbi.nlm.nih.gov/geo
EBI Expression Atlas	Gene Expression patterns under different conditions after initial analysis	http://www.ebi.ac.uk/gxa
GXD, The Mouse Gene Expression Database	Collection of gene expression data for developmental biology	http://www.informatics.jax.org/expression.shtml
TCGA- The Cancer Genome Atlas	Multidimensional analysis of molecular characteristics in human cancer data	https://gdc.cancer.gov/
LINCS – The Library of Integrated Network Based Cellular Signatures	Network data of gene expression and other cellular processes upon perturbation	https://clue.io/

(Table 3) cont.....

Name	Description	URL
CCLE: The Cancer Cell Line Encyclopaedia	A compilation of gene expression, chromosomal copy number and sequencing data from human Cancer Cell Line	http://www.broadinstitute.org/ccle
PRIDE Proteomics IDEntification	Reposatory of proteomics data	https://www.ebi.ac.uk/pride/archive
COPaKB	Proteome Biology Platform specifically for Cardiovascular Disease	http://www.heartproteome.org

A large amount of data is available in different databases on gene, protein, pathways, and molecular interactions. The list of databases is tabulated in Table **4**.

Table 4. Overview of databases containing biomedical knowledge (Kramer *et al.*).

Name	Description	URL
Molecular Information		
GenBank	DNA sequence database	http://www.ncbi.nlm.nih.gov/genbank/
UniProt	Composite database of protein with link to other relevant databases	http://www.uniprot.org/
Ensembl	A genome browser for genomics and transcriptomics study	http://www.ensembl.org/
Signaling Pathways		
Reactome	Network data repository integrated with cell line information	http://reactome.org/
NDEx – the Network Data Exchange	A genome browser for genomics and transcriptomics study	http://www.ensembl.org/
WikiPathways	A database of biological pathways	http://www.ndexbio.org/
Metabolic Pathways		
MetaCyc	Curated database of metabolic pathway from different organisms	http://metacyc.org
KEGG - Kyoto Encyclopedia of Genes and Genomes	Includes graphical diagrams and data of biochemical pathways	https://www.genome.jp/kegg/pathway.html
Protein-Protein Interaction		
IntAct Molecular interaction database	Open source database system with analysis tools of molecular interaction data	http://www.ebi.ac.uk/intact

(Table 4) cont.....

Name	Description	URL
Molecular Information		
STRING protein Protein interaction networks	Database of known and predicted protein-protein interactions	http://string-db.org
BioGRID – biological general repository for interaction datasets	Interaction repository	http://thebiogrid.org
Other Interaction Knowledge		
DrugBank	Information on approved and trial drugs and their targets with	http://www.drugbank.ca/
PharmGKB Pharmacogenetics	Database on Pharmacogenetic studies	http://www.pharmgkb.org/
Knowledge Base		
DiseaseConnect	Webserver for visualization and comprehensive analysis of disease mechanism	http://disease-connect.org/
OMIM – Online Mendelian Inheritance in Man	A comprehensive knowledge base of human genes and genetic disorders compiled to support human genetics research and education.	http://www.ncbi.nlm.nih.gov/omim/

Many of these databases can be integrated using different software packages like R, BioPAX-ontology, Systems Biology Markup Language (SBML), *etc*. Those packages are listed in Table **5**.

Table 5. Overview of standards and tools for encoding and working with pathway knowledge (Kramer *et al.*).

Name	Description	Software Tools
R studio	Statistical framework	Different packages like Bioconductor
BioPax	A standard language that aims to visualize and analyze the biological pathway data	Biopax Paxtools
SMBL- The Systems Biology Markup Languages	An XML based format for storing and Communicating Computational Models of Biological Pathways and Processes	LibSBML
SBGN-The Systems Biology Graphical Notations	A visual language to encode the relationship between different molecular entities	LibSBGN

(Table 5) cont.....

Name	Description	Software Tools
HUPO -PSI Molecular Interactions Format	A community standard data model for proteomics data that facilitate analysis, exchange and verifications	PSICQUIC
Cytoscape	An open-source platform for complex network analysis. CX data model for network exchange. It is designed for modularity and flexibility	Cytoscape

In combination with mapping services, for example, BioMart, these packages enable the integration and merging of prior knowledge for further analyses. Integrated omics have the potential to open new avenues in disease analysis, diagnostics, and drug discovery.

A large amount of biomedical knowledge is available from online databases. This ranges from genetic sequence information on GenBank to protein information on UniProt, and the various sites of knowledge on molecular interactions, many of which are collected on the Pathguide.org website, which currently enlists over 600 resources related to a biological pathway and interaction knowledge. The most prominent pathway databases are Reactome, the Network Data Exchange (NDEx), the Kyoto Encyclopedia of Genes and Genomes (KEGG), and WikiPathways as well as disease-specific databases such as the Online Mendelian Inheritance in Man (OMIM) resource. Databases focusing on molecular interactions include BioGRID, IntAct and STRING. Further knowledge sources include drug-target databases, which connect therapeutic and targeted proteins and disease-target databases, which contain diseases known to be associated with a specific mutation. Table **2** enlists several well-known databases containing knowledge about molecular interactions.

CONCLUSION

Biological components such as transcripts, proteins, and metabolites do not function alone in an isolated manner, rather they form networks. If the co-expressed gene networks are combined with the GWAS data of cardiovascular disease, a new causal gene can be identified which was earlier not known to have direct consequences. However, there are many challenges, *i.e.* **1)** translation of research into clinical relevance, **2)** big data handling and storage, **3)** biobanking: harmonization and standardization, **4)** ethical data protection and sharing issues and, **5)** communication in a multidisciplinary team. Different kinds of large omics data can be put together in a network context that enables pathophysiological understanding of the disease. Diagnostics have been evolved in such a manner that no more only a single entity is responsible, instead, a subnetwork can be considered as a biomarker or drug target. We are on the path to understanding the system medicine, as a formula, instead of only a single drug molecule. Investigation of complex changes, interactions in an interdisciplinary team, and integration of the industry into the system medicine workflow can be advantageous for translating the knowledge into clinical trials.

CONSENT FOR PUBLICATION

Not applicable.

CONFLICT OF INTEREST

The author declares that there is no conflict of interest in this chapter.

ACKNOWLEDGEMENTS

The authors are thankful to Mr. Nanda Gopal Saha, Head of Nutrigenomics Lab, Camillotek, India Pvt Ltd for encouraging to work on system medicine.

REFERENCES

[1]   Peter AK, Bjerke MA, Leinwand LA. Biology of the cardiac myocyte in heart disease. Mol Biol Cell 2016; 27(14): 2149-60.
        [http://dx.doi.org/10.1091/mbc.E16-01-0038] [PMID: 27418636]

[2]   Yoshida Y, Yamanaka S. Induced pluripotent stem cells 10 years later: for cardiac applications. Circ Res 2017; 120(12): 1958-68.
        [http://dx.doi.org/10.1161/CIRCRESAHA.117.311080] [PMID: 28596174]

[3]   Brandão KO, Tabel VA, Atsma DE, Mummery CL, Davis RP. Human pluripotent stem cell models of cardiac disease: from mechanisms to therapies. Dis Model Mech 2017; 10(9): 1039-59.
        [http://dx.doi.org/10.1242/dmm.030320] [PMID: 28883014]

[4]   Ramsey SA, Gold ES, Aderem A. A systems biology approach to understanding atherosclerosis. EMBO Mol Med 2010; 2(3): 79-89.
        [http://dx.doi.org/10.1002/emmm.201000063] [PMID: 20201031]

[5]   Evandro TM, Eduardo NS, Antonio José LJ. The paradigm of systems biology applied to cardiovascular diseases Int J of cardiac Sc 2015; 28: 78-86.

[6]   Louridas GE, Kanonidis IE, Lourida KG. Systems biology in heart diseases. Hippokratia 2010; 14(1): 10-6.
        [PMID: 20411053]

[7]   Kramer F, Just S, Zeller T. New perspectives: systems medicine in cardiovascular disease. BMC Syst Biol 2018; 12(1): 57.
        [http://dx.doi.org/10.1186/s12918-018-0579-5] [PMID: 29699591]

[8]   MacLellan WR, Wang Y, Lusis AJ. Systems-based approaches to cardiovascular disease. Nat Rev Cardiol 2012; 9(3): 172-84.
        [http://dx.doi.org/10.1038/nrcardio.2011.208] [PMID: 22231714]

[9]   Louridas GE, Lourida KG. Conceptual Foundations of Systems Biology Explaining Complex Cardiac Diseases. Healthcare (Basel) 2017; 5(1): 10.
        [http://dx.doi.org/10.3390/healthcare5010010] [PMID: 28230815]

[10]   Sperling SR. Systems biology approaches to heart development and congenital heart disease. Cardiovasc Res 2011; 91(2): 269-78.
[http://dx.doi.org/10.1093/cvr/cvr126] [PMID: 21527437]

[11]   Zhang L, Chen Q, An W, *et al.* Novel Pathological Role of hnRNPA1 (Heterogeneous Nuclear Ribonucleoprotein A1) in Vascular Smooth Muscle Cell Function and Neointima Hyperplasia. Arterioscler Thromb Vasc Biol 2017; 37(11): 2182-94.
[http://dx.doi.org/10.1161/ATVBAHA.117.310020] [PMID: 28912364]

[12]   Musunuru K, Strong A, Frank-Kamenetsky M, *et al.* From noncoding variant to phenotype *via* SORT1 at the 1p13 cholesterol locus. Nature 2010; 466(7307): 714-9.
[http://dx.doi.org/10.1038/nature09266] [PMID: 20686566]

[13]   Schunkert H, König IR, Kathiresan S, *et al.* Large-scale association analysis identifies 13 new susceptibility loci for coronary artery disease. Nat Genet 2011; 43(4): 333-8.
[http://dx.doi.org/10.1038/ng.784] [PMID: 21378990]

[14]   Romanoski CE, Lee S, Kim MJ, *et al.* Systems genetics analysis of gene-by-environment interactions in human cells. Am J Hum Genet 2010; 86(3): 399-410.
[http://dx.doi.org/10.1016/j.ajhg.2010.02.002] [PMID: 20170901]

[15]   Gargalovic PS, Imura M, Zhang B, *et al.* Identification of inflammatory gene modules based on variations of human endothelial cell responses to oxidized lipids. Proc Natl Acad Sci USA 2006; 103(34): 12741-6.
[http://dx.doi.org/10.1073/pnas.0605457103] [PMID: 16912112]

[16]   Goh KI, Cusick ME, Valle D, Childs B, Vidal M, Barabási AL. The human disease network. Proc Natl Acad Sci USA 2007; 104(21): 8685-90.
[http://dx.doi.org/10.1073/pnas.0701361104] [PMID: 17502601]

[17]   Li X, Xu X, Wang J, *et al.* A system-level investigation into the mechanisms of Chinese Traditional Medicine: Compound Danshen Formula for cardiovascular disease treatment. PLoS One 2012; 7(9)e43918
[http://dx.doi.org/10.1371/journal.pone.0043918] [PMID: 22962593]

[18]   Kendir C, van den Akker M, Vos R, Metsemakers J. Cardiovascular disease patients have increased risk for comorbidity: A cross-sectional study in the Netherlands. Eur J Gen Pract 2018; 24(1): 45-50.
[http://dx.doi.org/10.1080/13814788.2017.1398318] [PMID: 29168400]

[19]   Shameer K, Dow G, Glicksberg BS, *et al.* A Network-Biology Informed Computational Drug Repositioning Strategy to Target Disease Risk Trajectories and Comorbidities of Peripheral Artery Disease. AMIA Jt Summits Transl Sci Proc 2018; 2017: 108-17.
[PMID: 29888052]

[20]   Johnson KW, Shameer K, Glicksberg BS, *et al.* Enabling Precision Cardiology Through Multiscale Biology and Systems Medicine. JACC Basic Transl Sci 2017; 2(3): 311-27.
[http://dx.doi.org/10.1016/j.jacbts.2016.11.010] [PMID: 30062151]

SUBJECT INDEX

A

Acid 79, 90, 91, 92, 97, 111, 176, 177, 187
  arachidonic 79, 90, 176, 177
  citric 115
  dihydrocaffeic 90
  dihydroguaiaretic 92
  glycyrrhetinic 97
  nitrooleic 111
  propanoic 187
  rosmarinic 97
  shikimic 91
Acroischaemic syndromes 172
Actin cytoskeleton 198
Activation 80, 81, 110, 112, 116, 117, 129, 131, 177, 185, 192, 193
  receptor-mediated 177
Activity 69, 74, 76, 85, 125, 144, 145, 177, 213, 214, 215, 216, 217
  amidolytic 85
  cardiac pacemaker 125
  cardioprotective 213, 214, 215, 216
  diuretic 217
  fibrinolytic 74, 76, 177, 216
  locomotor 144
  metabolic 145
  phospholipase 177
  plasmin 74, 76
  proteolytic 69
Adipogenesis 115, 134, 135, 137, 138, 139, 141, 145, 146
  gene expression 139
  inhibiting 146
Adipogenic differentiation 135, 139, 141
Adiponectin production 134, 139, 144
  stimulate 144
ADP-induced platelet aggregation 77, 89
Aggregation 70, 171, 184, 193, 235
  inhibited 70
Agonists 37, 112, 115, 135, 136, 144
  endogenous 115
  synthetic 136
Alzheimer's disease 6
American diabetes association (ADA) 50

Amino acid 109, 186
  homologies 109
  residues 186
Aminotransferases 187, 188
  hepatic 187
Anaemia 175, 188
Angina 13, 19, 20, 48, 169, 173, 179, 212, 213, 215, 218, 221
  cardiac 218
  stable 169
  unstable 19, 20, 48, 179
  vasospastic 169
Angiogenesis 111, 225
  impaired 225
Angiotensin-converting enzyme (ACE) 43, 52, 189, 194, 197
  inhibitors 189
  receptor blocker 43, 197
  receptor neprilysin inhibitor (ARNI) 52
Antagonists 37, 96, 113, 115, 128, 137
  endogenous 115
  mineralocorticoid receptor 37
  synthetic 113
Anticoagulant 65, 72, 77, 90, 92
  agents, effective 65
  properties 72, 77, 90, 92
Anti-diabetic agents 37, 53
  evaluating novel 37
  novel 37
Antithrombotic agents 65, 92, 97
  effective 67
Anti-TNF-alpha antibody 226
Anxiety 174, 191
Apolipoprotein 241, 244, 245
Apoproteins 4, 5
Apoptosis 38, 122, 126, 128, 131, 132, 134, 138, 144, 226
  doxorubicin-induced cardiomyocyte 131
  increased cellular 226
  mediated cardiomyocyte 132
  myocardial 131
Apoptotic genes 142, 213
  expression 142

Atta-ur-Rahman & M. Iqbal Choudhary (Eds.)

Arterial hypertension 109, 169, 179, 190, 191,
    227
  pulmonary 179, 227
  secondary 190
  systemic 109
Assays 75, 77, 78, 82, 226
  chromogenic substrate 82
  luciferase 226
  molecular docking 77
  protease inhibition 75
  silico docking 78
Atherosclerosis 4, 11, 15, 23, 212, 213, 215,
    216, 217, 218, 225, 226, 228, 235
  coronary 217
  prevention and treatment of 216, 218
  progression of 11, 15
  risk factors 23
ATP 19, 114, 120, 171, 172
  binding cassette (ABC) 19
  in neonatal rat cardiomyocytes 120
  increased erythrocyte 171
  level depletion 171
Atrial natriuretic peptide (ANP) 117, 120,
    122, 125, 128

B

Balance 137, 145
  negative energy 145
  positive energy 137
Baseline 9, 11, 21, 23, 44
  cholesterol 9, 11
  CV disease 44
  inflammation 23
  LDL-cholesterol 21
  measurements 9
Basilar artery 223
BAT activation 141, 145
Beer belly syndrome 109
Beta-adrenergic receptors property 214
Beta cell transplant 42
Beta-oxidation 53
  hepatic 53
Beta-thromboglobulin 184
Bile acids 3, 12, 13
  binding gut 12
  sequestrants 12, 13
Bile salt export pump 186
Bis-substituted urea 96
Blood 4, 183, 212, 216, 217, 218, 219, 221

  healthy 219
Blood cholesterol levels 4
Blood clotting 218
Blood coagulation 72
Blood flow 171, 172, 175, 177, 190, 198, 212
  blood cell rigidity compromises 171
  peripheral 172
  reduction 190
  renal 177
Blood glucose 36, 53, 142, 146
  levels 53
Blood pressure 6, 8, 9, 12, 36, 41, 126, 130,
    170, 172, 177, 214, 219, 220, 228
  arterial 177
  decreasing 41
  diastolic 8
  healthy 219
  systolic 8, 12, 41
Body weight (BW) 6, 131
Botulinum toxin 164, 197, 198
Bradycardia 180, 221, 224
Brain natriuretic peptide (BNP) 43, 47, 117,
    118, 120
Brown adipocytes 137, 140, 144
  differentiation 137, 140
Brown adipose tissue (BAT) 113, 114, 132,
    134, 136, 137, 138, 140, 141, 143, 145,
    147
Buerger disease 165

C

Caffeine consumption 166
Calcium channel blockers (CCBs) 164, 167,
    169, 170, 174, 195, 197
Calcium channel-modulatory 215
Calcium levels 40, 177
  cytosolic 177
  increasing mitochondrial 40
Capsaicin 114, 115, 122, 128, 130, 131, 140,
    141, 143, 145, 146, 147
  activation member 114
Captopril prevention project (CAPP) 9
Cardiac 119, 224
  adverse effects (CAE) 224
  arrhythmias 119
Cardiac dysfunction 40, 128, 130, 131
  doxorubicin-induced 128, 131
  obesity-mediated 40
Cardiac events 17, 20

composite major adverse 20
developing major adverse 20
Cardiac hypertrophy 108, 116, 117, 118, 119,
    120, 122, 125, 129, 130, 131
  development of 129, 130
  diet-induced 128
  pathological 116, 118
  prevented TAC-induced 122
Cardiac injury 40, 123, 126, 132, 147
  doxorubicin-induced 126
  morphogenesis 113
  prevented doxorubicin-induced 132
Cardiac myocytes 117, 119, 132, 211, 225,
    235
  rod-shaped freshly-isolated 225
Cardiac remodeling 108, 116, 117, 131
  adaptive 117
Cardiogenesis 127
Cardiometabolic 109
  diseases, combat 109
Cardiomyocyte hypertrophy 118, 120
  attenuated 118
  induced 118
  mild hypoxia-induced 120
Cardiomyocytes 116, 117, 119, 120, 122, 128,
    129, 131, 235
  cell-derived 120
  primary neonatal 129
Cardiomyopathy 42, 43, 120, 123, 127, 128,
    212, 213
  cardiac dystrophic 123
  hypertrophic 120, 128, 213
  obstructive 43
  restrictive 42
Cardio-renal protection 39
Cardiotoxicity 123, 126, 127, 131, 132
  attenuated doxorubicin-induced acute 123
  doxorubicin-induced 123, 126, 127, 131,
    132
Cardiovascular disease 2, 214, 217, 219
  prediction 2
  treatment of 214, 217, 219
Cerebrovascular disease 6, 65, 171, 173, 213
Cervical 196, 197
  dystonia 197
  sympathectomy 196
Chemerin adipokine 226
Chemo-genomic enrichment analyses (CGEA)
    244
Chinese 80, 90, 211, 217, 218, 221, 228

herbal medicine 218, 221, 228
lacquer tree 80, 90
magnoliavine fruit 217
polyherbal formulations 211
Cholesterol 1, 2, 3, 4, 6, 9, 12, 13, 16, 19, 22,
    214, 215, 216, 241
  dietary 3
  elevated serum 3
  low-density lipoprotein 241
  structure of 3
Cholesterol levels 4, 8, 13, 14, 192, 215, 216,
    219
  reducing 4
  serum 4, 219
Chronic 22, 41, 42, 45, 46, 50, 51, 116, 197,
    212, 215, 217, 218, 236
  cardiac diseases 236
  cystitis 42
  headaches 197
  hemodynamic alterations 116
  kidney disease (CKD) 22, 41, 45, 46, 50,
    51, 212
  myelogenous leukemia (CML) 217, 218
  respiratory disease 215
Cinnamaldehyde supplementation 143
Clindamycin 196
Coagulation 69, 72, 117
  fibrinogen 69, 72
Coagulation 68, 69, 98
  cascade 68, 98
  phenomena 69
Collagen 69, 70, 72, 80, 84, 87, 90, 92, 93, 96,
    97, 118, 130, 228
  deposition 118
  replacement 130
  synthesis 228
Combination therapy 196, 197
Comorbidities 109, 132, 133, 138, 145, 234,
    243, 244, 245
  cardiovascular 234
  random 243
Competitive thrombin inhibitor 85
Compound danshen formula (CDF) 243
Computational flow dynamics 23
Concentrations 40, 41, 172, 181
  increased glucose 41
  maximum plasma 181
  plasma fibrinogen 172
  plasma glucose 40
Connective tissue 119, 165

disease 165
   growth factors (CTGF) 119
Consolidated standards of reporting trials
      (CONSORT) 11
Constipation 171, 191
Contractile function 116, 120, 122, 123, 128
Contractility 40, 125
   resulting improved cardiac 40
Contraction 41, 198
   decreased vascular smooth muscle cell 198
   intravascular volume 41
Coronary artery diseases (CAD) 20, 38, 211,
      212, 234, 240, 243
   angiographic 20
   microvascular 38
Coronary heart disease (CHD) 1, 2, 6, 7, 8, 9,
      11, 12, 16, 18, 20, 23, 179, 215, 218
Cough 174, 190, 218, 219
   dry 190
Counter cardiac arrhythmia 215
Crataegus pinnatifida 77, 78
   seeds 78
Creatinine 43, 44
CVD 2, 10, 18, 51
   atherosclerotic 10, 51
   significant reductions in 2, 18
CV death 36, 37, 42, 43, 44, 45, 46, 47, 48,
      50, 51, 54, 55
   and all-cause mortality 47
   decreased 46
   reduced 47, 48
   reductions in 47
CV diseases 37, 41, 44, 45, 49, 51
   atherosclerotic 45
   pre-existing atherosclerotic 45
CVD 3, 5, 22, 66, 243
   pathogenesis 22
   prevention 3
   related deaths 66
   risk factors 5
   treatment 243
CVD risk 7, 24
   function scores 7
   reduction 24

D

Damage 184, 186, 211
   hepatocellular 186
   irreversible DNA 211

   vascular 184
Data 235, 238, 242, 245, 246, 248
   mass spectrometry 245
   miRNA 245
   multifaceted 235
   proteomics 246, 248
   transcriptomics 238, 242
Death 2, 16, 17, 19, 20, 23, 44, 46, 54, 235
   cardiac 16
   cardiovascular 16, 17, 19, 20, 23, 54
   coronary 17
   leading cause of 2, 235
   renal 44, 46
Decreasing uricemia 41
Deficient oxygen supply 211
Deletion 119, 123, 124
   single channel gene 119
Dense single-nucleotide polymorphism 241
Depletion, platelet serotonin 184
Depression 184, 191
Diabetes mellitus (DM) 18, 36, 38, 40, 41, 43,
      48, 50, 51, 54, 55
Dialysis 1, 17, 18, 24
Diarrhoea 173, 174, 179, 180, 182, 183, 191
Dietary monoacylglycerols 145
Diet-induced obesity 108, 134, 136, 141, 143,
      145
   high-fat 136
Digital 165, 194, 195
   gangrene 194, 195
   ulcerations 165
Digital ulcers 164, 165, 167, 168, 169, 174,
      176, 177, 180, 186, 187, 190, 194, 195,
      196, 197, 198
   active SSc-related 186
   intractable 198
   scleroderma-related 196
Disease 110, 113, 218, 234, 241, 242
   causing genes 242
   comorbidities 234
   chronic 218
   neurodegenerative 113
   respiratory 110
   susceptibility 241
Disorders 5, 65, 109, 110, 173, 211, 213, 214,
      216, 218, 220, 224, 244, 247
   bladder 110
   blood clotting 213
   cardiovascular 214
   chronic kidney 244

coronary artery 224
  genetic 247
  menstrual 218
  metabolic 109, 216
  myocardial 224
  peripheral vascular 173
Dispelling rheumatism 217
Dizziness 171, 173, 182, 189, 191
DM 38
  cardiomyopathy 38
  induced cardiomyopathy 38
DNA 13, 238, 246
  binding domains 13
  methylation 238
  sequence database 246
Downstream effector 198
Doxorubicin 131
  induced cell atrophy 131
  metabolites 131
Dysfunction 40, 45, 108, 110, 121, 126, 127,
    128, 129, 131, 132, 174, 186, 221, 225
  contractile 132
  diastolic 131
  erectile 129, 174
  hepatic 186
  human cardiac myocyte 225
  left ventricular systolic 40
  mitochondrial 121, 126
  moderate renal 45
  sinus node 221
Dysfunctional glucose metabolism 135, 139
Dyslipidaemia 14, 21, 23
  atherogenic 21
Dyslipidemia 38, 109, 214
  atherogenic 109

E

Effects 41, 91, 130, 173, 177, 190, 192, 244
  antagonistic 244
  antiaggregatory 177
  anticoagulant 91
  cardiac 130
  dermatological 173
  hypotensive 190
  natriuretic 41, 177
  nephroprotective 41
  pleiotropic 192
Electrical pain signals 110
Electrophoresis 4

Emblica officinalis 216
Endocytosis 5
Endothelial 120, 164, 166, 168, 175, 199
  independent manner 175
  injury 164, 166, 168, 175, 199
  nitric oxide synthase 120
  human aortic 225
Endothelin 169, 184, 185, 186, 187, 188, 195,
    197
  pathway 184
  receptor antagonist (ERAs) 169, 184, 185,
    186, 187, 188, 195, 197
  receptor antagonists 169, 184
End-stage renal disease (ESRD) 42, 43, 44,
    45, 46
Engineered heart tissues (EHTs) 235
Enzymes 13, 99, 173, 183, 189
  angiotensin-converting 189
  phosphodiesterases 173
Epoprostenol therapy 180
ERAs, nonpeptide 185
Erythema 174, 179
Established CV disease 42
European association for the study of diabetes
    (EASD) 50, 51
Events 12, 13, 17, 22, 38, 44, 45, 54, 55, 114,
    134, 234
  hypoglycemic 44
  macrovascular 38
  major cardiovascular 17, 22, 45
  recurrent hospitalization 54, 55
  severe vascular 234
  vesicular trafficking 114
Expression 115, 116, 117, 118, 119, 121, 122,
    137, 138, 145, 146, 193, 226, 227, 239,
    241, 242
  module 241
  of platelet activation markers 193
  profiles 239
Extracts 68, 72, 77, 79, 80, 81, 82, 85, 90, 91,
    97, 111, 164, 167
  crude 97
  herbal 164, 167
  hydrophilic 77
Extra-terminal protein 227

F

Factors 7, 36, 119, 120, 122, 128, 185
  connective tissue growth 119

epigenetic 7
hypoxia-inducible 120, 128
profibrotic 185
prognostic 36
tumor necrosis 122
Fascaplysin 72
Fasting-induced hyperphagia 144
Fat oxidation 139, 141, 145
Fatty acids 3, 139, 144, 215
    bound polyunsaturated 215
    polyunsaturated 144
FDA-approved combinations 52
Fibroblasts 110, 116, 117, 119, 124, 184, 185,
        194, 235
    cardiac 124, 235
    interstitial 184
    sensitivity 194
Fibrosis 40, 117, 118, 119, 122, 123, 126, 127,
        128, 130, 131, 184, 185, 194, 240
    attenuated interstitial 117
    cardiac 123, 240
    myocardial 122, 126, 130
    tissue 184, 185
Food and drug administration (FDA) 37, 47,
        49, 53, 54, 179, 187, 221, 224, 225
Framingham heart study 1, 2, 6, 7, 8, 9, 22,
        24, 38
Function 19, 23, 108, 109, 114, 121, 126, 133,
        146, 215, 218, 219, 222, 238, 239, 240,
        242, 243, 248
    defective lysosomal 114
    endothelial cell 23
    healthy brain 219
    mediating adipocyte 133
    metabolic 109
    stomach 218
    tissue 146
    vascular smooth muscle cell 240
Functional enzymatic domains 112

G

Gastro-esophageal reflux disease 174
GC-MS analysis 213
Gene-encoded potassium ion 224
Gene expression 118, 134, 136, 139, 143, 245,
        246
    inflammatory 139, 143
    lipolytic 139, 143
    present reduced 134

patterns 245
Genes 116, 135, 136, 137, 139, 146, 226, 234,
        235, 238, 239, 241, 242, 244, 245, 246,
        248
    adipogenic 136, 146
    expressed 238
    hypertrophic 116
    tumour suppressor 226
Genetics 241
Genome 238, 241, 248
    organelle 238
Genome-wide association studies (GWAS)
        234, 241, 242
Ginkgo biloba 164, 167
GLP-1 and insulin secretion 143
Glucose 39, 40, 41, 134, 135, 139, 140, 142,
        143, 144
    fasting 139, 142
    homeostasis 39, 41, 134, 135, 143, 144
    intolerance 135, 140
    metabolism 140, 144
    reabsorption 41
    transporter, low-affinity 39
Glycosides 77, 215
    monoterpenoid 77
Gonadal white adipose tissue (GWAT) 240
Good manufacturing practice (GMP) 217
GRid-INdependent Descriptor (GRIND) 223
Guidelines, cardiovascular prevention 5
Gummi Olibanum 220

H

Haematological malignancies 165
Haemodialysis 17, 18, 21
Haemostasis 177, 184
HDL-cholesterol 21, 22
    and triglyceride values 21
    raising agents 22
Heart 111, 112, 113, 116, 117, 118, 120, 121,
        122, 123, 124, 125, 212, 213, 220, 224,
        238
    arrhythmia 212, 224
    arteries 221
    ischemic 238
    rheumatic 212
Heart disease 1, 2, 6, 8, 12, 20, 36, 55, 65,
        110, 179, 212, 213, 214, 215, 216, 217,
        218, 221
    congenital 65, 212, 213

coronary 1, 2, 6, 20, 65, 179, 215, 218
  hypertensive 212
  ischemic 216, 217, 221
  rheumatic 65, 213
  severe coronary 179
  structural 55
Heart failure 7, 43, 44, 51, 54, 55, 179, 212,
    215, 217, 220, 221, 238
  chronic 55, 179, 221, 238
  congestive 7, 217, 220
  hospitalization for 43, 44, 51, 54, 55
  refractory chronic congestive 215
  systolic 212
Heart weight (HW) 131
Hemostasis cascade 68
Heparin 72, 179, 194, 195
  low molecular weight 194, 195
  therapy 194
Hepatic injury 186, 187
High-fat diets display 134
High-throughput technologies 235, 238
Histopathological evaluations 213, 214
HMG-CoA reductase 13
  genes encoding 13
Homeostasis 112, 114, 211, 214
  disturbed antioxidant 211
  intracellular antioxidant 214
  lysosome ion 114
Homocysteine 16
Human 119, 121, 122, 225, 226, 228
  aortic endothelial cells (HAEC) 225
  atrial cardiomyocytes 122
  atrial myocytes 121
  coronary artery endothelial cells
    (HCAECs) 226
  dermal microvascular endothelial cells
    (HDMECs) 228
  pluripotent stem cell 119
Human cardiac 124, 128, 225, 227
  fibroblasts 124
  microvascular endothelial cells (HCMECs)
    227
  myocytes (HCM) 124, 128, 225
Human pulmonary 226, 227
  artery endothelial cells (HPAECs) 226
  microvascular endothelial cells (HPMECs)
    227
Hyperglycemia 40, 142
Hyperhidrosis 197

Hypertension 7, 11, 38, 129, 212, 214, 215,
    217, 219, 225, 238, 243
  pulmonary artery 129
Hyperthermia 130
Hypertrophy 40, 116, 117, 118, 123, 124, 125,
    128
Hypoglycemia 40, 43, 53
Hypotension 42, 171, 172, 176, 179, 191
  and decreased vascular tone 172
  pronounced 176
Hypothyroidism 165
Hypotonic cell swelling and heat 112
Hypoxia up-regulates chemerin expression
    226

I

Immunofluorescent staining 225, 226, 227,
    228
Infections 53, 54, 180, 196, 244
  catheter-associated 180
  fungal genital 54
Inflammation 22, 38, 41, 112, 115, 122, 123,
    131, 132, 134, 137, 139, 141, 192, 195
  monthly reducing 22
Inflammatory cytokines 225
Information 97, 222, 234, 244, 247, 248
  genetic sequence 248
  toxicological 222
Infusion 119, 177, 178, 179
  single monthly 178
Inhibiting oxidative stress 131
Inhibition 40, 41, 69, 71, 72, 73, 74, 78, 79,
    81, 86, 87, 93, 94, 95, 96, 123, 124, 125,
    128, 129, 132, 133, 171, 172, 173
  of platelet aggregation 78, 86, 87, 93, 94,
    95, 96, 172
  of platelet integrin 73
  of proteolysis and protection 69
  of thrombin activatable fibrinolysis
    inhibitor 74
  of thrombin-induced fibrin polymerization
    81
Inhibitors 77, 79, 164, 171, 197
  non-selective phosphodiesterase 171
  phosphodiesterase 164, 197
  plasminogen-activated 79
  serine protease 77
Insomnia 173, 174, 217, 220
  treating 220

In-stent restenosis 130
Insulin 49, 53, 133, 138, 142, 145
Insulinemia 40
Insulin release 108, 138, 141, 142
    glucose-stimulated 138
Insulin resistance 108, 109, 132, 134, 137,
        138, 140, 141, 144
    development of 132, 137
    syndrome 108
Insulin secretion 40, 133, 135, 136, 138, 142,
        143, 144, 145, 147
    ameliorate 147
    glucose-induced 135, 144
    glucose-stimulated 142, 143
    stimulated 133, 135
Intermediate density lipoproteins (IDL) 4
Intravenous iloprost 178, 179
    infusions 178
    therapy 179
Intravenous infusion 178, 180
    prolonged 178
Intravenous prostanoid therapy 176
Ischaemia 165, 193, 197, 214
    intractable 197
    peripheral vascular 193
Ischaemic 16, 112, 172, 215, 223
    lesions 172
    cardiomyopathy 215
    disease 16, 223
    reperfusion injury 112, 215
ISPH-induced 213
    myocardial necrosis 213
    oxidative stress 213
    up-regulation of apoptotic genes 213

K

Kidney disease 22, 41, 45, 51, 114, 212, 234
    autosomal dominant polycystic 114
    chronic 22, 41, 45, 51, 212
    diabetic 50
Kyoto encyclopedia of genes and genomes
        (KEGG) 246, 248

L

Lactate dehydrase 131
LDL-cholesterol 2, 5, 6, 8, 10, 11, 12, 14, 15,
        16, 19, 20, 21, 24

and HDL-cholesterol values 8
    decreased 12
    efficacy 5
    increased 6
    reduction 11, 14, 20, 21, 24
    reducing 14, 24
    target 20
Left main coronary artery (LMCA) 120
Leptin levels 143
Lesions 3, 167, 187
    necrotic 167
    vascular 3
Leucocyte filterability 172
Leukocyte adhesion 225
Ligands 108, 112, 113
    endogenous 108, 112
    exogenous activator 110
Lipid 15, 21, 225, 244
    homeostasis 244
    lowering agents 21
    lowering treatment 15
    phosphate phosphatase 225
Lipophilic efficiency 223
Lipoprotein 4, 6
    fractions 6
    lipase 4
Liver 17, 177, 186, 187, 188, 193
    cirrhosis 177
    damage 187
    enzymes 188
    toxicity 186
    transaminases 187, 193
Liver disease 42, 193, 218
    chronic 218
    nonalcoholic fatty 193
Logistic regression analysis 9
Low density lipoprotein (LDL) 1, 2, 4, 5, 10,
        215, 216
Low-density lipoprotein receptor 240
LV 118, 123, 126
    dysfunction 118, 126
    hypertrophy 123
Lysosomal storage disease 114

M

Macrovascular diseases 36
Mechanisms 2, 5, 24, 38, 40, 55, 123, 130,
        167, 170, 192, 194, 224
    biochemical 224

calcineurin-dependent 130
  insulin-independent 40
Medications 45, 48, 49, 50, 51, 53, 54, 190
  anti-diabetic 45, 49
  diuretic 53
  first-line anti-diabetic 51
  nephrotoxic 54
  second-line anti-diabetic 50
Medicine 216, 211, 217, 228, 243
  ayurvedic 217
  herbal 216, 228
  therapeutic 217, 228
  traditional Indian 243
  traditional system of 211
Melanocytes 110, 112
Membrane 19, 40, 171, 172, 215
  basolateral 40
  bound phosphodiesterase 172
  jejunal brush border 19
  myocardial 215
Metabolism 4, 146, 211, 238
  altered energy 238
  dynamic cellular 211
  lipoprotein 4
Molecules 3, 65, 66, 69, 71, 72, 73, 98, 99,
    110, 114, 121, 132, 144, 147, 178, 185,
    224, 236
  adhesion 178
  anticoagulant 69, 73
  anti-inflammatory 132
  enhancing survival signaling 121
  natural non-caloric sweet-tasting 144, 147
  reactive electrophilic 110
  synthetic 66
  vascular cell adhesion 178
Monthly pregnancy tests 187
Morbidity 65, 108, 212
  cardiometabolic 108
mRNA expression 117, 120, 223, 226
  increased 120
  levels 226
Multiplex immunoassays 238
Mutations 4, 114, 242, 248
Myocardial 10, 43, 44, 45, 46, 48, 49, 117,
    120, 122, 126, 129, 130, 179, 223, 224,
    241
  development 122
  infarction (MI) 10, 43, 44, 45, 46, 48, 49,
    117, 120, 129, 130, 179, 223, 224, 241
  isoproterenol-induced 216

Myocardial 16, 211, 216, 217
  ischemia reduction 16
  necrosis 211, 216, 217
Myocardium 108, 117, 121, 122, 215, 216
  adult ventricular 121
  hypoproliferation 121
  ischemia-reperfusion 117
Myxobacterial strains 76

N

Natural product androgapholide 96
Natural products 66, 67, 77, 97, 98, 80, 98
  antithrombotic activity of 66, 67
  isolated 80
  marine-based 98
  microorganism-based 98
  plant-based 77, 97, 98
Natural products and semi-synthetic
    molecules 65
Natural scaffolds 65, 96, 97, 98
Nausea 173, 179, 180, 182, 187, 191, 218
Neonatal rat cardiomyocytes 120
Neonate hearts 118
Nervous system 3
Network data exchange (NDEx) 246, 248
Neuromuscular junction 197
Nitroglycerin 176
  gel vehicle 176
Nitroglycerin ointments 176, 197
  topical 197
Nodularia spumigena 94, 96
  cyanobacteria 96
NO-mediated pathway 197
Non-coding regions elucidate 242
Non-selective ion channel sensors 109
Nucleic acids 236

O

Obese 135, 136, 137
  diet-induced 137
Obesity 139, 140
  counteracting 140
  and dysfunctional glucose metabolism 139
Observation 3, 187
  post marketing 187
Oedema 180, 188, 191
  peripheral 188

pulmonary 180
Oral 115, 243
   bioavailability screening 243
   cavity 115
Organic synthetic methods 66
Original cohort aging 6
Orthostatic hypotension 179, 191
Osmotic changes 115
Osteomyelitis 195, 196
Osteoporosis 6
Overexpression 119, 120, 125
   cardiac 119
Oxidative stress 38, 40, 41, 117, 120, 122,
   123, 126, 213, 215, 216
   hypoxia-induced 117
   markers 213

P

PAF-induced platelet aggregation inhibition
   88
Pain 110, 174, 179, 180, 187, 188, 196, 198,
   215, 217, 221
   abdominal 187, 193
   chest 174, 179, 180, 188, 215
   chronic 110
   jaw 180
   leg 217
Pancreas 39, 40, 42, 108, 110, 114, 116, 133,
   136, 138, 143, 147, 218
   adipose tissue and endocrine 116, 143, 147
   inflamed 218
Pancreatic β-cells 113, 133, 134, 135, 136,
   138, 141, 144, 145
   human 136
   inflammation 144
   isolated 135
Pancreatitis 40
Parathyroid hormone 115
Parkinson's disease 6, 111
Pathology 165, 175, 235, 238
   non-rheumatic 165
   well-recognized 175
Pathophysiology 212, 227
   of CVD 212
Pathways 4, 14, 71, 72, 79, 90, 123, 173, 185,
   188, 214, 234, 235, 244, 246
   extrinsic coagulation 79, 90
   intrinsical coagulation 98
   intrinsic coagulation 71, 72, 90

lipid transport 4
   signalling 214
   susceptible 234
Peptide 43, 47, 37, 51, 71, 72, 98, 117, 128,
   130, 184
   amino-acid 184
   atrial natriuretic 117, 128
   brain natriuretic 43, 47, 117
Percutaneous coronary intervention 43
Peripheral 47, 48, 54, 65, 213, 234, 243, 244
   arterial disease (PAD) 47, 48, 54, 65, 234,
      243, 244
   venous disease 213
Phenotypes 23, 130, 139, 140, 144, 240, 244
   atherogenic lipoprotein 23
   lipolytic 139, 144
   vascular smooth muscle 130
Plasma insulin 142, 143
   secretion 142
Plasma protease 72
Platelet aggregation 69, 72, 80, 81, 85, 86, 87,
   90, 91, 92, 93, 94, 95, 96, 97, 98
   collagen-induced 85, 91
   factor (PAF) 87, 92
   inhibited thrombin-induced 72
   inhibiting thrombin-induced 97
Platelet-leukocyte aggregates (PLA) 70, 72
Platelet-rich plasma (PRP) 70
Pluripotent stem cell (PSC) 118, 119, 129, 235
Post-translational modification 192
Pravastatin in ischemic disease 16
Primary uncorrected valve disease 42
Progesterone 3, 112
Prognosis 4, 166
Proinflammatory cytokines 136
Proline-rich tyrosine kinase 121
Prostacyclin 164, 176, 180, 182, 185
   synthetic 180
Prostacyclin receptor agonist 183
Prostaglandins 111, 141
   cyclopentenone 141
Proteases 13, 197
Protein kinase 129, 172
   G (PKG) 129
Protein-Protein Interaction 246
Proteins 13, 19, 109, 110, 119, 120, 122, 234,
   236, 239, 240, 241, 242, 246, 248
   low-abundant intracellular 122
   mammalian TRP channel 109
   sterol response element binding 13

Protein synthesis 130
Protein tyrosine kinase 129
Proteolysis 69
Prothrombin time (PT) 78, 79, 81, 83, 85, 90,
    91
Pulmonary 37, 174, 179, 180, 183, 185, 187,
    213, 223, 226, 227
    arterial hypertension (PAH) 179, 180, 183,
        185, 187, 227
    congestion 37, 179
    hypertension (PH) 174, 223, 226, 227
    stenosis 213
Pulmonary thrombus 74, 76
    degrading 76

R

Reaven's syndrome 109
Receptors 72, 78, 111, 112, 119, 134, 135,
    184, 185, 186, 187, 192
    proliferators-activated 192
Regular hemodialysis 15
Regulating feeding behavior 135
Release 117, 132, 172, 183, 184, 194, 198,
    225
    cytokine 225
Renal 15, 16, 44, 177
    failure, chronic 177
    replacement therapy 44
    transplantation 15
    transplant recipients 16
Renal disease 21, 42, 43, 44, 45, 51
    chronic 21
    progression of 44, 51
Rhabdomyolisis 193
Rheumatic diseases 165, 199
    systemic 199
    systemic autoimmune 165
Rheumatoid arthritis 165
Rheumatologists 165, 169, 199
Rho-kinase Inhibitors 198
Risk factors 5, 6, 7, 9, 12, 23, 51, 212, 235,
    244, 245
    cardiovascular 235
Rosuvastatin therapy 18

S

Salt 7, 90, 182

quaternary ammonium alkaloid 90
Saponin 66, 67, 91, 97
    natural 97
    triterpenic 91, 92
Saposhnikoviae root 221
Sarcolemma 120, 126
Sarcomeric alpha-actinin 225
Sargassum micracanthum 93
Scavenging 167, 217
    effects, radical 167
    property, radical 217
Secondary 165, 167
    raynaud's phenomenon 167
    RP in rheumatic diseases 165
Secretion 39, 41, 53, 79, 81, 83, 132, 225, 241
    glucagon 39
    induced 79, 81, 83
    uric acid 41
Semi-synthetic anticoagulant compounds 93
Serotonergic neurons 183
    peripheral 183
Serotonin 164, 183, 184, 193, 194
    inhibition 183
    reuptake inhibitor 184
    transporter 183
Serum creatinine 44, 45, 46
Severe peripheral vascular syndrome 196
Single-nucleotide polymorphism (SNP) 241
Skin keratinocytes 115
Sphingosine 113
Statins 20, 192, 193, 198
    high intensity 20
    hydrophilic 192
    lipophilic 192
    pleiotropic effects of 192, 193, 198
Statin therapy 18, 19, 20, 192
    high intensity 20
    intensive 19
Sterol response element binding protein
    (SREBP) 13
Store-operated channels (SOCs) 111
Stroke 2, 7, 17, 20, 43, 44, 45, 46, 48, 49, 193,
    212, 213, 218, 220
    acute ischemic 218
    cold 220
    fatal 17
    haemorrhagic 17, 193
    ischaemic 2
Subcutaneous infusion 180
Surgery 13, 196

coronary bypass 13
Syndrome 16, 17, 19, 20, 23, 36, 43, 108, 147,
        165, 197, 219, 220
    acute coronary 16, 17, 19, 20, 36, 43
    cardiometabolic 108, 147
    carpal tunnel 165
    kidney yang deficiency 219
    metabolic 23
    piriformis 197
    post-concussion 220
Synthesis 96, 97, 172, 173, 184, 192, 194, 198
    extracellular matrix 184
    stimulate prostacyclin 172
    thromboxane 172
Systemic 42, 164, 165, 167, 172
    lupus erythematosus 165, 172
    sclerosis 164, 165, 167
    steroids 42
Systems biology 236, 247
    holistic strategy 236
    markup language (SBML) 247

T

TCA-cycle enzymes 213
Teratogenicity 187
Testosterone deficiency 24
Therapeutic effect of Ginkgo biloba 167
Therapeutics 97, 213, 228
    cardiovascular 213
    nature-derived 228
Therapies 13, 21, 22, 23, 42, 48, 55, 146, 164,
        179, 187, 193, 195, 236, 243, 245
    adjunctive 193
    anti-inflammatory 22, 23
    disease-modifying 55
    fibrate 21, 23
    immunosuppressive 42
    novel cardiovascular 245
Thermogenesis 108, 141
Thermogenic genes expression 140, 144
Thrombin activatable fibrinolysis inhibitor
        (TAFIa) 74, 77, 94, 97, 98
Thrombin-induced fibrinogen clotting 85
Thrombin 76, 77, 79, 81, 83, 95, 96, 99
    induced fibrin polymerization 81
    inhibitors 76, 77, 95, 96, 99
    production 79, 83
Thrombolysis 43, 45
    in myocardial infarction (TIMI) 43, 45

Thrombosis 77, 216, 225
Thrombotic complications 235
Tissue 114, 117, 185, 194, 215
    biopsies 117
    expression 114
    fibroblasts 185
    injury 215
    ischaemia 194
Total cholesterol 1, 2, 6, 7, 8, 13
    reducing 13
Toxicodendron vernicifluum 80, 90
Tradicional chinese medicine (TCM) 90, 218,
        220, 243
Transcriptome 238, 241
    profiling 241
Transcriptomics 224, 235, 245
Transforming growth 116, 184
Transient mobilization 193
Translocation 39, 191, 198
    cold-induced 198
    tissue glucose 39
Transport, high-affinity glucose 39
Transverse aortic constriction (TAC) 117,
        118, 122, 123, 124, 125, 127, 128, 129,
        130
Triglycerides 4, 7, 15, 21, 22, 215, 216
Tumorigenesis 112
Tumor suppressor 112

U

Ulcers 182, 190, 195
    active 182
    chronic 195
    infected 190
Umbilical cord veins 188
Underlying pathogenesis 164
Urinary 40, 43
    excretion 40
    glucose excretion 40
    tract infection 43

V

Vascular 38, 167, 169, 170, 179, 182, 194,
        213, 226
    complications 179, 182
    disease 38, 213
    endothelial growth factor expression 226

injury 194

  pathology 167

  smooth muscles 169, 170

Vasoconstriction 184, 185, 190, 191, 198

  cold-induced 191

  decreased 198

Vasomotor reactions 174

Vasospasm 130, 164, 166

  coronary 130

Vasospastic attacks 165, 167, 170, 172, 180, 181, 189

Venous infusions 172

Ventricular 127, 221

  hypertrophy 127

  remodelling 221

Ventricular tachycardia 122, 127, 223

  lethal 223

Very low density lipoprotein (VLDL) 4

Vomiting 173, 179, 180, 187, 218

W

Wall shear stress 23

Weight gain 138, 143, 145, 146

  high-fat induced 143

Well-tolerated drugs 164, 167

White adipocytes 132, 140, 141, 144

  cultured 144

  human 140, 144

White atractylodes rhizome 220

Wild type (WT) 118, 120, 128, 129, 143, 225

World health organization (WHO) 66, 183

X

Xanthomatosis 4

Z

Zebrafish caudal vessels 78